Mammography Screening

Truth, lies and controversy

PETER C GØTZSCHE
MD, DrMedSci, MSc
Professor of Clinical Research Design and Analysis
Director, The Nordic Cochrane Centre
Chief Physician
Rigshospitalet and the University of Copenhagen
Denmark

Forewords by

IONA HEATH
President of the Royal College of General Practitioners
London

and

FRAN VISCO
President of the National Breast Cancer Coalition
The United States

Radcliffe Publishing
London • New York

Radcliffe Publishing Ltd
33–41 Dallington Street
London
EC1V 0BB
United Kingdom

www.radcliffepublishing.com

British Library Cataloguing in Publication Data

A catalogue record for this book is available from the British Library.

ISBN-13: 978 184619 585 3

Supported by KræftFonden (The Cancer Foundation)

The paper used for the text pages of this book is FSC® certified. FSC (The Forest Stewardship Council®) is an international network to promote responsible management of the world's forests.

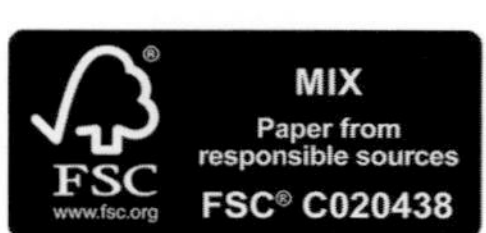

Typeset by Darkriver Design, Auckland, New Zealand
Printed and bound by Hobbs the Printers, Totton, Hants, UK

Contents

Foreword by Iona Heath

Advanced breast cancer is a terrible disease which takes a huge toll of the lives of too many women. And so it is very easy to understand the motivation that drives scientists, doctors and policy-makers to try and prevent it through early diagnosis and screening. Sadly, the whole field has become pervaded by good-intentioned wishful thinking which has seemed to blind too many people to the problems inherent in this approach. There is a conundrum intrinsic to the whole endeavour which is the impossibility of clearly distinguishing between benign and malignant cells on histological examination. There are cells which are definitely benign and others which are unequivocally malignant but in between there is a grey area populated by abnormal cells which may or may not progress to cancer. If such cells are classified as benign, some cases of early breast cancer will be missed; if they are classified as malignant, some patients will be labelled as having cancer and will be subjected to invasive and sometimes mutilating treatments when the cells were never going to progress to symptomatic cancer in the lifetime of the affected patient. The latter is the problem of overdiagnosis which has become more and more clear since screening was introduced in relatively affluent countries across the world.

If Peter Gøtzsche did not exist, there would be a need to invent him. He is a committed and meticulous scientist who has worked as a clinician and who delights in numbers and mathematics and what they can tell us, to an extent that is rare among doctors. He is also tenacious and refuses to tolerate the foolishness of wishful thinking, however well-intended. In 1999, he and his colleague Ole Olsen in The Nordic Cochrane Centre embarked on a Cochrane review of mammographic screening for breast cancer and documented both the poor quality of many of the trials on which the policy was founded and the extent of subsequent overdiagnosis. Those responsible for breast screening programmes in the UK and elsewhere have been very slow to appreciate the significance of these findings and to inform women invited for screening of the implications of overdiagnosis.

Those committed to mammographic screening programmes face a number of problems. Firstly, the programmes are extremely expensive and healthcare resources are increasingly stretched; secondly, if the possibility of overdiagnosis is acknowledged and properly communicated to the women invited for screening, uptake is likely to drop, undermining the utilitarian calculus and reducing the effectiveness of the programme. Finally, as treatment for symptomatic breast cancer improves, as it has done enormously over the last two decades, the effectiveness of screening is further eroded. However, there are huge vested interests at work and it may still take time for the limitations and harms of screening to be properly acknowledged and for women to be enabled to make adequately informed decisions. When this happens, it will be almost entirely due to the intellectual rigour and determination of Peter Gøtzsche.

Iona Heath
President of the Royal College of
General Practitioners
London

Foreword by Fran Visco

In May 2001, Peter Gøtzsche stood at the podium during a plenary session of the National Breast Cancer Coalition's annual Advocacy Training Conference in Washington D.C. The audience was about 700 mostly women from across the United States and a few from other countries. They were primarily breast cancer survivors, their friends and families, representing various organizations serving women with breast cancer, raising awareness, supporting research and health care. We invited Peter to speak, along with Anthony Miller, lead investigator of the Canadian National Breast Screening Study, and Stephen Feig, a radiologist and screening proponent. Peter had recently published the meta-analysis of the trials in the *Lancet*. As he states in this book, he looked around for an exit because he was about to bring a controversial message to the group: that the evidence behind mammography screening is questionable and that screening has doubtful benefits and causes harm. We could see the surprise in his reaction when a majority of the audience rose to give him a standing ovation.

Wait. Breast cancer advocates applauding Peter Gøtzsche's work that would undermine years of awareness and marketing messages about mammography screening saving lives? How did that happen? For decades the public in the United States has been given one message about breast cancer: Early detection saves lives and women should be screened for breast cancer every year. But the goal for all of us who care about breast cancer cannot be finding more of it, or figuring out how best to detect it, it has to be to end breast cancer so that women no longer die of the disease or are no longer harmed by the treatments for it. That is why the advocates in the audience that day in May 2001 rose to applaud Peter's seminal work. Because we care about the truth. We care about scientific evidence. We care about why we are being told to do something. We had educated ourselves to understand that the evidence was questionable and that at most screening benefited a small fraction of women with breast cancer and harmed many more.

If you care about breast cancer, and we all should, you must read this book. Breast cancer is complex and we cannot afford to rely on the popular media, or on information from marketing campaigns from those who are invested in screening.

We need to question and to understand. The story that Peter tells matters very much: that there are questions being asked about the evidence for mammography screening. It matters whether a statement in support of screening is based on an observational rather than a prospective, randomized trial; it matters who does the trials, how they are designed, and what biases remain. This book puts those scientific details into a real world setting. It describes the intrigue, the infighting, the maneuvering within the community of science journals where decisions made have significant impact on the health care we receive. It pulls back the curtain and lets us see the reality of science. And it allows us to understand that much of the world of mammography screening has lost sight of the goal: to save lives, not careers or reputations.

As Peter describes throughout this book, questioning mammography screening, even through science, can have severe ramifications. Attacks are usually pointed, personal and emotional. In 2009, when the United States Preventive Services Task Force looked carefully at the trials of mammography screening and revised their guidelines, recommending that women between the ages of 50 and 74 have a screening mammography every other year and that women 40–49 make individual decisions, they were vilified and completely misrepresented to the public. Dr. Otis Brawley, medical director for the American Cancer Society, said, 'With its new recommendations, the USPSTF is essentially telling women that mammography at age 40 to 49 saves lives; just not enough of them.' Some physicians took to the airwaves and internet to proclaim that the guidelines represented a major setback, wiping out decades of progress, that the USPSTF questioned the value of life, and that thousands of women would die as a result of their actions. How can the public believe otherwise when they are told women will die by people with many initials after their names and known organizations behind them?

This book is particularly timely. There is a push to bring screening to developing countries and to younger and younger women. We need to dispel the illusion that bringing widespread mammography screening with its harms, significant cost and limited benefit to developing countries will decrease burden and improve health outcomes for women. We need to take the time to understand the science and the basis for health recommendations we receive, both in the healthy population and in those diagnosed with breast cancer. This book will help us get there.

Fran Visco
President of the National Breast Cancer Coalition
The United States

Acknowledgements

My sincere thanks to Cornelia Baines, co-principal investigator of the Canadian National Breast Screening Study, for explaining the intricacies of English grammar and colloquialisms and for suggesting ways in which content and style could be strengthened. I also thank Richard Horton, editor-in-chief of the *Lancet*, for his strong support in getting unwelcome data published and in helping resolve our conflict with the Cochrane Breast Cancer Group; Drummond Rennie, editor of the *Journal of the American Medical Association*, for helpful advice in the same conflict; Kay Dickersin, director for the US Cochrane Center, for her great help in her capacity as Cochrane publication arbiter; and Karsten Juhl Jørgensen, researcher at The Nordic Cochrane Centre, for our long-standing and fruitful collaboration.

I also thank Stephen Morrell for providing me with original graphs for Figure 16.4; the *British Medical Journal* for permission to reproduce Figures 15.1, 16.1, 16.2, 19.4, 19.5; and John Wiley & Sons for permission to reproduce Figure 25.1. Publication of this book was supported by KræftFonden (The Cancer Foundation).

Peter C Gøtzsche MD, DrMedSci, MSc
Professor of Clinical Research Design and Analysis
Director, The Nordic Cochrane Centre
Chief Physician
Rigshospitalet and the University of Copenhagen
Denmark

Books by the same author

Gøtzsche PC. *Rational Diagnosis and Treatment: evidence-based clinical decision-making*. 4th ed. Chichester: Wiley; 2007.

Wulff HR, Gøtzsche PC. *Rationel klinik. Evidensbaserede diagnostiske og terapeutiske beslutninger*. 5. udgave. Copenhagen: Munksgaard Danmark; 2006.

Gøtzsche PC. [On safari in Kenya] [Danish]. Copenhagen: Samlerens Forlag; 1985.

1

Introduction

SOMETIMES YOU CAN'T BELIEVE THAT WHAT YOU'VE JUST SEEN IS actually true. And sometimes it isn't. An example of this could be if you saw a magician suspend a person in the air without support. However, what I describe in this book *is* true, although much of it goes far beyond what most people would think scientists were capable of doing, not only to each other but also, more importantly, to the public they are supposed to serve.

Like other people, scientists are often driven by emotions, career aspirations, strong beliefs, money and fame rather than facts and logic. This is not unexpected. However, when it comes to mammography screening, the extent to which some scientists are ready to deny what they see – and here I am not talking about magic – and sacrifice sound scientific principles in order to arrive at politically acceptable results in their research is astounding. I have a vague hope that it might be better in other disciplines, but I doubt it, as it all comes down to human psychology.

This book gives plenty of examples of *ad hominem* attacks, intimidation, slander, threats of litigation, deception, dishonesty, lies and other violations of good scientific practice. For some years I kept a folder labelled *Dishonesty in breast cancer screening* on top of my filing cabinet, storing articles and letters to the editor that contained statements I knew were dishonest. Eventually I gave up on the idea of writing a paper about this collection, as the number of examples quickly exceeded what could be contained in a single article.

In November 2009, I attended a meeting in London on cancer screening. The exaggerated claims about mammography screening that I heard at this meeting triggered something for me. Retired breast surgeon Michael Baum also attended the meeting and, finding ourselves thinking along similar lines, we agreed to write a book together. Once having started writing – actually in the middle of the meeting – I just couldn't stop. I also realised it would be much easier to write the book alone, which Baum happily accepted. He published his own book, *Breast beating: A personal odyssey in the quest for an understanding of breast cancer, the meaning of life and other easy questions*, on screening in 2010, which is also an autobiography.

Sweden has been a major player in research on mammography screening, encouraging the implementation of screening all over the world. Much of the brouhaha our research on screening has created has occurred in Sweden and Denmark. I believe an account of the events in these countries has wider interest and, as few people can read Swedish and Danish, this book describes these events in English. The book also describes research and events in other countries, with an emphasis on the United States, the United Kingdom and Australia.

My interest in research misconduct began early. I studied biology and chemistry at the universities of Copenhagen, Uppsala and Lund and I acquired a full academic education both in Denmark and in Sweden. Uppsala is the home town of Carl von Linné, the famous taxonomist who gave Latin names to so many of our plants and animals, and the surroundings of the city were ideal for bicycle excursions into the wilderness.

A newly qualified biologist, I was employed by the Swedish drug company Astra in Copenhagen in 1975. In the beginning, I worked as a drug representative and product manager, but I quickly moved into clinical research and established a medical department at a new joint venture company, Astra-Syntex, where I handled regulatory affairs and was responsible for clinical trials.

I knew a good deal about insects, which was my speciality in biology, but virtually nothing about drugs. However, it didn't take long before I learned there were also plenty of bugs in drug research. I was relatively free to work as I wished at Astra-Syntex and I wasn't forced to do things against my principles, but I knew this luck couldn't last forever. The working practices of the drug industry, both in research and in marketing, are problematic, and the industry's priority is profit-making, which often leads to untoward consequences for the patients and for our national economies. Therefore, I wanted to leave. As I was attracted to the challenges in healthcare, I decided that, rather than going back to biology, where there were few career options, I would study medicine.

I asked for my director's permission to attend courses in 10% of my full working time, which later became 33% and then increased to 50% during the final years. During this time, I was offered an attractive job as clinical research director for the Nordic area, located at the headquarters of Astra in Sweden, which would have earned me the largest and most well-equipped Volvo that money can buy, and a corresponding salary, but I preferred to finish my studies. It is surprising how effective one can be when there is little time. I finished medical studies in 6½ years, in 1984, left the company and started clinical work at hospitals in Copenhagen. Then came two revelations that influenced me greatly.

The first occurred right after my final exams, during my first appointment. The head of endocrinology suggested my thesis subject should be insulin antibodies, and I collected about 500 scientific articles on the subject. However, I couldn't make much sense of them. I tried to construct dose-response curves on the effects of insulin using published data, but some of the papers were so incompatible that I realised that not all researchers had been entirely honest.

The next revelation came a year later when I conducted a study where I had carefully worked out the dose of insulin for a physiological experiment, based on a graph from a paper published in the prestigious *New England Journal of Medicine*. I studied the cardiovascular effects of insulin, and I thought it wouldn't be possible for any of our diabetes patients to get a dose that was too high. It was pretty shocking, therefore, that the very first patient developed symptoms of hypoglycaemia to such an extent that I needed to give a rescue dose of intravenous glucose. When an endocrinologist external to our research group heard who the first author was of the paper I had trusted, he asked me if I didn't know him. I didn't. The endocrinologist explained that the graphs this person published were too good to be true. Thus, it seemed that my patient and I had fallen victims to fraud.

I published our study[1] but I wasn't proud of it. It had eight patients, but also eight authors, which was a bit much considering only three people did the research. Our study wasn't particularly useful and I wondered whether we should refrain from asking patients to participate in such studies.

The two revelations about insulin research indicated that not only were serious manipulations with the data common in the drug industry but also that they occurred in research led by academics. I shall never forget how happy I was when I dumped the 500 insulin papers in the rubbish. Goodbye insulin and goodbye endocrinology. I decided to turn my negative experience into a positive one by embarking on a very different project for my thesis: bias in clinical research.

I also decided to work alone. I wasn't happy with the prevailing tradition of having many authors on papers that only few people had contributed to, often including the chair of the department for no other reason than being the chair of the department. Some doctors' creative ideas about authorship made one of my colleagues remark that if a doctor had lent Shakespeare a pencil, he would have become co-author of *Macbeth*. And it led to an amusing letter in the *New England Journal of Medicine* with the title 'Et al. gets Nobel Prize'[2] (when there are many authors on a paper, it is customary to mention only the first few and to group the rest as '*et al.*', which means 'and others'). I was inspired by Charles Darwin, who had written *On the Origin of Species* alone, which I consider the most important piece of research that has ever been done, and I was also inspired by a relative of mine who was sole author of the six papers that comprised his thesis.

I wrote a protocol for the thesis and assembled 244 reports of trials that had compared one anti-arthritis drug with another. The thesis, 'Bias in double-blind trials',[3] which was based on six papers,[4–9] was defended in 1990. It was the first time a whole therapeutic area had been so thoroughly investigated, and the thesis changed my career. The ink was hardly dry before UK statistician Douglas Altman picked it up at the library, read, and sent it to the director of the National Perinatal Epidemiology Unit, Iain Chalmers, in Oxford, urging him to read it. I didn't know who Iain Chalmers was, but my ignorance didn't last long. He invited me to Oxford in 1992 when the British minister of health opened the UK Cochrane Centre. I opened The Nordic Cochrane Centre in Copenhagen in 1993 and abandoned clinical work in 1997.

Iain Chalmers started The Cochrane Collaboration in 1993 and was later knighted for his outstanding achievements. It built on a common frustration among researchers and others that much medical research was of poor quality and was biased, and on the realisation that we lacked updated, reliable systematic reviews of the randomised trials that could tell us what the benefits and harms of our interventions were. We couldn't offer our patients the best treatments, as the medical research literature was such a mess that we didn't know which treatments were best.

Once established, The Cochrane Collaboration caught on and grew quickly. It is a registered charity and represents the state of the art for the conduct and dissemination of systematic reviews, as described in the 649-page *Cochrane Handbook*.[10] The collaboration currently involves more than 25 000 people. The reviews are published electronically in *The Cochrane Library*, and there are more than 4000 such reviews, which are regularly updated. Half of the world's population have free access to the full reviews through national subscriptions financed by their national governments; the other half have access to the abstracts.

My thesis had other ramifications. It led to an invitation by statistician David Moher in Ottawa to attend a workshop in 1993 aimed at defining criteria for scoring the reliability of randomised trials. A few hours into the workshop, the late Thomas C Chalmers suggested that it was futile to try to agree on a quality score for assessing trials. It wouldn't work and we should rather focus on the various biases, one by one. All agreed to his proposal, and the agenda was changed into one of suggesting a set of guidelines for transparent reporting of trials that enabled the readers to assess their reliability. I co-authored the CONSORT guidelines for good reporting of randomised trials that most top journals refer to in their instructions to authors, as well as co-authoring similar guidelines for observational studies (STROBE) and systematic reviews (PRISMA). Currently, the research groups I am a member of work on guidelines for writing protocols for trials (SPIRIT) and protocols for systematic reviews (PRISMAP).

My thesis focused on statistical issues. What I particularly love about mathematics is that, in contrast to medicine, where one has to learn so much by heart, it isn't necessary to remember much, as one can deduce what is needed based on rather few premises. At the exam in mathematics at the university, I drew a question, started in the upper left corner of the green-board and ended in the lower right corner after having filled it entirely with formulae. The only comment from my examiners was 'Thank you'. They gave me the highest mark on an elaborate scale where this mark was used only in exceptional cases.

The reason I tell you this is to provide a little balance. My opponents in the scientific debates about mammography screening have often accused me of having made numerous errors in my calculations. As far as I know, I haven't made any, and I shall show in this book that those accusations that were concrete, and not just mere utterings and condemnations, were wrong. I shall also explain why so many of the analyses performed by professors of statistics in the area of breast screening are wrong. This raises an interesting question:

> *Why is it that all gross calculation errors made by screening advocates favour screening?*

What it really means to be 'controversial'

'How do you wish me to introduce you?' asked the chairman. As we knew each other well, I replied that he could say whatever he pleased, as long as he didn't say I was controversial.

When it became my turn to give a talk, the chairman said in his introduction – with a broad teasing smile – that I was controversial. So I started my talk by explaining to the audience that if it was controversial to tell the truth . . . well . . . then I was controversial. I added that I'd noticed that my results were often unpopular with some people, particularly those with financial interests in the issue I had researched.

This was in 2007, at a scientific meeting in Amsterdam, and my talk was about selective reporting of research results. Our research group had shown that there was poor agreement between research protocols for randomised trials and what was subsequently published.[11] It was particularly shocking that at least one primary outcome was changed in two-thirds of the trials studied and that this was not acknowledged in any of the published reports. Primary outcomes, e.g. death or myocardial infarction in a trial of a cholesterol-lowering drug, are the most important, whereas secondary outcomes could be admission to hospital or serum cholesterol.

The changes we found were not exactly minor. For example, a new primary outcome appeared in one-third of the publications that had not been mentioned in the protocol, although trial protocols are usually very lengthy and detailed. The reason why it is deceptive to make changes in primary outcomes without telling the readers about it can be illustrated by the 'Texas sharpshooter'. If a cowboy fires a gun at a large, white wall, draws the target around the bullet hole in the wall and then claims he hit the bullseye, he would obviously be cheating.

There is much secrecy in healthcare research, particularly when the commercial interests of drug companies are involved, and it was therefore difficult to do the study. Douglas Altman and the Canadian Rhodes scholar An-Wen Chan had tried to do the study in the United Kingdom and had acquired permission to look at a set of trial protocols from research ethics committees when a lawyer got wind of the project and sabotaged it, claiming that the protocols contained confidential information. Altman and I were both members of the editorial advisory board for the *British Medical Journal* (*BMJ*) and, during a farewell dinner in London, I explained that such a study could be done in Denmark. We did the study together, with three other researchers from Canada and Denmark, and published it in the *Journal of the American Medical Association* (*JAMA*) in 2004.[11] Two years later, we published another study in *JAMA* based on the same material, this time about constraints on publication rights for academic researchers participating in industry-initiated trials.[12] This study was also revealing. Half of the protocols explicitly described that the industry sponsor either owned the data or needed to approve the manuscript, or indeed both, and the fact that the academics had their hands tied in their collaborations with the drug industry was not revealed in any of the publications.

When I translated this paper into Danish and published it in the *Danish Medical Journal* (*Ugeskrift for Læger*),[13] the Danish pharmaceutical industry association (Lif) said in a Danish newspaper that it was 'shaken and enraged about the criticism' that it could not recognise. This statement was astounding. We had merely reported what the international drug companies wrote in their trial protocols, which Lif could easily have verified for themselves. We also assumed Lif was well aware that our findings were correct, in contrast to its public statement.

Lif subsequently filed a groundless case against us, alleging we had committed scientific misconduct. Meanwhile, a *BMJ* editor visited me and when I told her about the 'case' she burst into laughter. She couldn't imagine why anyone would be foolish enough to accuse Altman and me of scientific misconduct. She asked to have a paper about the affair when we had been acquitted, and I submitted one. However, the *BMJ*'s lawyer was worried about possible litigation. Therefore, our paper was transformed into the article 'Industry attack on academics', written by one of the *BMJ*'s journalists, which started thus:[14]

> An apparently uncontroversial study of potential industry influence on sponsored drug trials resulted in the authors facing accusations of misconduct.

This encapsulates what I mean about being called controversial. When powerful people don't like the results but cannot dispense with them using academic arguments, they shoot the messenger instead and they also call him controversial. Unfortunately, being 'controversial' carries a negative connotation. We often say that a piece of research is controversial when we really mean we don't have confidence in it.

I believe all types of misconduct in science should be publicly exposed, not only to deter others from behaving similarly but also because we may learn from it. Lif abused a well-functioning system that deals with accusations of scientific misconduct, and I exposed Lif's misconduct and explained in the *Ugeskrift for Læger* why Lif's attack on us couldn't possibly be based on an honest suspicion of scientific misconduct but, rather, was an attempt at intimidation and harassment.[15]

Journalists sometimes ask why I look for controversies. I don't; they come looking for me. An important reason for this is that digging deeply into the substance often produces interesting findings, even in well-researched areas where one would not have expected surprising discoveries. Most of the research we undertake at The Nordic Cochrane Centre stems from our own ideas, but even when we're asked by others to do a particular piece of research we regard as routine work, it often ends up being 'controversial', in the sense that the results are unwelcome to some people. As an example, my wife, clinical microbiologist Helle Krogh Johansen, and I once performed a systematic review of the randomised trials that had compared two antifungal agents – an old drug, amphotericin B, and Pfizer's new drug, fluconazole. The aim of the review was to find out which drug was best, as these two agents were the two most promising ones of those we had previously studied.

We learned that Pfizer had manipulated several of its trials, biasing both their design and the statistical analysis in a way that favoured their own drug over the old, cheaper comparator. Some of the trial reports were rather obscure, but the primary investigators were unable to answer our questions and referred us to Pfizer, who didn't answer them, however. One of the problems was that patients appeared in various publications on the same trial so confusingly that we couldn't tell whether we had inadvertently counted the same patients twice in our review. Another problem was that Pfizer had used oral doses of amphotericin B, although it should be given intravenously, and had lumped the results for the handicapped comparator drug with those for nystatin, which doesn't work at all.

Thus, the trials were, in effect, rigged. Pfizer is the world's largest pharmaceutical company, and our findings appeared in *JAMA* in 1999[16] alongside an editorial[17] and they also became front-page news in the *New York Times*.[18]

In 2001, The Nordic Cochrane Centre was on the front page of the *New York Times* again.[19] We had published a study on the effect of placebo in the *New England Journal of Medicine*,[20] which was considered 'controversial' by many placebo researchers. For about 50 years, researchers had believed that placebos were highly effective in treating subjective symptoms, but most of the research underlying this belief was flawed. It had estimated the effect of placebo as the before–after difference in a group of patients receiving a placebo. With this approach, the effect of placebo cannot be distinguished from the natural course of the disease, which often leads to spontaneous improvement, and the effects of other factors.

Our placebo work was initiated and led by a talented young researcher, Asbjørn Hróbjartsson, who did his PhD on this subject and still works with me, now as senior researcher. Through a highly elaborate searching process, he retrieved trials where the patients had been randomly assigned to either placebo or no treatment. He even convinced the US National Library of Medicine to rewrite its software so that he could search on 'no treatment', which wasn't possible as the word 'no' was not searchable in the database. Experts had thought there were few such trials, but Hróbjartsson included 130 in the review, most of which had a third group that received an active intervention, often similar in appearance to the placebo. We started the project believing there were important placebo effects, but when we finished, there wasn't much left. The review showed that the belief that placebos generally have powerful clinical effects was wrong. The only thing we found was a possible small effect of placebo on pain, but we couldn't exclude the possibility that this result was caused by bias and not by the placebo.

The review sent shock waves throughout the placebo research community and we needed to publish several additional papers to show that our critics were wrong when they interpreted our results in inappropriate ways or made errors in their calculations. We have also updated the review, most recently in 2009.[21] One of the criteria for judging the usefulness of a research paper is the amount of previous papers it renders superfluous. On that count, I would say that our placebo review is one of the most useful papers we have ever written.

Our research on mammography screening also made headlines, in the *New York Times* and elsewhere. Because of my repeated appearances in the *New York Times*, one of its reporters, Donald G McNeil, visited me in my home and wrote an article in 2002 in the series, 'Scientists at work'.[22] He called his article 'A career that bristles with against-the-grain conclusions' and started thus:

> Seated at an eerily neat desk in a modern office on the grounds of Denmark's state hospital, Dr. Peter C. Gotzsche does not seem a man whose bite is much worse than his very gentle bark.
>
> But this tall, gray-haired statistician is sending some eminent doctors into fits of apoplexy as he quietly implies that they've wasted their lives defending old wives' tales, maltreated their patients or assisted in frauds that perhaps ought to land them in jail.

One of the greatest joys of doing research is its unpredictability. Little did I know how fruitful our collaboration would turn out to be when, also in 2002, a medical student, Karsten Juhl Jørgensen, wrote to me that he wished to do a meta-analysis as his special subject.

We nearly missed the opportunity. As Karsten's final exam was just 6 months away, there wasn't enough time to do a meta-analysis, and I therefore advised him to ask my senior researcher, Asbjørn Hróbjartsson, whether he had a relevant project on stock that Karsten could finish in so little time. He hadn't, but Karsten was determined to work with us and he approached me again. I like determined people, and I suggested Karsten study the information on mammography screening provided by consumer organisations and compare it with that from cancer charities. This idea was pretty far from doing a meta-analysis, but Karsten accepted it, did the study, got his exam and published his survey of websites in the *BMJ*.[23]

After a couple of clinical years, Karsten enrolled as a PhD student at our centre, and he later expanded on his research portfolio in order to become a doctor of medical science instead. By the end of 2009, he had eight papers for his thesis, five of which were in the *BMJ*. This was a remarkable achievement, and although he had not yet defended his thesis, he succeeded in obtaining a 3-year postdoctoral grant from the Danish Research Council and also was one of only five young elite researchers in healthcare that year.

In 2007, Karsten and I were awarded the first prize from the Society of Medical Writers, for a *BMJ* paper on the content of invitations to publicly funded screening mammography.[24] There are three other awards I have been particularly happy to receive in relation to my work on mammography screening, as they carry the names of great men. I received the Skrabanek Foundation Prize in Dublin in 2001; the Niels A Lassen Award in Copenhagen in 2001; and the Michael Berger Award in Düsseldorf in 2009. Petr Skrabanek was anything but mainstream and opportunistic: he was a thinker. When he wrote a detailed and instructive review in the *Lancet* on breast screening in 1985,[25] a critic used not only a tactic that is common in politics, the 'if you can't beat them, lie about them' trick, but also the 'you're not one of us' trick. Skrabanek was accused of being an armchair scientist. Skrabanek responded to the untruthful statements and added, 'people who sit are not necessarily less often right than those who walk about: Einstein did no more than "armchair" research'.[26] The Niels A Lassen Award was special; although his research was in physiology, which is quite far from the research I do, the chairman of the award committee said that the motivation for giving me the award was that, like Lassen, I challenged traditional beliefs and stuck to my findings under pressure, as long as I hadn't been proven wrong. As will be apparent in this book, my research has not been similarly praised by screening advocates.

Our collaboration with the media

Battles of the hearts and minds of the public and the politicians take place in the media, also when these battles are about science. The media have almost always treated The Nordic Cochrane Centre fairly, valuing that the centre is free from political, financial and other conflicts of interest. It is very rare in healthcare that people do not have conflicts of interest, and we talk to journalists every week who seek advice related to stories they are working on.

In 2008, journalists Jeanne Lenzer and Shannon Brownlee wrote an article in the *BMJ* titled 'Naming names: is there an (unbiased) doctor in the house?'[27] which reminded their readers that journalists often forget that conflicts of interest may bias the opinions of expert sources. Another key point was that medical stories are often unbalanced or wrong because journalists fail to seek out sources who can offer an independent perspective.

Lenzer and Brownlee published the names of about 100 people whom they felt could be trusted and who were not on the take.[27] I happily agreed to appear on their list, which was enthusiastically embraced by other reporters, and many people requested copies of it. In contrast, it was roundly condemned by colleagues who are paid allies of the drug industry (the so-called industry apologists), and there have been attempts at smuggling moles onto the list under false pretences. A list of honest people is obviously too dangerous for the drug industry.

There is a built-in problem in the way journalists deal with controversies. Very often, the media give equal coverage to opposing views even when it is pretty clear that one side is right and the other wrong. Therefore, people wishing to spread doubt about an issue are often tremendously helped by journalists who perhaps rather naively do their work as they learned it at journalist school. As an infamous example, fraudulent research by Andrew Wakefield was published in the *Lancet* in 1998 that claimed to have found a relation between vaccination against measles and development of autism. The *Lancet* later retracted the paper,[28] but the media coverage might have given parents the impression that the scientific evidence for and against a link was equally strong.

The oddest thing about this false balance is that even when journalists know that one side is lying, they may still write articles that leave their readers in total limbo about who is right and who is wrong.[29] Journalists have a major responsibility in shaping public opinion, and they should do better than this.

Working with the media can be useful for getting important scientific messages out to the public. It can also have its amusing moments. A reporter from Canada's major newspaper wished to write a story about the mammography screening controversy and asked me in an email where I was sitting when I decided to 'pursue this idea?' Baffled, I replied 'I'm sorry, I don't understand. On my chair?' The reporter then asked whether I was in my lab, office or home: 'Describe the room, what was happening at the time. Were you looking out the window, sitting in your kitchen drinking coffee one Saturday morning?' This style of journalism doesn't win many bonus points with scientists.

References

1 Gøtzsche PC, Kelbæk H, Vissing SF, *et al*. Acute cardiovascular effects of insulin in hyperglycaemic type I diabetics. *Scand J Clin Lab Invest*. 1991; **51**(1): 93–7.
2 Hecht F. Et al. gets Nobel Prize. *N Engl J Med*. 1977; **296**(4): 234.
3 Gøtzsche PC. Bias in double-blind trials. *Dan Med Bull*. 1990; **37**(4): 329–36.
4 Gøtzsche PC. Reference bias in reports of drug trials. *Br Med J (Clin Res Ed)*. 1987; **295**(6599): 654–6.
5 Gøtzsche PC. Patients' preference in indomethacin trials: an overview. *Lancet*. 1989; **1**(8629): 88–91.
6 Gøtzsche PC. Methodology and overt and hidden bias in reports of 196 double-blind trials of nonsteroidal, antiinflammatory drugs in rheumatoid arthritis. *Control Clin Trials*. 1989; **10**(1): 31–56 (erratum in *Control Clin Trials*. 1989; **50**(9): 356).
7 Gøtzsche PC. Multiple publication of reports of drug trials. *Eur J Clin Pharmacol*. 1989; **36**(5): 429–32.
8 Gøtzsche PC. Review of dose-response studies of NSAIDs in rheumatoid arthritis. *Dan Med Bull*. 1989; **36**(4): 395–9.

9 Gøtzsche PC. Meta-analysis of grip strength: most common, but superfluous variable in comparative NSAID trials. *Dan Med Bull*. 1989; **36**(5): 493–5.
10 Higgins JPT, Green S, editors. *Cochrane Handbook for Systematic Reviews of Interventions: version 5.1.0 [updated March 2011]*. The Cochrane Collaboration, 2011. Available at: www.cochrane-handbook.org (accessed 22 May 2011).
11 Chan AW, Hróbjartsson A, Haahr MT, *et al*. Empirical evidence for selective reporting of outcomes in randomized trials: comparison of protocols to published articles. *JAMA*. 2004; **291**(20): 2457–65.
12 Gøtzsche PC, Hróbjartsson A, Johansen HK, *et al*. Constraints on publication rights in industry-initiated clinical trials. *JAMA*. 2006; **295**(14): 1645–6.
13 Gøtzsche PC, Hróbjartsson A, Johansen HK, *et al*. [Constraints on publication rights in industry-initiated clinical trials: secondary publication] [Danish]. *Ugeskr Læger*. 2006; **168**(25): 2467–9.
14 Gornall J. Research transparency: industry attack on academics. *BMJ*. 2009; **338**: 626–8.
15 Gøtzsche PC, Johansen HK, Haahr MT, *et al*. [Scientific misconduct] [Danish]. *Ugeskr Læger*. 2009; **171**: 1206–9.
16 Johansen HK, Gøtzsche PC. Problems in the design and reporting of trials of antifungal agents encountered during meta-analysis. *JAMA*. 1999; **282**(18): 1752–9.
17 Rennie D. Fair conduct and fair reporting of clinical trials. *JAMA*. 1999; **282**(18): 1766–8.
18 Grady D. Drug studies said to magnify benefit. *New York Times*. 1999 Nov 10: A1, A18.
19 Kolata G. A study casts doubt on the placebo effect. *New York Times*. 2001 May 24.
20 Hróbjartsson A, Gøtzsche PC. Is the placebo powerless? An analysis of clinical trials comparing placebo with no treatment. *N Engl J Med*. 2001; **344**(21): 1594–602.
21 Hróbjartsson A, Gøtzsche PC. Placebo interventions for all clinical conditions. *Cochrane Database Syst Rev*. 2010; (1): CD003974.
22 McNeil DG Jr. Confronting cancer: scientist at work – Peter Gotzsche; a career that bristles with against-the-grain conclusions. *New York Times*. 2002 Apr 9.
23 Jørgensen KJ, Gøtzsche PC. Presentation on websites of possible benefits and harms from screening for breast cancer: cross sectional study. *BMJ*. 2004; **328**(7432): 148–51.
24 Jørgensen KJ, Gøtzsche PC. Content of invitations to publicly funded screening mammography. *BMJ*. 2006; **332**(7540): 538–41.
25 Skrabanek P. False premises and false promises of breast cancer screening. *Lancet*. 1985; **2**(8450): 316–20.
26 Skrabanek P. Breast cancer screening. *Lancet*. 1985; **2**(8461): 941.
27 Lenzer J, Brownlee S. Naming names: is there an (unbiased) doctor in the house? *BMJ*. 2008; **337**: 206–8.
28 Dyer C. *Lancet* retracts MMR paper after GMC finds Andrew Wakefield guilty of dishonesty. *BMJ*. 2010; **340**: 281.
29 Caplan PJ. *They Say You're Crazy: how the world's most powerful psychiatrists decide who's normal*. Cambridge, MA: Da Capo Press; 1995.

2

Important issues in cancer screening

'CATCH IT EARLY', 'IT'S BETTER TO FIND A SMALL TUMOUR THAN A big one', 'By finding the tumours early, more women will avoid a mastectomy', 'Mammography screening saves lives'. You've probably seen or heard some of these slogans. They appear convincing, and as they come from cancer charities, information material from screening centres, or national boards of health, you might not have thought much about whether they are correct but, rather, have just accepted them on their face validity. They are all wrong, misleading or doubtful, and I'll show why in this book.

To make it easier to understand the issues, I have written a general outline of them in this chapter. However, please note, as a general precaution: don't believe in slogans about cancer screening.

What it means 'to have cancer'

Cancer is a malignant disease that consists of abnormal cells with uncontrollable growth spreading throughout the body until they kill the patient. This is the picture of cancer most people have. But the picture is only partly correct.

The paradigm that cancer is always lethal originated in France at the beginning of the nineteenth century, at which time the so-called Paris School of pathological anatomy was flourishing.[1] Anatomical and clinical observations were correlated, and it became the task of the clinician by means of the physical examination to make those diagnoses that were known from autopsy studies. When people had died of an emaciating disease that wasn't tuberculosis, it was usually cancer. Therefore, it is not surprising that cancer was considered uniformly deadly.

Such observations were very useful, but they contained an element of circular reasoning. They originated from corpses and the conclusion was about lethality of a disease. This isn't really possible, as it cannot tell us whether some people with cancer have been cured.

As a matter of fact, this happens. Recent data have suggested that a substantial fraction of detected cancers are of no threat to the person,[2] and regression of untreated cancers or precursors of cancer have been described for many cancers, including cervical cancer,[3] colon cancer,[4,5] renal cell cancer,[6] melanoma,[7] breast cancer[8,9] and neuroblastoma.[10]

Cancer is so common that it is likely that *all* middle-aged people have cancer somewhere in the body.[10,11] We know this from autopsy studies, and thyroid cancer is a particularly illuminating example. Very few people have heard about anyone dying from thyroid cancer. Yet, in a Finnish autopsy study of 101 people who died from other diseases, thyroid cancer was detected in 36, and the researchers calculated that if they had cut the thyroid in thinner slices, they would have expected to detect cancer in most, if not all, of them.[10,12]

Given this information, it is very difficult to condone an advertising campaign, 'Don't forget to check your neck', which ran in the United States in 2009 and that encouraged people to visit doctors for clinical exams to detect thyroid cancer.[13] There is no evidence whatsoever that this would do more good than harm, but it seems that in the United States, nearly every body part susceptible to cancer has an advocacy group, politician or athlete with a public awareness campaign and slogans to promote screening.[13]

It is a biological fact of life that we cannot avoid getting cancer as we get older, and this has been explained at the molecular level. Our DNA contains telomeres, which protect us from development of cancer, but with time, this 'repair kit' runs out of supplies, and transformed cells can then continue their growth.

In common usage, the term 'having cancer' means being ill with cancer. However, it means something entirely different in a screening setting. As it is possible to detect cancer in virtually everybody over a certain age, if only we are investigated carefully enough, 'having cancer' may mean nothing other than harbouring harmless cell changes that will not give any symptoms for the rest of our lives.

Discussions often go astray because people – including professionals who work with cancer – do not distinguish between the two meanings of 'having cancer'. Old habits die slowly and, although we have now screened for cancer for about half a century, we still tend to think that 'having cancer' means being ill with cancer, just as the doctors thought in Paris 200 years ago.

This misconception brings me to another illuminating example, neuroblastoma, which is a cancer mainly seen in children. In Japan, screening for neuroblastoma was introduced in 1985 without any evidence from randomised trials that it would do more good than harm. The number of diagnoses rose markedly, which concerned some physicians. Since the treatment – surgery and chemotherapy – could kill the children, a group of paediatricians offered watchful waiting to parents of children with a cancer smaller than a tennis ball. The parents of 11 children accepted this, and the cancer disappeared in all of them without treatment.[10]

Overdiagnosis and overtreatment

The purpose of screening for a particular cancer is to lower mortality from that cancer in the population, which is usually expressed as the annual number of deaths per 100 000 people. Cancer is a group of diseases, each of which is very heterogeneous, and many cancers grow very slowly or not at all. Hence, the first thing we know about cancer screening is that it inevitably leads to harm in the form of overdiagnosis and subsequent overtreatment. Overdiagnosis is the detection of cancers that would not have been identified clinically in someone's remaining lifetime.

The problem is that we cannot distinguish between these harmless cancers that wouldn't have given any symptoms or presented any difficulty for the bearer and those that are dangerous. Therefore, the standard is to treat all of them. For example, virtually all overdiagnosed breast cancers are treated by surgery, many with radiotherapy and some with chemotherapy.[14]

As cancer screening always causes harm, the important question is whether screening reduces mortality from the cancer and, if so, whether the reduction is large enough to justify the harms inflicted on the healthy population. This is a judgemental issue that I shall come back to later.

Even today, I often need to explain what overdiagnosis is when I talk to journalists, and they get surprised when I say that it is inevitable with cancer screening. Their immediate reaction typically is that the pathologists must have made a wrong diagnosis, but that is not what it is about. Health professionals may make the same mistake. When I recently lectured at a meeting for pathologists and explained about overdiagnosis with breast screening, a pathologist said that they didn't make so many erroneous diagnoses. No, they don't. The diagnosis is correct most of the time, but the cancer is inconsequential.

There is a curious divide betwen the different types of cancer. As it has been known for decades that it is impossible to screen for prostate cancer without causing considerable harm in healthy males, it is strange that it has been possible for screening advocates to make people believe for so long that overdiagnosis isn't a problem with breast cancer.

Erroneous diagnoses and carcinoma *in situ*

Erroneous diagnoses cause much less harm than overdiagnosis, but they are still an important cause of harm with screening. This problem has received very little attention in the scientific literature and virtually none in the debates about breast screening. This is unfortunate, as both laypeople and physicians tend to overestimate grossly how accurate diagnostic tests are.[15]

A mammogram is an X-ray film, and it is difficult to interpret X-ray films. Many lesions are overlooked and many normal films are considered to be abnormal. One of the best studies on X-ray films dates back to the 1950s.[1,16] Ten doctors read almost 15 000 small chest films taken as part of a screening programme for tuberculosis among college students. One or more observers interpreted 1307 films as positive, meaning that more investigations were needed, but in the end, only eight students were found to have active tuberculosis. For tuberculosis, it is easy to decide whether or not a person with suspicious findings on the film also has the disease, as the presence of tubercle bacilli in a sputum sample establishes the diagnosis.

With breast cancer, we don't have such a convenient and reliable gold standard as the presence of tubercle bacilli. Instead, we have a pathologist who examines biopsies under the microscope to decide whether the cell changes should be called breast cancer. This can be a challenging task, and the difficulty and uncertainty are best illustrated when different pathologists evaluate the same biopsies independently of each other.

A very large observer variation study was based on the National Health Service (NHS) Breast Screening Programme in the United Kingdom and involved about 200 pathologists and 17 000 readings.[17] It showed that when a pathologist had decided that a patient had invasive breast cancer, the consensus was that it was *not* breast cancer in 3.1% of the cases, and that it was carcinoma *in situ* (including microinvasive cancer) in another 4.7%.

Carcinoma *in situ* is actually a misnomer. Cancer is an invasive disease and carcinoma *in situ* is Latin for cancer at the site. But carcinoma *in situ* is *not* invasive: the cell changes remain where they originated.

Words create what they describe, and names and classifications are important for our views of things. A pathologist once wrote a paper with the title 'Carcinoma-in-situ of the breast: have pathologists run amok?'[18] By calling it cancer, although it is *not* cancer, the pathologists contribute to the decision-making process in a way they should not, as the anxiety and the likelihood of treatment increases when patients and doctors hear the word *cancer*. Virtually all cases of carcinoma *in situ* in the breast are treated as if they were cancer. As fewer than half of these lesions ever develop into breast cancer, their detection through screening contributes substantially to overdiagnosis (*see* Chapter 16).

The disagreements among pathologists are particularly pronounced for carcinoma *in situ*.[17,19] In a study that included 17 cases of epithelial proliferations of the breast, five expert breast pathologists diagnosed 0, 1, 2, 3 and 9 cases as carcinoma *in situ*.[19]

Even so, the first uncertainty in breast screening – reading the mammogram – is considerably greater than the second – interpreting biopsies – as the level of agreement when two or more observers evaluate the same mammograms independently is so poor.[20–23] I shall return to this problem in some detail in Chapter 25 when discussing what the effect of screening is today.

The two uncertainties involved in deciding whether a woman has breast cancer, reading the mammogram and interpreting the biopsy, mean that some women who are diagnosed with breast cancer at screening do not have breast cancer. Errors of this kind cannot be avoided, but they are far less likely to occur when patients consult a doctor because of symptoms, e.g. the finding of a hard mass in the breast, than when the whole population in a certain age group is invited to screening. This is explained by the low disease prevalence in a screened population. A test that performs relatively well when patients consult a doctor because of symptoms will often perform poorly when used for screening healthy people. Clinicians are used to seeing patients with symptoms, and therefore get it wrong when asked about screening. A study showed that most gynaecologists think the risk is greater than 80% that a woman with a positive mammogram at screening has cancer, but it is actually only 10%.[24] Statisticians express the difference in this way: the a priori likelihood that a woman with symptoms has breast cancer is vastly greater than the likelihood that a woman invited to screening has breast cancer. Therefore, it is inevitable that many more erroneous diagnoses are made relative to the number of correct diagnoses when people are screened, compared with usual clinical practice, even if the same test is used, with the same criteria for a positive and a negative finding.[1]

I have not come across any publications estimating how commonly women are wrongly diagnosed with breast cancer, and so I have tried to work it out myself. Since there is a rather strong suspicion that a woman referred for biopsy has cancer – as the mammogram suggested this – the pathologist may tend to label borderline cases as cancer, particularly in the United States, where doctors fear being sued if they overlook a cancer (so-called defensive medicine). Therefore, whenever in doubt, it is tempting to say 'cancer'. If we assume that 10% of biopsies involve some degree of doubt,[17] and that half are true-positives and half are true-negatives, but that the pathologist says 'cancer' for them all, then 5% will have been diagnosed as cancer erroneously. This corresponds to about 1000 women every year in the UK breast screening programme.[25] Therefore, it is clear that, whatever the true rate of erroneous diagnoses is, the problem cannot be ignored.

More generally, considering diseases other than cancer, results from quite a few diagnostic tests are indeterminate, i.e. neither clearly positive nor clearly negative. But the answer given to the clinician is almost always that the patient either does or does not have the disease, not 'I don't know'. I once asked a pathologist why this was so and, to my surprise, he replied that clinicians cannot deal with uncertainties. They cannot act on a 'maybe'.

This black-and-white tradition has reinforced the terribly wrong idea that diagnostic tests are generally accurate and unambiguous. Patients – and also many doctors – don't realise that for almost all tests, there is a continuum from being clearly healthy to being clearly diseased, with a grey zone in the middle.[1] We have to make a decision where to split the grey zone into those we declare ill and those we declare healthy. No matter which cut-off point we choose, some of those we declare ill are healthy, and vice versa. The media contribute to the confusion by crying 'scandal' when cancer diagnoses have been missed and politicians look for scapegoats.

A study from the United Kingdom illustrates the problem of the grey zone in reading mammograms. Two radiologists looked at 33 734 mammograms independently and disagreed considerably as to who should be recalled for further testing.[26] If the women had been recalled whenever one of the radiologists recommended this, the recall rate would have been 9.9%. However, the radiologists discussed their findings and could also consult with a senior radiologist, which resulted in a recall rate of only 4.2%. This study shows why screening without meticulous quality control procedures and double readings, such as can occur in private practice, results in poor performance.

Erroneous diagnoses, and correctly diagnosed but overdiagnosed cases, provide the background for the saying that a healthy person is one who has not been subjected to enough diagnostic tests. They also explain why routine health checks applying many tests may do more harm than good. A mileage check-up may work well for cars, but not for humans.

Basic issues in cancer epidemiology

You need not know much about epidemiology to be able to follow the arguments in this book. However, there are a few essential issues.

The *incidence* of a disease is the number of new cases occurring in a certain time period,[27] often the calendar year. If we wish to compare the incidence of cancer in different countries, or changes in incidence in the same country, we use a common denominator, usually 100 000 people. For example, the incidence of invasive breast cancer in the United States was about 300 per 100 000 women aged 50 years or older in 1984.[28]

The *prevalence* of a disease is the proportion of a population that has the disease at a given point in time, e.g. on 1 January 2006. The prevalence encompasses all cases, including those that have existed for many years. Like incidence, it is usually expressed per 100 000 people and for a certain age group.

In relation to cancer screening, these concepts have been further refined. The *prevalence screen* is the first screen in a population. The idea is to detect cancers that have not yet been found as they have not given rise to symptoms. The *incidence screens* are those screening sessions that come after the prevalence screen; therefore, they detect new cancers that were not detected at the previous screen. Finally, cancers that pop up between two screening sessions because of clinical symptoms are called *interval cancers*.

For purely mathematical reasons,[10] screening primarily detects slow-growing cancers. This is because the longer the cancer has existed, the greater the chance that it will be picked up at a screening session. In contrast, a cancer that grows very quickly is much more likely to be detected clinically, between two screening sessions. Interval cancers are therefore more dangerous than cancers detected at screening.

As screening increases the prevalence of cancers with an excellent prognosis through overdiagnosis, and primarily picks up slow-growing cancers, cancers diagnosed in a region with screening will have a more favourable prognosis, on average, than cancers in a region without screening. This cannot say anything, of course, about the effect of screening, as the number of breast cancer cases in the screened region has been 'boosted' with many harmless cancers that weren't detected in the other region, as they don't give any symptoms. This fundamental problem is called *length bias*. Some of the slow-growing cancers in the screened region would have surfaced and caused symptoms at some later time, but those that wouldn't have surfaced are the overdiagnosed cancers. Overdiagnosis is therefore a special form of length bias.

Another fundamental problem that may lead to biased comparisons between screened and non-screened regions or countries is *lead-time bias*. The idea with screening is to detect cancers earlier than without screening; therefore, it is obvious that even if there wasn't any length bias (and therefore there weren't any overdiagnosed cancers), comparisons of regions or countries with and without screening will be biased if we use the number of years the patients have survived from the date of diagnosis as the outcome.

Comparisons within the same country made between a period before screening and a period with screening will suffer from the same two biases as comparisons between two countries. Awareness of these two biases is fundamental for those involved in cancer screening. However, misleading comparisons of the type I have just described abound in the breast cancer screening literature. What makes such deceptions particularly depressing is that they are easy to avoid. We only need to look at mortality instead of survival, e.g the annual number of breast cancer deaths per 100 000 in the population, which is not influenced by length and lead-time biases. People who are overdiagnosed won't die from their cancer, but this doesn't matter because we only count the number of deaths, not the number of those who live. The problem with counting those who are alive is that the denominator is not the entire population but, rather, the number of cases. This is where it all goes wrong.

These issues are so important that I shall explain them again below, with concrete examples, but first, a description of the difference between randomised trials and observational studies is needed.

Randomised trials, observational studies and a little statistics

A randomised trial is the most reliable method we have to study the effect of interventions. If we randomise a large number of people to receive or not receive an intervention, such as a series of screening mammograms, we can be confident that the two groups are very similar with respect to all known and unknown prognostic factors that may influence the risk of dying from breast cancer. For breast cancer, examples of such factors are age, socio-economic status, parity and the use of hormones.

However, if we see an effect, e.g. a difference in number of breast cancer deaths in the two groups, we cannot be certain whether it is real or just the play of chance. We use a statistical test to help us make an informed judgement about this, a so-called hypothesis test. Our null hypothesis is that there is no effect of screening, but if the observed difference is sufficiently large, it is unlikely that we would have seen it if there were no effect of screening. Traditionally, we reject the null hypothesis of no effect, if the chance of obtaining the difference we've seen in our trial, or an even larger difference, is less than 5%. We then say that the result is statistically significant at the 5% level, which is expressed as $p < 0.05$, where p means probability.

We may also address several similar trials in a systematic review and combine their results in a meta-analysis in order to see what the overall difference is between the intervention and no intervention in the trials. However, no matter how small the p-value is, we can never be certain that what we've seen in a trial or a meta-analysis is real. A better way of dealing with this inherent uncertainty in clinical research is to use the 95% confidence interval instead of the p-value. We don't know what the true effect is, but we are 95% confident that the true effect lies within the 95% confidence interval.

The 5% p-value and the 95% confidence interval are complementary, in the sense that $p < 0.05$ means that the 95% confidence interval does not include zero effect. As an example of this, the randomised trials showed that screening leads to a 35% increase in surgery (mastectomy or lumpectomy), with a 95% confidence interval ranging from a 26% to a 44% increase.[14] As the interval did not include 'no increase', this result must be statistically significant, and the p-value was actually < 0.00001. Therefore, we are 95% confident that the true increase in surgery lies between 26% and 44%.

This holds in an ideal world where the randomisation is performed correctly and where the researchers don't manipulate their data when they analyse them. This is not how the world is, however. Bias in analysis and reporting of results is very common, and there are far too many significant p-values in the literature.[29] Therefore, we always need to be careful when we interpret research findings.

In observational studies, we don't randomise people but we observe what happens, e.g. in a group that is screened and in a group that is not. Such studies are less reliable than randomised trials, as it is very likely that the two groups differ in other respects than whether or not they have been screened. We talk about confounding when a factor that increases or decreases the risk of dying occurs more or less commonly in screened people than in people who are not screened. The type of people who do not turn up for screening, for example, also tend to be those who don't follow other types of advice doctors give them, and if they experience a higher mortality, it might not have anything to do with screening but, rather, with their unhealthy lifestyles.

A good example of confounding comes from one of the screening trials, where the randomisation method was so poor that the two groups weren't similar. A trial from Edinburgh did not randomise women but, rather, randomised 87 general practices. With this cluster randomisation, all women attending a particular practice belonged to the same group, i.e. either they were all invited to screening or they were all not invited. It is a highly risky procedure and it failed. Only 26% of the women in the control group belonged to the highest socio-economic level, compared with 53% in the screened group.[14] Screening was associated with a 26% reduction in cardiovascular mortality and a 15% reduction in total mortality, which cannot have been caused by screening and merely shows that a high socio-economic level predicts a good life expectancy.

This doesn't mean that observational studies are useless. They can be very important for elucidating the harms of interventions, which are often insufficiently described in randomised trials. The researchers might not have looked for them or perhaps they randomised too few people to catch rare but important harms. The reason could also be that the follow-up was too short to capture harms that take a long time to develop, e.g. the cardiovascular harms of radiotherapy and the development of secondary cancers after chemotherapy and radiotherapy. Observational studies are also important for evaluating whether the beneficial effect seen in the trials can be reproduced in clinical practice. As I shall show in Chapter 15, this hasn't been the case for mammography screening.

Why screening leads to misleading survival statistics

The Malmö mammography screening trial is ideal for demonstrating in practice why screening leads to misleading survival statistics.[30] The trial ran for 9 years and during this period, 588 women were diagnosed with breast cancer in the screened group and 447 in the control group, i.e. there were 32% more cancers in the screened group. During this time, 63 of the 588 women (10.7%) with breast cancer in the screened group died from breast cancer, while 66 of the 447 women (14.8%) with breast cancer in the control group died. Thus, if we naively compare these death rates, the relative risk of dying from breast cancer is 10.7%/14.8% = 0.72, which means that screening has reduced breast cancer mortality by 1 − 0.72 = 28%.

If we look at all randomised women, which is what we should do, the relative risk of dying from breast cancer is (63/21 088)/(66/21 195) = 0.96, i.e. a 4% reduction in breast cancer mortality. This is the true result, which the Malmö trialists reported.[30]

What was wrong with the first analysis was that the denominator was not the number of randomised women, but the number of women with breast cancer.

The 32% additional women with breast cancer in the screened group have an excellent prognosis because of *length bias*. As my calculation was based on the number of deaths, length bias was the only bias operating, but it was large enough to yield a grossly misleading result.

If I had used survival time from the date of diagnosis, my result would have been even more misleading, as it would now also suffer from lead-time bias. The combined effect of these two biases and a third, very important, bias, the healthy screenee effect (those who attend are much healthier than those who do not accept the invitation), explains why women with screen-detected cancers have an excellent prognosis, e.g. in Malmö, 97% of these women were alive after 10 years.[31]

Why 10-year survival is also misleading

Survival from date of diagnosis is particularly misleading in a screening setting, as shown here in a fictitious example related to lung cancer screening with computerized tomography (CT) scan.[32] Imagine a group of patients with lung cancer currently diagnosed at age 67 years, all of whom die at age 70 years. Each survived only 3 years, so their 10-year survival rate is 0% (*see* Figure 2.1).

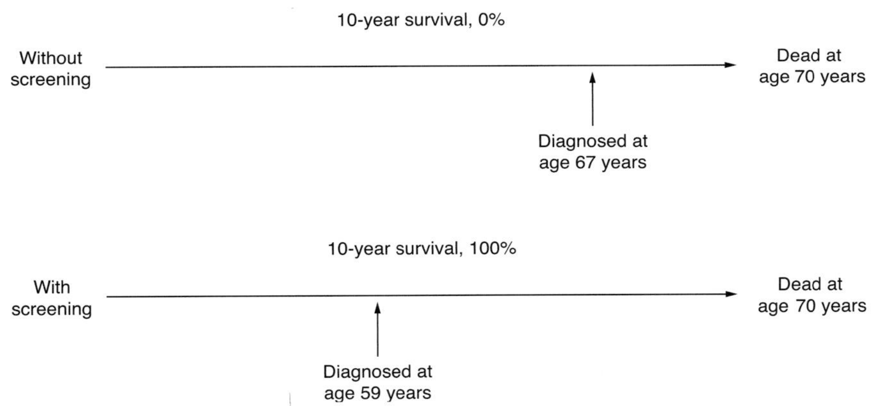

FIGURE 2.1 Lead-time bias. The 10-year survival is increased from 0% to 100% because the diagnosis is made earlier, but death is not delayed

Now imagine that the same group is diagnosed 8 years earlier by screening – at age 59 years – but they still die at age 70 years. As they have all survived 11 years, their 10-year survival rate is 100%. Even though the survival rates changed dramatically, nothing has changed about the time of death, as all patients died at age

70 years. This simple example of lead-time bias demonstrates how survival can be increased by advancing the time of diagnosis, even if no deaths were delayed.

Cancer charities and cancer researchers publish misleading survival analyses so often that it looks like a deliberate strategy to deceive the public into believing that important progress is being made in the fight against cancer. I shall give many examples of this in Chapter 19, and one example here.

Claudia Henschke and colleagues[33] published a study on CT screening for lung cancer in the *New England Journal of Medicine* in 2006. This study was totally unreliable.[32] The Achilles heel of their study was that it was not randomised but, rather, observational. However, the authors used it for a public relations campaign that was carefully planned.[34] Physicians giving media interviews had been instructed to conceal the study design by avoiding the use of terms such as 'observational' and 'non-comparative'. These tactics were seen as efforts to spin the results and deceive the public. A director of a health journalism graduate programme was shocked, as the scientists had urged each other to mislead journalists and to run from the truth.

Henschke denied that her study was observational and said there was no lead-time bias,[35] although both statements are untrue. She also viewed an ongoing randomised trial sponsored by the US National Cancer Institute as unethical, but what was unethical was the deceit practised by Henschke and her colleagues, which appeared to be effective. For example, the Lung Cancer Alliance, a patient group, declared that the verdict on CT scanning had been reached and called for action, although Henschke's paper gives no meaningful data about whether screening works and what its harms are. It was later revealed that two of the lead investigators of the study owned patents related to procedures for CT screening and that the study was partly funded by a tobacco company.[36]

Another interesting example is prostate cancer. It can be detected in most elderly males, but the vast majority of these cancers grow so slowly that they will not present any problems or come to the men's attention before they die from other causes. Thus, it is common to die *with* prostate cancer, i.e. a cancer that was first detected at autopsy and had never given any symptoms, whereas it is uncommon to die *from* prostate cancer. Autopsy studies have shown that invasive prostate cancer occurs in about 60% of men in their sixties, whereas the lifetime risk of dying from it is only about 3%.[10] It starts very early: prostate cancer was found in about 30% of men who died in their thirties in accidents.[11] Although this is fairly well known in the public at large, people still get it terribly wrong, as they don't distinguish between the two meanings of 'having prostate cancer'. For example, Republican Rudy Giuliani, former mayor of New York, used his experience of prostate cancer to political effect in a 2007 radio campaign advertisement.

Giuliani remarked, 'I had prostate cancer, five, six years ago. My chances of surviving prostate cancer and thank God I was cured of it, in the United States, 82 percent. My chances of surviving prostate cancer in England, only 44 percent under socialized medicine.'[37]

The sobering fact is that the incidence of prostate cancer pseudo-disease has exploded in the United States because of the unconscionable use of the prostate-specific antigen (PSA) test.[38] In the United Kingdom, far fewer males get tested. Therefore, it is totally misleading to compare the survival of people with the diagnosis in the two countries, as, because of overdiagnosis, many more males with the diagnosis in the United States have a harmless form of prostate cancer than those in the United Kingdom. In fact, the annual number of deaths from prostate cancer per 100 000 males shows that the death rate is the same in the United States as in the United Kingdom.[24] And what Giuliani calls socialised medicine in the United Kingdom is better than the US healthcare system, which costs nearly double that in Western Europe and yet US health outcomes are markedly poorer.[39]

Misleading survival analyses can also be produced without screening. At a meeting in 2004, Marianne Ewertz, a professor of oncology, talked about progress against cancer and presented the survival of women with breast cancer as of today and compared it with the survival half a century earlier. There was no hint in her presentation that such a comparison is misleading, because women were diagnosed much later in the course of their disease 50 years ago. This made a politician in the row behind me whisper to his neighbour: 'I think we are now moving away from evidence-based medicine!'

The term evidence-based medicine was coined by Gordon Guyatt from McMaster University in Hamilton, Canada, in 1991,[40,41] and it is now commonly used to say that our decisions should be based on the best available science. Instead of looking to authority when in doubt, we should identify the relevant studies, critically appraise them and apply the results to the problem at hand.

A paper in the *Journal of Clinical Oncology* reported in 2008 that among breast cancer patients of at least 80 years of age, the 5-year breast cancer–specific survival was 82% among women who were non-users of screening mammography, as opposed to 88% among irregular users and 94% among regular users.[42] The investigators noted that regular mammography may be beneficial for older women, without reservations.

With colleagues from Europe and North America, I commented that lead-time and length biases are elementary and fundamental in cancer epidemiology and observed that the journal's editors must have been unaware of these biases, otherwise they wouldn't have published the paper.[43] Moreover, we pointed out that credible evidence of a beneficial effect of breast cancer screening for older women doesn't exist, whereas there is solid evidence of harms.

But the damage had been done. The media coverage in the United States was considerable, with stronger conclusions than the authors intended. The American Society of Clinical Oncology fanned the flames with its totally inaccurate and misleading press release entitled *Women 80 and Older Benefit from Mammography, but Few are Screened*.[44]

There is no shortage of examples of invalid results receiving undue attention in the media. A particularly egregious one was published by Mike Richards and colleagues[45] in the *BMJ* in 2000. The authors wished to estimate the number of lives saved because of screening and improved treatment of cancer by comparing two time periods in England and Wales. That is very simple to do: count the number of cancer deaths in the recent period of interest for each cancer and compare it with the expected number, by extrapolating the time trend in cancer mortality in the earlier time period. However, the authors looked at 5-year survival rates and, unsurprisingly, their study was torn to pieces in the letters that followed.[46] People experienced in cancer surveillance, statistics and public health were among the authors of the article, and one came from a 'Cancer Intelligence Unit'. But their study wasn't intelligent. Their starting point was the government's target that by 2010 the mortality from cancer in people below 75 years of age should be reduced by at least 20%. It was curious, therefore, that the authors did not look at exactly that: mortality.

The following chapters describe the scientific evidence for the benefit and harms of mammography screening, the scientific and political controversies, and the way the public has been informed about screening. At the end of this book, I shall discuss which effect of screening we might have expected based on the tumour data from the screening trials, and which effect we may expect today.

References

1 Gøtzsche PC. *Rational Diagnosis and Treatment: evidence-based clinical decision-making*. 4th ed. Chichester: Wiley; 2007.

2 Newman DH. Screening for breast and prostate cancers: moving toward transparency. *J Natl Cancer Inst*. 2010; **102**(14): 1008–11.

3 Schlecht NF, Platt RW, Duarte-Franco E, *et al*. Human papillomavirus infection and time to progression and regression of cervical intraepithelial neoplasia. *J Natl Cancer Inst*. 2003; **95**(17): 1336–43.

4 Hofstad B, Vatn MH, Andersen SN, *et al*. Growth of colorectal polyps: redetection and evaluation of unresected polyps for a period of three years. *Gut*. 1996; **39**(3): 449–56.

5 Loeve F, Boer R, Zauber AG, *et al*. National Polyp Study data: evidence for regression of adenomas. *Int J Cancer*. 2004; **111**(4): 633–9.
6 Gleave ME, Elhilali M, Fradet Y, *et al*. Canadian Urologic Oncology Group. Interferon gamma-1b compared with placebo in metastatic renal-cell carcinoma. *N Engl J Med*. 1998; **338**(18): 1265–71.
7 Printz C. Spontaneous regression of melanoma may offer insight into cancer immunology. *J Natl Cancer Inst*. 2001; **93**(14): 1047–8.
8 Krutchik AN, Buzdar AU, Blumenschein GR, *et al*. Spontaneous regression of breast carcinoma. *Arch Intern Med*. 1978; **138**(11): 1734–5.
9 Zahl P-H, Mæhlen J, Welch HG. The natural history of invasive breast cancers detected by screening mammography. *Arch Intern Med*. 2008; **168**(21): 2311–16.
10 Welch HG. *Should I Be Tested for Cancer? Maybe not and here's why*. Berkeley: University of California Press; 2004.
11 Welch HG, Schwartz L, Woloshin S. *Overdiagnosed: making people sick in the pursuit of health*. Boston, MA: Beacon Press; 2011.
12 Harach HR, Franssila KO, Wasenius VM. Occult papillary carcinoma of the thyroid: a 'normal' finding in Finland; a systematic autopsy study. *Cancer*. 1985; **56**(3): 531–8.
13 Singer N. Forty years' war in push for cancer screening, limited benefits. *New York Times*. 2009 Jul 16.
14 Gøtzsche PC, Nielsen M. Screening for breast cancer with mammography. *Cochrane Database Syst Rev*. 2009; (4): CD001877.
15 Woloshin S, Schwartz L, Welch HG. *Know Your Chances: understanding health statistics*. Berkeley: University of California Press; 2008.
16 Garland LH. Studies on the accuracy of diagnostic procedures. *Am J Roentgenol Radium Ther Nucl Med*. 1959; **82**(1): 25–38.
17 Sloane JP, Ellman R, Anderson TJ, *et al*. Consistency of histopathological reporting of breast lesions detected by screening: findings of the U.K. National External Quality Assessment (EQA) Scheme; U.K. National Coordinating Group for Breast Screening Pathology. *Eur J Cancer*. 1994; **30A**(10): 1414–19.
18 Foucar E. Carcinoma-in-situ of the breast: have pathologists run amok? *Lancet*. 1996; **347**(9003): 707–8.
19 Rosai J. Borderline epithelial lesions of the breast. *Am J Surg Pathol*. 1991; **15**(3): 209–21.
20 Kerlikowske K, Grady D, Barclay J, *et al*. Variability and accuracy in mammographic interpretation using the American College of Radiology Breast Imaging Reporting and Data System. *J Natl Cancer Inst*. 1998; **90**(23): 1801–9.
21 Beam CA, Layde PM, Sullivan DC. Variability in the interpretation of screening mammograms by US radiologists: findings from a national sample. *Arch Intern Med*. 1996; **156**(2): 209–13.
22 Poplack SP, Tosteson AN, Grove MR, *et al*. Mammography in 53,803 women from the New Hampshire mammography network. *Radiology*. 2000; **217**(3): 832–40.
23 Sickles EA, Wolverton DE, Dee KE. Performance parameters for screening and diagnostic mammography: specialist and general radiologists. *Radiology*. 2002; **224**(3): 861–9.
24 Gigerenzer G, Gaissmaier W, Kurz-Milcke E, *et al*. Helping doctors and patients make sense of health statistics. *Psychol Sci Public Interest*. 2008; **8**(2): 53–96.
25 Patnick J, editor. *NHS Breast Screening Programme Annual Review 2008: Saving Lives through Screening*. Available at: www.cancerscreening.nhs.uk/breastscreen/publications/2008review.html (accessed 4 March 2009).

26 Warren RM, Duffy SW. Comparison of single reading with double reading of mammograms, and change in effectiveness with experience. *Br J Radiol*. 1995; **68**(813): 958–62.
27 Rothman KJ. *Modern Epidemiology*. Boston, MA: Little, Brown & Co.; 1986.
28 Gøtzsche PC. On the benefits and harms of screening for breast cancer. *Int J Epidemiol*. 2004; **33**(1): 56–64.
29 Gøtzsche PC. Believability of relative risks and odds ratios in abstracts: cross-sectional study. *BMJ*. 2006; **333**(7561): 231–4.
30 Andersson I, Aspegren K, Janzon L, *et al*. Mammographic screening and mortality from breast cancer: the Malmö mammographic screening trial. *BMJ*. 1988; **297**(6654): 943–8.
31 Janzon L, Andersson I. The Malmö mammographic screening trial. In: Miller AB, Chamberlain J, Day NE, *et al*., editors. *Cancer Screening*. Cambridge: Cambridge University Press; 1991. pp. 37–44.
32 Welch HG, Woloshin S, Schwartz LM, *et al*. Overstating the evidence for lung cancer screening: the International Early Lung Cancer Action Program (I-ELCAP) study. *Arch Intern Med*. 2007; **167**(21): 2289–95.
33 International Early Lung Cancer Action Program Investigators, Henschke CI, Yankelevitz DF, *et al*. Survival of patients with stage I lung cancer detected on CT screening. *N Engl J Med*. 2006; **355**(17): 1763–71.
34 Goldberg P. I-ELCAP 'soundbites' for investigators were a protocol for spin, critics say. *Cancer Lett*. 2006; **32**(42): 1–5.
35 Goldberg P. Lung screening advocates say verdict's in, attack NCI randomized trial as 'outdated'. *Cancer Lett*. 2006; **32**(39): 1–7.
36 Corrections. *N Engl J Med*. 2008; **358**(17): 1862, 1875.
37 Dobbs M. The Fact Checker: Rudy wrong on cancer survival chances. 2007 Oct 30. Available at: http://blog.washingtonpost.com/fact-checker/2007/10/rudy_miscalculates_cancer_surv.html (accessed 22 May 2011).
38 Jemal A, Tiwari RC, Murray T, *et al*. Cancer statistics, 2004. *CA Cancer J Clin*. 2004; **54**(1): 8–29.
39 Nolte E, McKee CM. Measuring the health of nations: updating an earlier analysis. *Health Aff (Millwood)*. 2008: **27**(1): 58–71.
40 Guyatt G. Evidence-based medicine. *ACP J Club (Ann Intern Med)*. 1991; **14**(Suppl. 2): A–16.
41 Evidence-Based Medicine Working Group. Evidence-based medicine: a new approach to teaching the practice of medicine. *JAMA*. 1992; **268**(17): 2420–5.
42 Badgwell BD, Giordano SH, Duan ZZ, *et al*. Mammography before diagnosis among women age 80 years and older with breast cancer. *J Clin Oncol*. 2008; **26**(15): 2482–8.
43 Berry DA, Baines CJ, Baum M, *et al*. Flawed inferences about screening mammography's benefit based on observational data. *J Clin Oncol*. 2009; **27**(4): 639–40.
44 American Society of Clinical Oncology. *Women 80 and Older Benefit from Mammography, but Few are Screened*. Available at: www.asco.org/ASCOv2/Press+Center/Latest+News+Releases/General+News+Releases/Women+80+and+Older+Benefit+from+Mammography,+but+Few+Are+Screened (accessed 22 May 2011).
45 Richards MA, Stockton D, Babb P, *et al*. How many deaths have been avoided through improvements in cancer survival? *BMJ*. 2000; **320**(7239): 895–8.
46 Baum M. Survival and reduction in mortality from breast cancer: impact of mammographic screening is not clear. *BMJ*. 2000; **321**(7274): 1470; author reply 1471–2.

3

Does screening work in Sweden?

THERE HAVE BEEN NINE MAMMOGRAPHY SCREENING TRIALS AND four of these have been carried out in Sweden. The Swedish trials have been hugely important for the introduction of mass screening in the United States, the United Kingdom, Australia, Europe and elsewhere. One trial in particular stands out: the Two-County trial from the Kopparberg and Östergötland counties.

The Two-County trial was published in the *Lancet* in 1985 and showed a 31% reduction in breast cancer mortality.[1] The fact that the trial was supported by the Swedish National Board of Health helped in getting a national screening programme established at an unprecedented speed for such major undertakings. It started in the same year, and by only 4 years after this, 85% of the Swedish women in the relevant age group (50–69 years) had been included in the programme.[2] In the United States and Australia, screening became more widespread at about the same time, and it was introduced in the United Kingdom in 1988.

Therefore, it was totally unexpected when a study in the *Swedish Medical Journal* (*Läkartidningen*) by general practitioner Göran Sjönell and clinical pharmacologist Lars Ståhle reported in 1999 that screening was ineffective.[2] The effect in the Two-County trial was so large that it should have been easy to see an effect of the programme in Sweden so many years later. But breast cancer mortality was only 1% lower than what it would have been without screening. Sjönell and Ståhle therefore called for a reassessment of the rationale for screening.

What ensued contained all of the ingredients that should prevail in the international debates about mammography screening during the following decade. Misleading statistical analyses, accusations of poor science when results are unwelcome, *'you're not one of us'* (and therefore not worth listening to), conflicts of interest, speculations about the motives of one's opponents, and poor understanding of the basics of cancer screening. If that wasn't enough, the screening advocates played the ultimate trump card, which I shall call the 'you are killing my patients' argument: that those who raise questions about screening are responsible for the death of many women.

The first letter was written by the director of the Swedish National Board of Health, Nina Rehnqvist, and two professors from the same institution, Måns Rosén and Ingvar Karlberg.[3] They pointed out it was inconsistent that Sjönell and Ståhle had excluded counties that introduced screening early or where randomised trials of screening had been performed, when they had nonetheless included Stockholm, reasoning that only 10% of the women had participated in the trial. They also criticised that Sjönell and Ståhle had extrapolated a historical mortality trend to see whether screening had lowered breast cancer mortality, compared with what was expected without screening. This criticism was less important, as one would not expect much change in a mortality trend that had been stable for decades.

Rehnqvist and colleagues[3] noted that the 10-year survival of patients with breast cancer was better in those counties that started screening early than in those that started late. They didn't present a statistical analysis of their data, which is poor science, as we can't know if the difference was statistically significant or if it could have occurred by chance. However, they made a far worse error, and Sjönell and Ståhle[4] pointed out what it was.

Ten-year survival is highly misleading in a screening setting because of lead-time and length biases. For example, Swedish counties starting screening early will have more overdiagnosed cases than counties starting late, i.e. they have included more women who will not die from breast cancer, which is a special case of length bias. These women will inflate the 10-year survival rate; therefore, the comparison Rehnqvist and colleagues[3] made is hopelessly flawed, also because earlier diagnosis inflates 10-year survival (lead-time bias). Sjönell and Ståhle[4] mentioned there was 30% overdiagnosis during the first 6 years after screening started, and when they adjusted the calculation for this problem, the counties in the Two-County trial had a 10-year survival that was *lower* than the average for the whole country.

The primary investigator for the Two-County trial, László Tabár,[5] and the chairman of the Swedish Cancer Foundation's Planning Group for Mammography Screening, Lars Erik Rutqvist,[6] also published criticisms. Two of them were particularly relevant; namely, that the follow-up after screening had started wasn't very long and that some of the deaths were caused by cancers detected before screening started, which would make it more difficult to see an effect if there was one.

However, the crux of the issue had nothing to do with methodology. It was that no one seemed interested in taking the observations seriously. People filter what they see through their belief system. According to an old adage, there is none so blind as he who *will* not see, and all the critics had vested interests in mammography screening. Eleven years later, in 2010, our research group confirmed the findings of Sjönell and Ståhle,[7] and I shall come back to this in Chapter 15.

When strong believers run out of good arguments, *ad hominem* arguments and bullying often take over. In *The Art of Always Being Right*, German philosopher Arthur Schopenhauer (1788–1860) calls this 'the ultimate strategy'.[8] When you perceive that your opponent has the upper hand, the only thing you can do is to attack the person rather than his arguments.

Måns Rosén and colleagues[9] from the Swedish National Board of Health published a second letter, which was not about whether screening was efficacious but about protecting the programme. The title was 'Women: continue to go to mammography!' and their remarks about Sjönell and Ståhle were derogatory, e.g. 'they totally lack insight into how epidemiological data can be used and interpreted'. Most astonishingly, Rosén and colleagues[9] criticised Sjönell and Ståhle for not having taken into account that the incidence of breast cancer influences the mortality of breast cancer. But Sjönell and Ståhle[4] had just explained why it is misleading to take the increased incidence of breast cancer into account. By definition, overdiagnosed women don't die from breast cancer.

Unfortunately, it is very common in scientific disputes for people to ignore what their opponents have already explained. Rosén and colleagues[9] noted, 'The agreement in the criticism is total and no international scientific journal with careful peer review and quality demands would accept such articles.' How could they know this? And the 'total' agreement was among a few people – six to be exact – with vested interests. I shall call this the 'everybody agrees' trick.

Finally, Rosén and colleagues[9] played the 'you are killing my patients' card. They mentioned that some women had cancelled their appointments for screening and they estimated that between 50 and 100 women would die prematurely every year for that reason. They also noted that this was an ethical question that Sjönell and Ståhle and the mass media should have considered.

Let us pause for a moment and think. If we generalised this argument to become a common ethical standard, it would mean that researchers could never question any intervention if it was believed that the intervention saved lives. Thus, we would probably still have performed bloodletting in our hospitals for all kinds of diseases, even for cholera, where such treatment is detrimental.

Tabár[10] also came back and criticised Sjönell and Ståhle for having sought publicity, for having held a press conference and for spreading their comments via newspapers and the Internet. Well, that is what universities recommend researchers do: to disseminate their findings also to the public. Tabár[10] remarked that the good reputation of Sweden had been damaged. That is quite an accusation, in the same category as the 'you are killing my patients' argument.

The tactic of creating pariahs was also used. Rutqvist[6] was astonished that Sjönell and Ståhle had explained that the lack of an effect in practice might be because the effect in the randomised trials had been overestimated due to methodological errors. He said that Sjönell and Ståhle were alone in the world literature with this idea, which wasn't true: the reliability of the randomised trials had been criticised many times before,[11–15] including in the *Läkartidningen*.[15]

References

1 Tabár L, Fagerberg CJ, Gad A, *et al*. Reduction in mortality from breast cancer after mass screening with mammography: randomised trial from the Breast Cancer Screening Working Group of the Swedish National Board of Health and Welfare. *Lancet*. 1985; **1**(8433): 829–32.
2 Sjönell G, Ståhle L. [Mammographic screening does not reduce breast cancer mortality] [Swedish]. *Läkartidningen*. 1999; **96**(8): 904–5, 908–13.
3 Rehnqvist N, Rosén M, Karlberg I. [The National Board of Health and Welfare on mammographic screening: mortality analysis requires completely different methods] [Swedish]. *Läkartidningen*. 1999; **96**(9): 1050–1.
4 Sjönell G, Ståhle L. [A reply on mammographic screening. How long do we have to wait to see the affect on survival?] [Swedish]. *Läkartidningen*. 1999; **96**(15): 1882–3.
5 Tabár L. [Assessment of the effect of mammographic screening can not be based on wrong data] [Swedish]. *Läkartidningen*. 1999; **96**(14): 1763–4.
6 Rutqvist LE. [Reduced mortality with mammographic screening: the natural course, too rough methods resulted in miscalculation on breast cancer] [Swedish]. *Läkartidningen*. 1999; **96**(10): 1210–1.
7 Jørgensen KJ, Zahl PH, Gøtzsche PC. Breast cancer mortality in organised mammography screening in Denmark: comparative study. *BMJ*. 2010; **340**: c1241.
8 Schopenhauer A. *The Art of Always Being Right*. London: Gibson Square; 2009.
9 Rosén M, Rehnqvist N, Stenbeck M. [A final comment from the National Board of Health and Welfare: women–do attend the mammographic screening! A new group for analysis of the effects is being set up!] [Swedish]. *Läkartidningen*. 1999; **96**(15): 1883.
10 Tabár L. [Mammography saves lives through early intervention in the natural course of breast cancer] [Swedish]. *Läkartidningen*. 1999; **96**(16): 1943.
11 Skrabanek P. False premises and false promises of breast cancer screening. *Lancet*. 1985; **2**(8450): 316–20.
12 Skrabanek P. Mass mammography: the time for reappraisal. *Int J Technol Assess Health Care*. 1989; **5**(3): 423–30.
13 Schmidt JG. The epidemiology of mass breast cancer screening: a plea for a valid measure of benefit. *J Clin Epidemiol*. 1990; **43**(3): 215–25.

14 Schmidt JG. Response to Dr Shapiro's dissent. *J Clin Epidemiol*. 1990; **43**: 235–9.
15 Isacsson S-O, Larsson L-G, Janzon L. [Is the documentation really sufficient? Don't promote screening without debate] [Swedish]. *Läkartidningen*. 1985; **82**: 2672–3.

4

Stonewalling the Cochrane report on screening

THE DISAPPOINTING RESULTS IN SWEDEN WERE ALSO NOTICED IN Denmark. One month later, the Danish Medical Association contacted the Danish National Board of Health with its worries about the lack of benefit, erroneous diagnoses and the overtreatment of harmless cases.

The letter from the association arrived at the the Board of Health's rather newly established Health Technology Assessment (HTA) agency at a delicate moment. In 1999, screening in Denmark took place in only two areas, corresponding to 20% of the population. Many people had doubts about screening, but a political majority was in favour of spreading it to the whole country. This went against the view held by the minister of health, and a voting about screening was just 5 weeks away.

Historically, the Board of Health had taken a zigzag course on mammography screening. In 1989, it issued a whole book[1] based on only three trials that recommended that all women aged 50–69 years should be offered regular screening.[2]

In 1994, additional trials had been published that were less convincing, and a new thick report appeared that was more undecided, with a vague and awkward conclusion.[3] The board could not counter the decisions made by those counties that had planned to introduce screening. But it said nothing about what the other counties should do. It mentioned that the trials didn't give an unambiguous answer, and it noted that the randomisation in the Two-County trial was not optimal, whereas the Canadian trials were well done and didn't suffer from the shortcomings of earlier trials.

Only 3 years later, in 1997, a third heavy report recommended screening in the whole country.[4] The doubt was gone, although no new results had been published and there was no attempt at quality assessment of the trials. The trial results were taken for granted, even the totally unreliable result from Edinburgh. It is a mystery what caused this change in policy and lack of a critical look at the evidence, but it is clear that the pro-screeners had won the power struggle.

The Danish Society of General Practitioners represents those doctors who will have to deal with all the negative consequences of screening. It participated in the working group but was overruled by the pro-screening lobby.[5] The society had wanted the following sensible statements to be included in the 1997 report's nine-page summary, but this request wasn't granted.

- Screening has not decreased total mortality.
- About 25% of all healthy women will be suspected of having cancer in the course of 10 screenings.
- About 24% of the cancers will not be detected at screening [these are the dangerous interval cancers].
- Screening reduces the risk of dying from breast cancer from 5% to 4% [this came from the 1997 report, but it was misleading; it should have been from 0.5% to 0.4%].[6]

The spokesperson for the society, Inga Marie Lunde, also wondered why a newspaper article from a leading person in the Danish Breast Cancer Group, Mogens Blichert-Toft, was emotional and revealed a lack of understanding of the uncertainties of screening. He described his own arguments as logical and factual, although they were surprisingly quite the opposite, and he consistently described other people's arguments as unfactual. Blichert-Toft also played the 'you are killing my patients' card, saying that opponents of screening wished that Danish women continued to die from the disease. That is certainly not factual. Ole Hartling, chairman of the Danish Council of Ethics, a parliamentary committee that initiates debates about difficult ethical issues in healthcare and gives advice to politicians, noted that it is outrageous to suggest that opposition against screening should be based on such evil thoughts.[7]

The hot potato from the Danish Medical Association didn't stay for long at the HTA agency. The agency had a collaborative agreement with The Nordic Cochrane Centre, and so the hot potato was passed on to me a week later. Statistician Ole Olsen and I told the Cochrane Breast Cancer Group the next day that we were interested in doing a Cochrane review on screening. As epidemiologist Lennart Nyström, who had previously published a meta-analysis of the Swedish trials,[6] had declared a similar interest, we contacted him, too, and agreed to do the Cochrane review together.

The Nordic Cochrane Centre was very small at the time. The few staff I had survived on grants and included Ole Olsen, who had mostly worked on pregnancy and childbirth and occupational medicine. In 1996, I published a report on the benefits of health technology assessment[8] on behalf of the Danish Council of Ethics, and a year later I shared a long taxi ride with the minister of health that gave me an opportunity to discuss the possible introduction of health technology assessment in Denmark. She was very keen to do this and she also realised that it was important to provide funding for my centre, as we knew how to evaluate the research literature critically. However, when the government bestowed its HTA agency with an annual budget of DKK25 million (about €3.3 million), a lot for a small country, we were forgotten.

Therefore, I was constantly on the lookout for funding opportunities and thought that if we did our job well, it might open up the money chest in the wealthy HTA agency for other projects we were more interested in. We didn't have the slightest interest in mammography screening, and the only thing we knew was that the Swedish trials had been criticised for using suboptimal randomisation methods.

It was a clear advantage that we knew so little about the subject and didn't know anyone involved with the trials or with running a screening programme. As soon as you know someone, it becomes more difficult to evaluate that person's research in an objective manner and to write about it in a straightforward manner. Furthermore, we didn't belong to any power or lobbying circles and our findings wouldn't be important for our careers. Or at least, so we thought. I had no idea that I would use much of my time over the next 10 years on mammography screening.

We took a break with our other projects and focused almost entirely on screening. We were baffled by what we found. We had expected the trials to be more convincing than they were, as screening seemed to be so popular, despite its high costs. The unexpected findings made us work very quickly, as it would have been rather futile to deliver our report after the politicians had voted about screening. Our report was finished in just 4 weeks, with the conclusion that the scientific basis for introducing mammography screening was very uncertain. We also noted that we could not exclude the possibility that screening did more harm than good.

The HTA agency had asked us to assess the systematic reviews and the relevant trials and to look not only at breast cancer mortality but also at total mortality. We found major problems with the randomisation procedures, e.g. the decriptions in the oldest trial, the Health Insurance Plan trial, which started in 1963 in New York, were very confusing, vague and contradictory, and we got the initial impression that it was a matched cohort study and not a randomised trial. Furthermore, we couldn't understand that the number of cancers was the same in the screened group as in the control group in this trial. As already explained, there will always be more cancers in a screened group than in a control group, and if the number of cancers is the same, there cannot be any effect of screening. However, the New York trial reported a 35% reduction in breast cancer mortality. This couldn't be a true effect. Furthermore, Petr Skrabanek[9] noted in 1989 that only 15% of the breast cancers in the screened group were detected by mammography and that the observed benefit was mainly seen in patients with metastases. This is also wholly unreasonable, but it required extensive detective work to find out exactly what was wrong with this trial (*see* Chapter 5).

I have already mentioned why the Edinburgh trial was also unreliable. This didn't matter for the screening advocates. It reported an effect on breast cancer mortality, which is what they wanted to hear, and they included it in their meta-analyses without reservations.

We also found serious problems with the Two-County trial. The population was divided into 45 clusters, which is only half as many as in Edinburgh, but in contrast to that trial, no baseline data have been published that can be used to judge whether or not the two groups were comparable apart from the age of the women. We observed that Nyström's meta-analysis of the Swedish trials from 1993 claimed that the Two-County trial wasn't biased,[6] but the reference to this claim was to a lecture that appears to have been unpublished. This had slipped under the radar of the *Lancet*'s editors, who would not normally allow a reference to unpublished material.

The other Swedish trials were carried out in Malmö, Stockholm and Gothenburg. We noted that the number of women in the Swedish trials was inconsistently reported, which is a very worrying observation. When trialists change the number of randomised women from report to report, it shows that they don't have the necessary expertise to carry out clinical trials. Later on, when we had had time to review the whole literature on the mammography trials, we found numerous additional discrepancies, both in number of women and in number of deaths, in the Swedish trials.

Adding to the confusion, the meta-analysis of the Swedish trials had not included the same women as those in the individual trial reports. It included women based on their exact age at randomisation, rather than the year when they were born. This led to a curious discrepancy for Stockholm where the number of women *fell* from 40 318 to 38 525 in the screened group, but *increased* from 19 943 to 20 651 in the control group. If the trials had been adequately randomised, the differences would have gone in the *same* direction. Reports on the Stockholm trial were terribly confusing, but we found out later that most women in the control group had been counted twice!

We commented on the poor randomisation methods in three of the Swedish trials and noted that the women in the screened groups and the control groups didn't have the same average age.

When we included all trials in our meta-analysis despite their shortcomings, we found a significant reduction in breast cancer mortality, but we were sceptical of this result for two additional reasons. First, because assessment of cause of death is difficult and inevitably leads to bias in favour of screening. Second, because screening increases the risk of death from causes other than breast cancer, e.g. the overdiagnosed healthy women in the screened group will be harmed by the unnecessary radiotherapy many of them received.

Total mortality is the only mortality outcome that is guaranteed free from bias in adequately randomised trials, and what we found was truly remarkable. In their meta-analysis of the Swedish trials, Nyström and colleagues[6] wrote – not in the results section but in the discussion – that the relative risk for total mortality was 1.00 (no confidence interval was shown). That was all. However, Skrabanek[10] reacted on this little piece of information, and Ole Olsen and I wrote about it in the *Lancet* 6 months later (we described the Two-County trial as two trials, which was sometimes done):[11]

> The credibility of the Swedish meta-analysis is greatly weakened because it did not report that there were important imbalances at baseline in four of the five trials; that there was increased mortality in the screened groups; and that an adjustment for age had been made without being described.[10] The last point is particularly important, since readers would not have expected any adjustment to have been made in a meta-analysis of hundreds of thousands of women in which adjustments would not change anything, provided that the trials had been properly randomised. Shortly after the publication of the meta-analysis, Skrabanek obtained the mortality rates from the primary author and drew attention to the increased mortality in the screened groups[36] (10.0% vs 9.4%; relative risk 1.06). In their response,[37] Nyström and Larsson did not mention the imbalance in age, but defended the relative risk of 1.00 reported in the meta-analysis by comparing the observed number of deaths in the screened groups with the expected number in the population (15,695 vs 15,710). They also noted that the relative risks for total mortality in the individual trials were 0.98, 0.98, 0.99, 1.00, and 1.00. It is quite impossible, however, to have such rates for the individual trials and then an increased mortality of 1.06 (as we calculated) for the pooled analysis. Swift[38] noted subsequently that 'a more precise and apt comparison is that between the mortality rates in the exposed and control groups.' In response to this indisputable fact Nyström and Larsson

> wrote that 'we prefer (see our response to Skrabanek) standardised relative risks to crude relative risks.'[39] This reply is remarkable since the whole idea of randomisation is to make unbiased analyses possible, but it was another 3 years before Nyström and colleagues admitted publicly that the analysis of total mortality had been adjusted for age.[35]

This suggests that Nyström and colleagues[6] tried to avoid admitting they had tuned their analysis without telling the readers about it. In randomised trials, the comparisons should of course be made between the two randomised groups. It is grossly inappropriate to compare a mortality rate in one of the two randomised groups with some 'expected number in the population'. It should be compared with the rate in the other group in the trial.

In our report to the Board of Health, we reported the 6% increase in total mortality in the Swedish trials but we also mentioned Nyström's estimate of no increase in mortality, pointing out that the difference in age had a major impact on the results. We cautioned that there must have been many other imbalances than that for age, and that adjustment for these would undoubtedly have yielded other relative risks for total mortality. In fact, a study of such problems that was based on individual patient data from two large randomised trials showed – contrary to conventional wisdom – that adjustments for imbalances often increase bias rather than reduce it.[12]

We also reported that, in contrast to what was usually claimed, screening doesn't lead to less radical treatments but to increased use of radical treatments because of an overdiagnosis of 25% to 35%. We furthermore noted that data from the United States had shown that 49% of screened women would experience at least one false positive mammogram during 10 screening rounds and that 19% would have a biopsy taken.[13] Finally, we mentioned that it is most relevant for the women to know the *absolute* effect of screening and not the *relative* effect. If one doesn't know what the risk of dying is, it is like seeing that a dress is for sale with a 25% discount without knowing what the original price was. We noted that the Swedish trials had reported a reduction in breast cancer mortality after 12 years from 0.5% to 0.4%,[6] i.e. an absolute reduction in risk of 0.1%, which meant that if there was any effect of screening, it must be very small. We also said we couldn't confirm the numbers in the 1997 report from the Danish National Board of Health that claimed a reduction from 5% to 4%.[4] This exaggeration of 10 times originated from a doubtful extrapolation to age 80 years, far beyond what the data allowed, and assuming that the women wouldn't die from anything else before that age, which is wrong. Another error was that as the 1% estimate was based on the lifetime risk of dying from breast cancer, it included young and elderly women outside the screened age groups who couldn't benefit from screening.

The erroneus 1% benefit would come up time and again, also in other countries. In Denmark, the Board of Health made precisely the same 'all-in' error in 2001 when it published an HTA report recommending screening for colorectal cancer.[14] The Board of Health never admitted its mistake, but after much pressure from independent scientists, a very long time and the assistance of a professor of biostatistics, Niels Keiding, the Board of Health issued a press release saying that it was possible to calculate the mortality reduction in other ways! The only time I have listened to a lecture on screening for colorectal cancer – which was in 2009, when it had still not been introduced in Denmark – the lecturer, surgeon Anders Fischer, showed the inflated number of preventable deaths, to the great surprise of some of the attendants.

We learned early on that politicians are often badly served by the institutions they have created and by the specialists whose salaries they provide. People tend to control and distort the information to serve their own interests. Unfortunately, this also applies to national boards of health and, not to forget, to the politicians themselves.

The Danish National Board of Health interferes with our report

Our 11-page report arrived at the Danish National Board of Health on 12 May 1999, a week before the voting in parliament on screening. The hot potato was quickly put on ice. The next day, we received instructions from Director Einar Krag to change our report. Our summary on page one was gone and had been replaced by a very short overall judgement, which was now on the last page, which is quite unusual and didn't apply to the board's own 1997 report. Furthermore, our conclusion, that we couldn't exclude the possibility that screening did more harm than good, had been edited away. There was nothing wrong with it, and we said the same in our Cochrane review 2 years later.

We were allowed to say that we could not exclude the possibility that screening had no effect and that total mortality was higher in the screened groups. But the conclusion now was that it was very important to perform a careful meta-analysis after Cochrane standards, seeking answers on the fundamental, outstanding questions through contacts with the trialists.

At a meeting on 14 May, we were told that our revised report was classified as a 'non-paper'. This meant that it was secret and could not be accessed through the Freedom of Information Act. I wondered whether this was legal. It later turned out that we had inadvertently sabotaged this ploy. As we had sent our report with a messenger to save time, it had been officially registered in the system and could not therefore become non-existent.

What made me even more uncomfortable was a letter to the head of the HTA agency, dated 14 May, which I didn't write, although I had to sign it in my name. It was drafted by Krag and was just *too* politically convenient, as it said something about 'misunderstandings'. There were absolutely no misunderstandings in our report, which was very clear. Therefore, I removed these sentences – which would have undermined our work – before I signed the letter.

This interference by a public agency with a scientific assignment went too far. We were forced to make a third version of our report. In it, our remark that the Board of Health's own 1997 report[4] had exaggerated the benefit by a factor of 10 was gone. Interestingly, in handwritten anonymous comments to our report, which I have saved, someone at the board had remarked that our statement about the exaggerated benefit undermined the credibility of the central health authorities. It surely did, but it was deserved. Our remark that it is usually claimed that screening with mammography leads to less radical treatments, which the board's own report also stated, was also rather conveniently removed.

I firmly believe that when authorities ask researchers to do research, they shouldn't interfere whatsoever with that research by demanding changes. Authorities have their own agendas, and in this case even their own report to defend; when they insist on changes, they overstep the boundary between science and politics. They must be kept totally apart.

Later, we acquired funding from the HTA agency to do a Cochrane review, but that was not the reason we complied with the demands for revisions. I had great respect for Krag, had worked at his department when we were both clinicians and understood that our report put the Board of Health in a difficult position *vis-à-vis* the politicians and the Ministry of Health. Furthermore, I did not want to become smashed between two elephants that constantly struggled over the right to set policies.

Krag promised to send our report to the minister, but on the day of the voting, the minister said in an interview that he had been informed that our report was only provisional. The board had dubbed it provisional and a 'working paper' after having seen our findings and conclusions, but there was nothing provisional about it. We called it a report and it was final.

There were other curiosities. According to a spokesperson from the Board of Health, the minister was informed about our report 3 days before the voting, but according to the minister, he first heard about it on the radio on the day of the voting.

We had doubted whether our report would make it to the ministry, as we criticised the Board of Health, which had invested a lot of prestige in recommending screening. But we kept quiet. We didn't know the rules of the game and we were afraid of making powerful enemies. I had no funding for our centre and I worked on getting it from the government.

We had told some of our colleagues about our findings and our troubles, and one of them informed a journalist. She wrote two front-page articles and mentioned that the Board of Health was in possession of a report that doubted the effect of screening,[15] accused the Board of Health of having shelved our report[16] and noted that 'Nothing hurts like the truth about health.'

This caused a leading speaker on health in parliament to speak of Machiavellian methods, asking who decided what politicians are entitled to know about. The president of the Danish Medical Association commented that when such results were available from The Nordic Cochrane Centre, the politicians should not vote without having heard about them. My two letters to the Board of Health, my own and Krag's redacted one, were reprinted in full length in the newspaper.

Three weeks later, the same journalist published a damning two-page article called 'Cheating with mammography'.[17] She told me that while working on it, a member of the advisory group the Board of Health had established on breast screening had told her that it would be dangerous to write about it and that she would be punished. What this punishment would consist of wasn't explained, and the threat had no effect on her.

As the cat was now out of the bag, so to speak, the HTA agency decided to send our original, non-redacted report to those who requested it. In a letter to the editor of the *Läkartidningen*, the agency stated that the report had never had a secrecy stamp on it. Well, perhaps not *literally*, but the Board of Health had done what it could to keep it secret and it was called secret in a Swedish newspaper a month later.[18] Elsebeth Lynge, main author of the Board of Health's 1997 report, described the confusion in a letter to us asking for 'a copy of the report, the expert opinion, the internal working document, or whatever the correct term is'.

Ole Hartling was quoted as saying there was no lobby for testicular cancer in parliament, perhaps because testicles are less poetic than breasts. Many critics noted that the Board of Health's 1997 report was constructed so that it would give the politicians the most positive impression of screening, and that the pages with the conclusions were particularly misleading. One remarked that it was comical to read that although false positive diagnoses could lead to temporary anxiety, this could not be detected in blood samples. He asked whether this was what the doctors intended to tell their anxious patients. But the propaganda had been effective. The politicians could all recite the exaggerated mantra of a 30% reduction in breast cancer mortality.

There was also the issue of conflicts of interest. Five of the six experts in the Board of Health's advisory group came from the Danish Breast Cancer Group, which had advocated screening since 1987 and which got an income of DKK1000 from the counties for every new breast cancer patient. The newspaper article reported that screening increases the number of women with breast cancer by 30%, and an economist from the advisory group remarked that she got angry when she learned that very favourable premises had been used for calculating the costs of screening. She had planned to protest, but the Board of Health's 1997 report was approved at a meeting in the middle of the summer holidays that was forewarned by only a week, so she couldn't come.

It is not an exaggeration to speak of Machiavellian methods. I was shocked by my new insight into how health policies are made, and several politicians expressed dismay about the way the Board of Health composes its advisory groups, which in reality have all the power. Top politicians in the counties didn't take the lack of independent advice lightly, and they asked what motivated the Board of Health to change its recommendations between its 1994 and 1997 reports, but they didn't get a satisfactory answer. One noted that the expert advice had been poor, and another that the advice on mammography screening couldn't be used for anything.[19] A year after these events, my own hospital, Rigshospitalet (Copenhagen University Hospital), which had introduced screening in 1991, wished to close it down,[20] but the politicians wouldn't allow it.

A month after we had finished our report, the HTA agency wrote to the Danish Medical Association explaining that our report had become publicly known via the press and noting that the agency had not asked The Nordic Cochrane Centre to summarise its findings as we had done. That was a pretty startling comment. Researchers *always* summarise their findings and make conclusions. And we had not overstepped the boundary between science and policymaking, as we did not suggest whether or not screening should be introduced. The agency also remarked that it couldn't give a reply to the Medical Association before the Cochrane review was finished, and this was expected to take quite a while . . .

> *How to discredit an unwelcome report. Stage one: Refuse to publish in the public interest saying . . . you are waiting for the results of a wider and more detailed report, which is still in preparation. (If there isn't one, commission it; this gives you even more time).*
>
> *Yes Minister* (BBC series)

At a meeting at the Board of Health with the breast cancer advisory group some weeks later, we were told rather bluntly that the credibility of our centre would hardly be supported by the report we had written, and we were urged to include surgical expertise when we evaluated the trials for our Cochrane review. We were under increasing pressure and were becoming increasingly irritated, so I replied that we didn't need surgeons, as we were not going to operate on the breasts ourselves. When the issue of including appropriate experts came up again, I responded that we had learned how to read and didn't need help with this. We explained that we had in fact already submitted our observations to an international scientific journal.[11] The draft minutes from the meeting said that we would do what we could to stop the public debate about our report and that we would not criticise the Board of Health's expert advice. We had not agreed to this during the meeting and these gagging statements were therefore modified in the final minutes.

Later, I wrote to the Board of Health and asked what evidence its working group had used when it declared in the summary of the report[4] that the number of women who will have a mastectomy will decrease. I explained that there was no reference for this pivotal statement and that we had found the opposite to be true in the randomised trials. I copied Finn Børlum Kristensen, head of the HTA agency, on my letter, and he wrote back declaring firmly that my request didn't fall under the agreement we had made with his institute to review the trials. He also questioned the appropriateness of a Cochrane centre contacting a country's uppermost scientific authority on health asking for the evidence behind a statement in a report, and he asked whether there was a need to discuss the activity profile of my centre with its advisory board.

There was a double irony in this. My letter to the Board of Health was prompted by a letter from a member of its own working group, Henning Mouridsen from the Danish Breast Cancer Group, who said I was wrong about screening leading to more mastectomies, but he didn't explain why. Second, the Board of Health had itself asked us to read their report when we reviewed the trials, which we had dutifully done. The board did not answer my letter.

I believe no one should be immune to questioning. Particularly not national boards of health, which are guided by specialists who have their own axes to grind.

The Board of Health's attempts at keeping the debate out of the public domain didn't stop there. In December 1999, I informed Kristensen that we would publish our findings in the *Lancet* and that we would hold a press conference 2 days before. Kristensen was very worried about this and referred to 'a common understanding' about mammography screening, arguing that the important scientific debate could not possibly be part of the public debate when our paper had not been published. We had merely planned the press conference for practical reasons, as we expected a lot of media attention, but we cancelled it, as we had sympathy with Kristensen's worries. However, this didn't help, as the *Lancet* published its own press release.

References

1 Sundhedsstyrelsen (National Board of Health). [*Mammography screening: usage and organization*] [*Danish*]. Copenhagen: Sundhedsstyrelsen; 1989.
2 Hartling O. [Encroachment on women] [Danish]. *Politiken*. 1998 May 25.
3 Sundhedsstyrelsen (National Board of Health). [*Breast cancer: early detection and diagnosis*] [*Danish*]. Copenhagen: Sundhedsstyrelsen; 1994.
4 Sundhedsstyrelsen (National Board of Health). [*Early detection and treatment of breast cancer. Status report*] [*Danish*]. Copenhagen: Sundhedsstyrelsen; 1997.
5 Lunde IM. [Screening as a favourite cause] [Danish]. *Berlingske Tidende*. 1999 Jun 23.
6 Nyström L, Rutqvist LE, Wall S, *et al*. Breast cancer screening with mammography: overview of Swedish randomised trials. *Lancet*. 1993; **341**(8851): 973–8.
7 Hartling O. [The difficult screening] [Danish]. *Berlingske Tidende*. 1999 Jun 19.
8 Gøtzsche PC. [*The scientific basis for health technology assessment*] [*Danish*]. Copenhagen: Det Etiske Råd; 1996. pp. 1–32.
9 Skrabanek P. Mass mammography: the time for reappraisal. *Intl J Technol Assess Health Care*. 1989; **5**(3): 423–30.
10 Skrabanek P. Breast cancer screening with mammography. *Lancet*. 1993; **341**(8859): 1531.
11 Gøtzsche PC, Olsen O. Is screening for breast cancer with mammography justifiable? *Lancet*. 2000; **355**(9198): 129–34.
12 Deeks JJ, Dinnes J, D'Amico R, *et al*. Evaluating non-randomised intervention studies. *Health Technol Assess*. 2003; **7**(27): 1–173.
13 Elmore JG, Barton MB, Moceri VM, *et al*. Ten-year risk of false positive screening mammograms and clinical breast examinations. *N Engl J Med*. 1998; **338**(16): 1089–96.
14 Brodersen J, Hartling O, Mäkelä M, *et al*. [Screening for colorectal cancer – is it worth it?] [Danish]. *Månedsskrift for Praktisk Lægegerning*. 2008; **86**: 1497–507.
15 Libak A. [New doubts about breast cancer screening] [Danish]. *Berlingske Tidende*. 1999 May 20: 1.
16 Libak A. [The Danish National Board of Health shelves report] [Danish]. *Berlingske Tidende*. 1999 May 23: 1.
17 Libak A. [Cheating with mammography] [Danish]. *Berlingske Tidende*. 1999 Jun 13: 11–2.
18 Atterstam I. [Mammography seriously criticised] [Swedish]. *Svenska Dagbladet*. 2000 Jul 20: 1, 4.
19 Felsby O, Ebdrup M. [Case about screening revealed poor expert advice] [Danish]. *Dagens Medicin*. 2000 Feb 3: 15.
20 Pedersen FS. [The Rigshospitalet will drop cancer screening] [Danish]. *Berlingske Tidende*. 2000 April 20: 1.

5

Troubling results in the *Lancet*

To say that screening mammograms don't save lives and might lead to unnecessary suffering or death borders on blasphemy. But that's exactly what some scientists have done.

Rita Rubin, *USA Today*

AT THE NORDIC COCHRANE CENTRE, WE HAD BEEN EXCITED ABOUT what we found and what we had described in our report to the Danish National Board of Health in May 1999; therefore, we were disappointed that the board preferred to deep-freeze our report like a corpse one wants to get rid of before others begin to notice the smell.

It did occur to us, of course, that screening believers may find it arrogant that two newcomers to the field concluded after only 1 month's work that the benefit of screening was uncertain and that it might do more harm than good. But we had no doubts about our findings or that they were important. Danes were not supposed to learn about our findings, but I decided that the whole world should know about them, and we therefore submitted a paper to the *Lancet* less than 4 weeks after the Danish National Board of Health had stonewalled our report.

David McNamee from the *Lancet* wrote to us, 'Your views on screening mammography certainly caused heads to turn here, and among our reviewers.' The comments were helpful and we improved our paper considerably during the autumn, adding information we had received from the trialists. The editors of the *Lancet* seemed in accord with our worries over screening and the Swedish data, as the next letter ended with: 'If you do not "end the tale", the commentator [who wrote an accompanying editorial] may ask why not.'

We explained to McNamee that various allegations had been raised against the Swedish trials but that we would prefer not to describe these in our paper. We also noted that some of the Swedish trialists had pointed out to us that there was little variation in breast cancer mortality rates in the screened groups from trial to trial but much more variation in the control groups,[1] and that this might be related to biased interpretations of the cause of death.

Surely, there were tensions between some of the Swedish trialists at the time. Another issue was that Tabár had withdrawn his data from further scrutiny by the Swedish Cancer Foundation. Kjell Asplund, chairman of the board of the Swedish Council on Technology Assessment in Health Care, had expressed serious criticism of the Two-County trial in the Swedish newspaper *Svenska Dagbladet*, and the chairman of the Swedish Committee on Scientific Dishonesty, Professor Lars Terenius, said that although the study could not be called directly fraudulent, it was an evident case of scientific misconduct.[2]

In the Two-County trial, there was very little difference in breast cancer mortality between the screened group and the control group until 4 years after randomisation. Then, there was an abrupt increase in deaths in the control group, whereas the trend in the screened group continued unchanged. Several people have expressed concern about this, also to us, as one would have expected to see an unchanged trend in the control group and a decreasing mortality trend in the screened group after some years because of the effect of screening, and not the opposite.

Possible errors could have been introduced in the Two-County trial for two reasons. First, the autopsy rate was low, only 36%, whereas it was 76% in the Malmö trial.[3] Second, cause-of-death assessments were performed blinded in the Malmö trial, i.e. without knowledge about whether a particular woman belonged to the screened group or to the control group, whereas they were not blinded in the 1985 report of the Two-County trial.[3] It is easy to make errors in an unblinded trial, and we therefore compared the cause of death for women diagnosed with breast cancer in the Two-County trial and in the Malmö trial (*see* Table 5.1).[4,5]

TABLE 5.1 Deaths among women diagnosed with breast cancer in two Swedish trials

	Two-County trial		Malmö trial	
	study group	**control group**	**study group**	**control group**
Breast cancer deaths	124 (60%)	119 (78%)	63 (64%)	66 (70%)
Other deaths	81 (40%)	34 (22%)	36 (36%)	28 (30%)
Total deaths	205 (100%)	153 (100%)	99 (100%)	94 (100%)

In the Two-County trial, only 22% of the women with breast cancer in the control group were assessed as having died from causes other than breast cancer, compared with 30% in the Malmö trial. If we apply 30% to the 153 deaths in the control group in the Two-County trial, we get 46 deaths from other causes, but only 34 were reported. Conversely, there would have been 12 more breast cancer deaths in the control group of the Two-County trial than in the control group in Malmö. This suggested to us that the cause-of-death assessment was likely biased in the Two-County trial.

The Swedish experts who have been critical of this trial have mostly aired their reservations in private, out of fear of being threatened or ridiculed. Some have wondered how it was possible that a physician from Hungary became the main investigator and was entrusted with carrying through the biggest research endeavour ever performed in Sweden. According to PubMed, Tabár had only five publications in English-language journals before he embarked on the trial, and he hadn't done a randomised trial before. He wrote the *Teaching Atlas of Mammography* with radiologist Peter Dean from Finland in the beginning of the 1980s, which may have played a role in his promotion as reader at the University of Uppsala.

The Swedish National Board of Health protected Tabár against criticism right from the beginning, which very likely also influenced people to keep quiet with their concerns. When the Malmö trial's negative results were published in 1988,[5] there were debates in the Swedish media about the value of screening. The previous director of the Board of Health, Barbro Westerholm, remarked that it was unethical that doctors and researchers commented in the mass media on a study they had not participated in.[6] This is an incredible attempt at stifling academic debate. I am sure the drug industry would love it if Westerholm's proposal came true, as it would give them complete control over the information flow. No critical views on drugs would reach the patients.

In Sweden, mammography screening became a feminist issue in the 1980s and women from all political parties joined ranks and demanded screening. This is not a setting that invites reasoned academic debate.

When our paper came out in the *Lancet* on 8 January 2000,[7] it was met with strong emotions. I think the reason for this is encapsulated in its summary, which carried a message that was threatening to the scientific foundation of screening.

Summary

Background A 1999 study found no decrease in breast-cancer mortality in Sweden, where screening has been recommended since 1985. We therefore reviewed the methodological quality of the mammography trials and an influential Swedish meta-analysis, and did a meta-analysis ourselves.

Methods We searched the Cochrane Library for trials and asked the investigators for further details. Meta-analyses were done with Review Manager (version 4.0).

Findings Baseline imbalances were shown for six of the eight identified trials, and inconsistencies in the number of women randomised were found in four. The two adequately randomised trials found no effect of screening on breast-cancer mortality (pooled relative risk 1·04 [95% CI 0·84–1·27]) or on total mortality (0·99 [0·94–1·05]). The pooled relative risk for breast-cancer mortality for the other trials was 0·75 (0·67–0·83), which was significantly different (p=0·005) from that for the unbiased trials. The Swedish meta-analysis showed a decrease in breast-cancer mortality but also an increase in total mortality (1·06 [1·04–1·08]); this increase disappeared after adjustment for an imbalance in age.

Interpretation Screening for breast cancer with mammography is unjustified. If the Swedish trials are judged to be unbiased, the data show that for every 1000 women screened biennially throughout 12 years, one breast-cancer death is avoided whereas the total number of deaths is increased by six. If the Swedish trials (apart from the Malmö trial) are judged to be biased, there is no reliable evidence that screening decreases breast-cancer mortality.

Our message was simple. If the readers believed the Swedish trials were unbiased, screening increased total mortality. If they believed they were biased, there was no reliable evidence that screening decreased breast cancer mortality. Michael Baum, who set up the first breast screening centre in the United Kingdom in 1988, understood this. He said to the *Guardian*: 'You cannot have it both ways. If those trials are unbiased, then you have to accept that for every one breast cancer death prevented by screening, there will be six extra all-cause deaths.'[8]

We mentioned that the number of randomised women varied between different reports on the same trial and wondered – but didn't write this – whether the researchers had been similarly sloppy when they counted the number of deaths and their causes. We also noted that the screened group and the control group were different at baseline in most of the trials, for example with respect to age, which is a sign of a suboptimal randomisation procedure. Therefore, we judged only the trials from Canada and Malmö to be unbiased.

The biased trials found a 25% reduction in breast cancer mortality, whereas the unbiased trials found a 4% *increase* in breast cancer mortality. This difference in results was expected, as poorly randomised trials tend to exaggerate the estimated effect.[9,10] The exaggeration is not necessarily a direct consequence of the randomisation method but can be related to other factors, as poor randomisation is often a marker for other problems.

We also reported that screening led to 35% more breast operations and 23% more mastectomies. This crucial finding, that screening leads to more breasts being removed, would be fiercely denied over the next 10 years by screening advocates. The first sentence in our discussion would also be ignored:[7]

> The effect of screening programmes, if any, is small and the balance between beneficial and harmful effects is very delicate. It is therefore essential that such programmes are rigorously evaluated in properly randomised trials.

The screening advocates would continue to lump all the trials together, including the flawed trials from New York and Edinburgh, but often excluding the two excellent trials from Canada that didn't tell them what they wanted to hear.

The Canadian trials

The two Canadian trials have been subjected to a lot of criticism, no doubt because they had the most negative results of the screening trials, but the criticism has been rebutted. It is ironic that these trials are those that are by far the best-documented ones.

A persistent criticism has been that it was difficult to find an effect because all women in the age group 50–59 years had their breasts physically examined. However, this is not important, because mammography finds many small tumours that cannot be detected on physical examination. Furthermore, the effect of physical examination is likely to be small, if any, as two large trials didn't find an effect of regular self-examination of the breasts.[11] What is disturbing about this criticism is that some of the critics must have known better. Physical examinations of screened women were performed in New York and Edinburgh, and screened women in the Two-County trial were encouraged to perform breast self-examinations once a month on a fixed date, which was Swedish policy generally.[3]

A nonsense argument is that the Canadian trials were not community based. Only in Canada were the women randomised after informed consent, which means that close to 100% received a mammogram in the first screening round. How this can be a problem is incomprehensible. It increases the chance of finding an effect, if there is one. In the other trials, segments of the population were randomised without having been asked, and not all attended.

Particularly the quality of the mammography has been criticised, but it is curious that the Canadian researchers have been punished for having published data on their quality control, as such data seem not to have been published for the other trials. Furthermore, this criticism would have been much more relevant if directed against the old New York trial, but it wasn't raised, as it yielded the effect people wanted to see. The Canadian trials are unique for their extensive quality control,[3,12] but screening advocates have propagated untruthful statements – including quite malicious ones – about the quality of the mammography repeatedly,[12–18] also after their errors were pointed out to them. The truth is that the tumours in the Canadian trials were smaller, on average, than those in the Swedish trials,[1] and it has been amply documented that the quality of the mammography was high and lived up to, for example, the standards set by Tabár, and they matched his own results.[18] Nonetheless, according to Cornelia Baines, co-principal investigator of the Canadian trials, Tabár said at a 1993 meeting that inadequate mammography diagnoses cancers that do not kill and that good mammography diagnoses cancers that will kill if not detected early.[18] It is difficult to believe that mammography can have such discriminating powers. One of the lies about the equipment used was circulated on the Internet in 2000: 'During that Canadian study the doctors were not even using mammography equipment but were using just regular X-rays. [US radiologist and hospital named] knows his stuff and will give you the correct information.'[12] Unfortunately, repetition renders falsehoods into received wisdom. I cannot recall having seen such lies about any other screening trial.

The Canadian trials were published in 1992, but on 29 June 1991, an anonymous editorial was published in the *Lancet* condemning the trial in those aged 40–49 years.[19] The protocol and the reliability of the data were said to have been 'fiercely criticised', with reference to a paper by US radiologist Daniel Kopans. This reinforces my view that *editorials should not be anonymous*. With publication comes accountability, but no one is accountable when their name is left out. The editorial built on a report in a newspaper, the *Sunday Times*, but Anthony Miller, co-principal investigator of the Canadian trials, regretted the appearance of the report and said that it included information not provided by himself or by Baines and that they had been unable to determine the source of the information.[14]

Radiologist Myron Moskowitz even went so far as to publish data in the *Journal of the National Cancer Institute* without the Canadian trialists' permission, although they were derived from a draft manuscript labelled 'Confidential not for publication or citation without prior permission of the authors'.[16]

What is true is that the randomisation could have been subverted, as the women's names were entered successively on allocation lists, in which the intervention – screening or control – appeared on each line. However, a forensic audit concluded that there could not have been enough cases of such subversion to affect the results. Furthermore, the screened and the control groups were very similar for important prognostic factors. This contrasted with all the other trials, none of which reported fully on any prognostic factor in the two randomised groups apart from age, and several of which had differences in age.

According to information I have received from the co-principal investigators, the coordinators were too busy to refer to the allocation lists when a woman came to the centre. And they had no direct contact with her or with the examiner who witnessed the consent process and conducted her examination until after the examination had been completed and the examination form filled out. Furthermore, they had no incentive to cheat, as any suspicion of cancer raised by the examiner would lead to mammography, also in the control group.

Media storm

We had expected some interest but were unprepared for the storm of debate and criticism that followed, which felt like a maelstrom. We found ourselves talking to radio and television stations from all over the world all the time. The *Lancet*'s press officer, Richard Lane, aptly described what happened.[20] We were blamed for the actions of others, for which we could have no responsibility:

> In January this year, Peter Gøtzsche and Ole Olsen from the Nordic Cochrane Centre in Copenhagen, Denmark, published a controversial meta-analysis in The Lancet. Their study, arrestingly entitled 'Is mammographic screening for breast cancer justified?', caused a media storm. Some sections of the press questioned The Lancet's judgement in publishing such a controversial review, which was roundly criticised by many 'experts'. As the press officer who put the press release on this paper into the hands of the media, I see this as a classic case-study of how science, and the publication of science in peer-reviewed journals, operates in an enormous goldfish bowl for all the world to see. The study, essentially a statistical exercise that consigned six previously published randomised trials to the dustbin because of methodological flaws, concluded that there was no evidence that mammographic screening for breast cancer saves lives.
>
> The headline on the BBC in the UK on the day the review was published was somewhat different from the authors' conclusion: 'New scientific study published today claims that mammography screening is a waste of time.'

> Similar headlines appeared in broadsheet and tabloid newspapers across the world. Just one short step from what was actually written in Gøtzsche and Olsen's article, to what a news editor wanted to say, and chaos ensued. For the record, in an interview on the BBC radio programme 'Today', Gøtzsche clearly stated that despite the BBC headline, he was not rubbishing mammography screening per se. If you read the press reports at the time, however, and some of the vitriolic comments from leading figures in the cancer organisations, you might have been forgiven for thinking that Gøtzsche had committed professional suicide. In this case, the spin came not from the scientists, but from certain areas of the media, who were helped on their way by 'expert' outside comment. These commentators, presumably for reasons of self-interest, had to condemn the study, even though they couldn't disprove it by offering alternative evidence.

A scientific analysis of the press coverage in the United Kingdom was also illuminating.[21] The contents of 148 articles in 113 newspapers were rather stereotyped. The main question was, 'Should the government abandon screening?' But each article had at least one reference to an 'expert' and the core content had little to do with our mortality analyses and was largely completely irrelevant, e.g. the data cited most frequently were number of cancers found, size of tumours at detection and mortality rates for the whole nation. Number of lives saved was also commonly reported, but as quoted in documents from the UK Screening Programme with no explanation how it was derived.

The most frequently cited information item from the *Lancet* was not even from our paper but from the opposing editorial by Harry de Koning,[22] who is a leading figure in the Dutch screening programme and a staunch supporter of screening. He said that we had ignored that other factors probably have a more important part in lowering the mortality rate through screening. It is not clear to me what exactly he meant by this cryptic remark, or how such other factors 'through screening' could change our negative result into a positive one.

There were also many testimonials from women, and many articles cited de Koning's statement that 'In the UK there has been a clear reduction in breast-cancer mortality due in part to screening.' This statement was not correct. It was not at all clear that screening had contributed.[23,24]

The first couple of days, cancer advocates and experts expressed 'dismay' and urged women to ignore our study, using theoretical arguments such as a better chance of recovery and sparing women disfiguring surgery. People with conflicts of interest were unquestioningly cited as authoritative, which is surprising, as journalists are usually critical about motives when they cite politicians.

In short, it was a remarkable defeat for evidence-based medicine. A lot of smoke, some errors and virtually no relevant substance in the comments from 'experts' and proponents for the programme.

The Department of Health issued a press release saying that the National Health Service (NHS) Breast Screening Programme is a success and that 'There is no new evidence in the report published today in *The Lancet*.' Pretty interesting that 'no news' can create such a fuss.

The director of the UK National Cancer Screening Programme, Muir Gray, said he walked from studio to studio and told the BBC that 'these two guys have the black belt in statistics'. If my memory doesn't fail me, Muir Gray has been the only official spokesperson saying he needed to look at what we had done, instead of offering hasty condemnations of our work, and a year later, he repeated that our paper was important.[25] We were therefore disappointed when he said in an interview with the *BMJ* that he suspected our paper had been rushed and not adequately peer-reviewed. He argued, 'the researchers stated that the meta-analyses were carried out only on 20 December 1999, yet the paper was published on 8 January 2000'.[26] I have no idea what made Muir Gray say this, and it isn't true. Our paper was submitted 6 months earlier, with the meta-analyses, and it was extensively peer-reviewed. I asked Muir Gray about this while writing this book, but he couldn't remember what the background was for his comment. I suspect he was misinformed by someone spreading lies about our research.

Other commentators were less forthcoming. Many comments were angry and derogatory, and if there was any scientific substance, it was misleading or false. It was not merely 'shoot before you ask', it was 'shoot in all directions and hope the monster goes away'. The most aggressive comments were from the United States. The head of a Long Island breast cancer advocacy group called '1 in 9' (the lifetime risk of getting breast cancer if you survive till age 85)[27] recommended women to get their mammograms and to do self-examinations, and added, 'To take away this tool – it's like murder'.[28]

Most comments were irrelevant. Harmon Eyre from the American Cancer Society stated that no other country was doing mammography screening as well as the United States.[29] This is not true, not only because screening is very poorly regulated[12] but also because many people cannot afford it, and I shall come back to this in Chapter 25. Muir Gray said that the UK programme was the best in the world,[30] which could be true, but that doesn't make the comment relevant. In a French journal, we were described as intellectual statistical masturbists,[31] which says more about the writer than about us.

Iben Holten of the Danish Cancer Society described our paper as an 'opinion piece' that expressed attitudes, called it unscientific in prime-time television news, and used the 'everybody agrees' trick.[30] She mentioned that she had recently attended a large meeting in Vienna about screening where everyone agreed that there was no doubt that mammography screening should be recommended.[32] I replied that in medical history, people had often agreed to make the same mistakes.[32] And I wondered what type of people show up at a screening meeting. Not a random sample of researchers, but a collection of screening enthusiasts.

The politician behind the proposal of introducing screening for all of Denmark declared that it would be sufficient for him if screening could improve the condition for only four patients.[30] With that type of prioritisation, we could easily spend more than our gross national product on healthcare.

The poorest argument, offered by cancer charities and politicians, was that the trials were outdated.[30] If that were the case, then logically, as we don't have evidence from trials we can trust, we would need to undertake new trials.

Spokespeople from the Swedish National Board of Health said that they could document that breast cancer mortality had fallen by up to 30%.[30,33] They published two studies within the next 2 months, neither of which, however, documented this. As I shall explain, the 30% estimate was nowhere to be found in their results,[34,35] neither at the time, nor later.

Email from researchers

In contrast to the public outcry, the email messages I received from researchers were supportive. Angela Raffle, consultant in public health for the national screening programmes in the United Kingdom, has written an excellent book with Muir Gray on screening,[36] and she congratulated us on our paper, which she felt brought very helpful simplicity and clarity, in plain English, for example, by talking about 'cell changes that may never develop into cancer' rather than using Greek and Latin. She considered this the only way we will ever get journalists and ordinary people to understand the issues. She also noted that everyone wants to make it a battle between enthusiasts and sceptics, as though it were some kind of religion, instead of taking the middle ground and saying screening is neither wonderful nor useless. It's complex, and facts are needed.

A biostatistician wrote that our results got a lot of attention in the United States, most of it furious denunciations by enraged oncologists, but he found their critique of our statistical methods amusing, 'since they are nearly all statistical illiterates'.

Cornelia Baines wrote that people never look closely at evidence that will undermine their beliefs and that she hadn't seen anything other than *ad hominem* attacks on our paper and on our 'flawed' study. She had listened to much of the media coverage and had realised that many of the US and Canadian screening experts who dismissed our research during media interviews – using every belittling adjective one can imagine – had not even read our paper. One of the things people said was that our paper was written by uninformed Danish mavericks who happened to be located at a Cochrane centre.

Baines also described her own experiences after she had reported the results of the Canadian trials. She received anonymous phone calls and letters telling her she was a murderer, that she should commit suicide and that she was personally responsible for the deaths of thousands of women.[17] At lectures sponsored by the American Cancer Society, she had been called a fraud, dishonest and unethical. She noted that people who believe in (or profit from) screening will defend it with a fury that is relentless and limitless. I agree with her. The rage and the *ad hominem* attacks were overwhelming.

A researcher told me he had contacted the *Australian*, the main national newspaper, and had asked their medical writer if she was going to write a similar piece about our review as one published in the *Sydney Morning Herald*. She replied 'probably not', as it would be difficult to write such a story without discouraging women from having mammograms. Pretty shocking, I would say. We know that decisions about news depend on their perceived effect on the population in dictatorship states and at Fox News in the United States, but in the main Australian newspaper?

A Norwegian colleague, Steinar Westin, told me a radiologist threatened to sue him after he gave an interview in a newspaper saying it would be unethical if specialists in private practice offered screening mammography. This was in 1989, when there was no screening in Norway. The radiologist complained to the Norwegian Medical Association, which ruled that Westin had done nothing wrong. There was never a court case, and it would have been highly 'un-Nordic' to sue anybody for their views on the ethics of screening.

Our collaboration with the trialists

Three days before our *Lancet* paper came out, we sent it to Lennart Nyström and the key investigators of the screening trials and invited them to participate in the Cochrane review. We had funding to cover the travel costs and suggested having a 2-day meeting in Copenhagen.

Anthony Miller was very keen to participate but he feared the key people might not wish to attend, as they had much to lose and nothing to gain by allowing others access to their secrets. Freda Alexander from Edinburgh and Philip C Prorok from New York also wished to come.

László Tabár declined our invitation. I didn't hear from the other Swedish investigators, but Ingvar Andersson from Malmö informed me that we would be invited to a meeting in Stockholm in the spring with the Swedish trialists, apart from Tabár, who had refused further collaboration with the other trialists and the Swedish Cancer Foundation, which sponsored an update of the Swedish trials. Tabár had said that he 'did not want his good results to be destroyed by the others' data'.[2]

Tabár had declined collaboration before. Following a consensus conference at the National Institutes of Health (NIH) in 1997, the US National Cancer Institute offered the trialists the opportunity to participate in a worldwide overview of the screening trials. Prorok informed me that 'some of the Swedish investigators' refused to participate. Miller said that Nyström was keen to participate, but that the NIH initiative had failed because of Tabár, which was confirmed in an article in the *Cancer Letter*.[37] Miller had visited Tabár in Sweden many years ago, when they were still on speaking terms, and his visit had worried him greatly. He was convinced that the cause-of-death ascertainment was biased.

Miller also doubted that the clusters in the Two-County trial were randomly selected. Baines recalled that Tabár said very bluntly that he would never let his data be contaminated by association with the trials carried out in Canada, New York and Edinburgh, as they were hopelessly flawed. She felt it was breathtakingly rude and arrogant and that there was a degree of territoriality among some of the male trialists that the females attending the US meeting deplored.

Nyström gave other arguments for the failure to collaborate in his thesis. He wrote that the Swedish trials evaluated the effect of invitation to mammography only (and not physical examination) and that they were population based.[38] I have already explained that both arguments are invalid.

Statistician Donald Berry from the MD Anderson Cancer Center in Texas noted, 'The credibility of these studies is very severely lacking, and it could be repaired simply by having the studies audited.'[39]

As Nyström had previously accepted to work with us on our Cochrane review, we felt we would succeed, but we didn't. The same day I talked to Andersson, who was positive, we received a letter from Lars Rutqvist, chairman of the Swedish Cancer Foundation's planning group for evaluation of mammography screening, which noted that he didn't 'find a collaboration with [us] worthwhile at this point in time'. He mentioned that he would be happy to invite us to one of their own meetings but that he preferred to wait till the update of the meta-analysis of the Swedish trials had been published. This was an effective brake, as it took 2½ years before it appeared in print.

Although no meetings could be arranged with the mammography screening trialists, we received replies to our questions about the trials from all the primary investigators, apart from Tabár.

Ten letters to the editor

After our paper was published, a female editor sent us 10 letters we should respond to. Back then, all letters in the *Lancet* started with 'Sir'. I reacted to this chauvinism by asking her whether we needed to reply with 'Sir' when we wrote to a lady and when the debate was about a disease in women. The editors were not moved, but the century-long habit of using 'Sir' disappeared from *Lancet* letters 3 years later.

The letters and our reply took up six pages,[40] which is more than our article. The Canadian trialists defended themselves against the routine but unjustified allegation of poor-quality mammograms, which de Koning had raised in his editorial.[22] They noted that the sensitivity and specificity of the Canadian mammograms were as good as those in any other trial, as were other indicators of performance, and they took issue with de Koning's claim that breast screening in the United Kingdom and the Netherlands had reduced breast cancer mortality. They explained that the reductions in the United States, the United Kingdom and the Netherlands were very likely caused by the widespread adoption of adjuvant chemotherapy and tamoxifen for node-positive disease (cancer that had spread to the lymph nodes) in the 1980s and noted that there had been no reduction in Sweden.

Michael Baum alerted the readers to the fact that the decline in breast cancer mortality in the United Kingdom had started *before* the screening programme was introduced, and he also credited adjuvant therapy for the decline.

Statistician Stephen Duffy, professor of cancer screening and a leading figure in the UK Screening Programme, and Tabár wrote that our paper was not 'worth a moment's consideration'. They also played the 'you are killing my patients' card, albeit indirectly, when they noted that:

> the morale of those who work hard to provide an effective mammographic screening service is needlessly damaged by high profile but inaccurate publications such as this. The second group is the millions of women faced with the decision whether to attend for screening.

They denied there were inconsistencies in numbers in the Two-County trial, although there are numerous inconsistencies, both in numbers of randomised women and in numbers of breast cancer deaths.[41,42]

A comment by Malcolm Law, Allan Hackshaw and Nicholas Wald was particularly interesting. They provided a meta-analysis in their letter, which included the seriously flawed Edinburgh trial and excluded the Canadian trials, and ended it by writing that:

> what is of concern is that a single dissenting paper can so readily undermine a well-researched conclusion endorsed by many international expert committees, because of the standing of the medical journal that published the paper. Such publications, and the publicity generated as a result, can erode public confidence, both in the medical activity in question and in scientific publications.

There are several issues here. First, expert committees have often been proven wrong when the scientific evidence was scrutinised by people without conflicts of interest. Second, their comment hints at censorship, as it indicates that our paper shouldn't have been published because of its perceived consequences. Third, they threw a boomerang. As I shall show in Chapter 20, Wald and Law later contributed substantially to eroding public confidence in research by publishing grossly erroneous estimates of the balance between the benefits and harms of mammography screening.

We rejected the statement by Duffy and Tabár that one of the Canadian trials was biased because there were more advanced cases of breast cancer in the screened group. This was not a sign of poor randomisation, but a result of the intervention, because the screening process increases the likelihood of detecting small cancers with positive nodes in the screened group.

We also dismissed the criticism of the Malmö trial by Sue Moss and colleagues that 24% of the women in the control group had undergone mammography. They failed to note that also in the other trials, such contamination had occurred.

Finally, we noted that Nyström had failed to mention that there had been a steady decline in breast cancer mortality in Sweden for 30 years, with no departure from this trend despite introduction of screening in 1985, and that it is irrelevant that the incidence of breast cancer has increased, which will always occur because of overdiagnosis.

A year later, Duffy published an invited paper in the *Breast* commenting on our *Lancet* article.[43] As its name suggests, the *Breast* is not a journal that bulges with papers critical of mammography screening, and Duffy's comment is now mainly of historical interest, as the issues he raised have been thoroughly dealt with in later papers. His conclusions were similar to those in his *Lancet* letter, but with more superlatives. Now people didn't just work hard; they worked extremely hard:

> Those clinical and related personnel who work extremely hard to provide high-quality screening, however, should not have their morale damaged by ill-considered publications such as those of GO [Gøtzsche and Olsen]. Similarly, women faced with the decision of whether to be screened should not be put off by hysterical headlines related to such high profile but inaccurate and flawed publications.

This rang a bell with me. Women with menstrual cramps were called hysterical before we knew that these pains were caused by prostaglandins and could be treated with prostaglandin inhibitors. So, people who think differently are hysterical and women should not ask questions, just attend screening. I doubt the women are grateful for Duffy's unsolicited paternalism. He thanked Tabár and Peter Dean for helpful discussion. I am sure it was helpful. But for whom?

Creative manipulations in Sweden

In January 2000, Måns Rosén from the Swedish National Board of Health and five others published a most curious five-page paper in the *Läkartidningen*. Apparently, the authors didn't know our *Lancet* article, which came out 3 weeks earlier, when they wrote their paper. They said there had been a reduction in breast cancer mortality of 20%–30% in the randomised trials and that – *mirabile dictu* – there had also been a reduction in breast cancer mortality of 20%–30% in those Swedish counties that introduced screening early.[34]

That was just too good to be true. If the effect is 30%, one would expect to see a reduction of only 8%–9% in the screened age groups after 10 years of screening (*see* Chapter 9). Although three of the authors were statisticians, there was no statistical analysis in support of the 20%–30% reduction and no confidence interval. Only some graphs were presented. It is very poor science to claim a positive effect without documenting it.

The authors noted that the mortality from breast cancer had increased in most countries, whereas it had decreased in Sweden, the Netherlands and the United Kingdom, where screening started in the 1980s. The documentation they provided was virtually non-existent and there were no references to their data, which is strange for a scientific journal. Further, when authors speak of trends, it is odd to show data for only 1 year for some of the included countries, and to show data for the 0- to 64-year age group, and not for those screened.

This paper was totally misleading. A year earlier, Levi and colleagues[44] had published trends for breast cancer mortality from 24 European countries, and it was impossible to see on the trends which countries had introduced screening and which hadn't. Levi published another paper in 2001 with additional data, and it was striking that the trend in Sweden in the age group 20–69 years was unchanged over almost 40 years, whereas there was a trend change for the better in several countries that had *not* introduced screening.[45] Furthermore, the average decline in Europe from 1988 to 1998 was substantially *larger* in the young age groups that had generally *not* been invited to screening (20–49 years) than in the relevant age groups (50–69 years). Levi updated these numbers in 2005 and in 2009, with similar results.[46,47] In a 10-year period, from 1990–94 to 2000–04, breast cancer mortality in the EU had declined by 25% for ages 35–44 years, 17% for ages 35–64 years, and only 6% for those aged 65 and above. This doesn't suggest an effect of screening but of better treatment, which benefits everyone, also those who are not screened.

We wrote an editorial in the same issue and noted that Rosén's paper wasn't a scientific article but rather an unsystematic review.[48] We quoted the authors for a 30% reduction in breast cancer mortality, which was what they had written in the manuscript we were asked to comment on, but in the published version, this had become 20%–30% without our knowledge.

Rosén and colleagues[35] seemed to have run out of arguments when they replied. They used a persuasive headline, 'The knowledge has been strengthened in favour of mammography screening' and intensified their cherry-picking and exaggerations. They now said that non-randomised studies (in three very small geographical areas, Florence, Nijmegen and Utrecht) had found a *decrease of 50%* in breast cancer mortality among those who participated in screening, again without references.

I knew this wasn't true. I had peer-reviewed the study from Nijmegen, which reported a non-significant 6%–16% reduction.[49] Rosén and colleagues[35] also played the 'you are killing my patients' card:

> That women as a result of these erroneous speculations become uncertain and perhaps do not attend screening is a consequence that Olsen and Gøtzsche should have thought about. How many deaths that occur too early will be caused by this?

Finally, they used the 'everybody agrees' trick, saying, 'Expert groups in the whole world agree about the effects of screening.' It is plain silly to say this, as experts never agree on anything, unless self-interest is involved. Sjönell and Ståhle had similar criticisms as we had.[50]

Rosén's next move was to publish the most peculiar analysis I have ever seen.[51] Rosén had five co-authors on his first comment, two on the next and now only one. I fully understand if none of the three statisticians on the first comment would have wanted to co-author Rosén's last piece. To accomodate the criticisms, Rosén and Stenbeck showed what the results were in those counties that had introduced screening early, middle and late. But it must have caused them difficulties to show what they wanted and I couldn't help thinking of an editorial in the *New England Journal of Medicine* that was about torturing the data until they confessed.[52]

What was so remarkable was that they used a *fourth-grade polynomial* to control for age effects in their logistic regression models. Further, they wrote nothing about their model, its assumptions or coefficients, whether it provided a good fit with the data, or why they didn't use simple regression (or a second- or third-grade polynomial).

With a fourth-grade polynomial, one can get almost any result one wants. One can, for example, take a straight line and bend it in almost any fashion, by choosing appropriate coefficients. I will illustrate this by means of a simple example. A fourth-grade polynomial has this formula:

$$y = ax^4 + bx^3 + cx^2 + dx + e, \text{ where } a, b, c, d \text{ and } e \text{ are constants.}$$

Let us assume that the x-values go from 1 to 10, corresponding to 10 years of observation. I now construct two sets of coefficients that are very similar, the only difference being that b is 0.05 in the first row and 0.02 in the second:

TABLE 5.2 Coefficients for a fourth-grade polynomial

a	b	c	d	e
–0.01	0.05	1	–2	6
–0.01	0.02	1	–2	6

This little difference has a major impact on the location of the two curves that I constructed using the coefficients and x-values from 1 to 10 (*see* next page).

This was just an example, with invented coefficients, but it illustrates the point. A small change in one of the coefficients had a dramatic effect on the results. If the two curves had illustrated projected revenues for a company, one of the curves

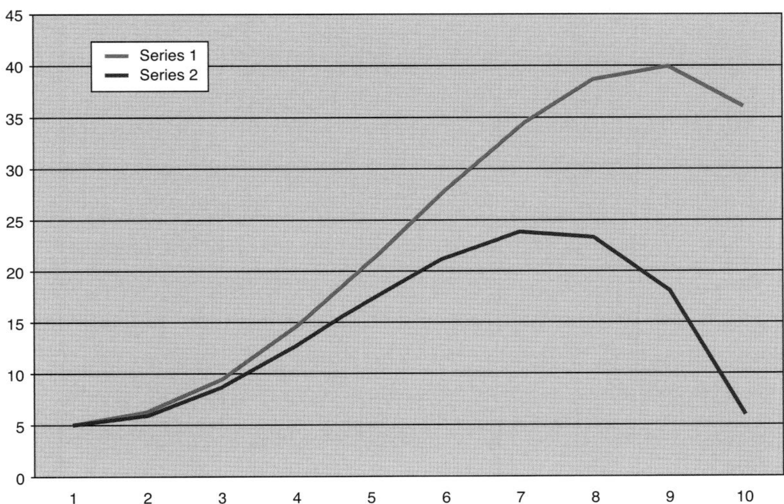

FIGURE 5.1 Two curves constructed from two fourth-grade polynomials with closely similar coefficients

shows a 620% increase in revenues, from 5 to 36, whereas the other shows a 20% increase, from 5 to 6, in the same time span of 9 years, a pretty big difference.

With this amazing technique, Rosén and Stenbeck showed that early adopters had an annual reduction in the risk of dying from breast cancer of 1.4%; middle adopters a reduction of 0.9% and late adopters a reduction of 0.4%. As their methods were completely obscure, they were impossible to criticise, step by step. Pretty smart, I would say, as people tend to believe what they cannot understand.

Peter Dean, a remarkable character

Peter Dean's approach came close to the 'if you can't beat them, lie about them' trick.[53] He said that our editorial in the *Läkartidningen*[48] and our *Lancet* paper both gave the false impression that they were official reports of The Cochrane Collaboration. This wasn't true. There is no such thing as an official report of The Cochrane Collaboration, and we had explained that we had invited the trialists to contribute to the Cochrane review we were working on.

In the lack of good arguments, Dean used superlatives: 'Gøtzsche and Olsen's heavily criticised reports give us no reason to doubt the results published from the highly respected Swedish mammography screening trials.'[53]

We replied that a scientific paper should be judged solely by its scientific merit and also wondered why one of these 'highly respected trials' was attacked by the

Swedish Medical Research Council and the Swedish Council on Technology Assessment in Health Care with allegations of scientific misconduct.[54]

Dean threw in additional troops in his reply.[55] He quoted an editorial by Nicholas Wald, 'Populist instead of professional', in the pro-screeners' favourite journal, *Journal of Medical Screening*, declaring that our *Lancet* paper 'lacks scientific merit' and that the *Lancet* 'should not have published this paper'.[56]

Dean also falsely accused us of not having used Cochrane principles. We wrote in the *Lancet*: 'We focused on the three most important sources of bias in randomised trials: suboptimal randomisation methods, lack of masking in outcome assessment, and exclusion after randomisation',[7] which were the three key Cochrane principles for reducing bias in systematic reviews. He also noted, 'All but one correspondent disagreed with the conclusions of the study.' I wonder if Dean believes that editors publish a random sample of the letters they receive. Editors tend to avoid letters that praise a study and focus on those that are critical and can stimulate debate.

Dean tried to get around the possible misconduct in the Two-County trial by saying that the Swedish Council on Technology Assessment in Health Care had not evaluated whether mammography screening was of value. Finally, he used an *ad hominem* argument, saying that we had limited experience and knowledge of the complex issue of breast cancer screening.

But there was another side to the story. We explained that our paper had made many researchers and people involved with screening all over the world doubt its value.[53] This had mainly been communicated to us personally, very likely for political reasons and for self-protection, but the doubt had also been made public.[40,57]

In Sweden, the spokespeople were also divided. It had been predicted that a substantial decline in breast cancer mortality would be seen around the turn of the century, but in 1999, Nina Rehnquist, director of the Board of Health, admitted that it was difficult to explain the lack of a visible effect of screening.[58] Ingvar Andersson, lead investigator of the Malmö screening trial, also expressed disappointment.[58] He hoped for a real break in the mortality trend when numbers became available for 1998, but to this day, such a change hasn't occurred.

Dean continued his campaign, usually copying a lot of people on his email messages, apart from us who received them from other people. In May 2000, he wrote to the editors of a national Swedish newspaper, *Svenska Dagbladet*, and complained about journalist Inger Atterstam, saying that he would no longer trust anything she claimed, as he had reservations about the way she had dealt with our *Lancet* paper. There was nothing wrong with that. Atterstam was a fine journalist.

The same month, Finn Børlum Kristensen wrote to Dean that for reasons unknown to him, the Danish HTA agency had been put on a list of recipients of email copies, and he wasn't comfortable with the style and content of the correspondences. He furthermore declared his confidence that The Cochrane Collaboration would ensure the quality of our systematic review before it was published in *The Cochrane Library*.

This clear message didn't stop Dean. He complained to Kristensen that what we had published in the *Lancet*, and which Kristensen had funded, had done no credit to Kristensen's institution, and remarked that the attention our report had received came more from the Cochrane name and reputation than it did from our name or reputation. He felt The Cochrane Collaboration should release a public statement, just as he had urged the editors of *Svenska Dagbladet* to react, and expressed disappointment that the Cochrane Breast Cancer Group believed that Ole Olsen and I were capable of performing an unbiased Cochrane review on mammography screening. Finally, we had lost credibility in the eyes of most of the serious investigators in the field and he wanted to know whether Kristensen's institution was still funding our work.

Kristensen calmly replied that he didn't necessarily agree with Dean on the issue of credit to Kristensen's institution in relation to our paper, which he saw as a contribution to science.

In November 2000, Dean was on the warpath against the Finnish Office for Health Technology Assessment, headed by Marjukka Mäkelä, who is also director of the Finnish Branch of The Nordic Cochrane Centre. Mäkelä is very careful to minimise the impact people with conflicts of interest have on technology assessment reports, but Dean wanted it otherwise. The agency had produced a draft report on screening that didn't recommend screening in those under 50 years of age, much to Dean's chagrin, although this is standard in Europe. Dean, who is an American radiologist working in Finland, wrote a letter to Mäkelä in which he advised:

> **Rather than publish a discussion of past mistakes, I would hope that you would be more careful in the future about your public statements on breast cancer, a subject on which you have no refereed publications.** Indeed, your immediate superior in the Cochrane hierarchy [Peter Gøtzsche] had no previous publications on breast cancer or even on cancer, but that did not prevent him from rushing to publication with an article (in which he evidently still believes) which, although published earlier this year in a reputable journal, is full of elementary errors and serious flaws. Is this a new 'Cochrane syndrome'? [bold type as in original]

Logic doesn't seem to be at the forefront in Dean's way of arguing. If those without prior publications on cancer are not allowed to publish on cancer, how can newcomers then get started? He added: '**I would greatly appreciate the opportunity to review your report before it is finally released.**' And he also asked for the names of those responsible for writing the final version and their knowledge and experience with the issues involved.

Dean doesn't exactly conceal his wish to be a policymaker, in fact *the* policymaker, on mammography screening.

Bad manners also in Norway

Pathologist Jan Mæhlen invited me to give a lecture on mammography screening at the annual meeting for the Norwegian Society of Pathologists in Oslo in November 2000, which led to violent attacks from those responsible for screening, both during the meeting and afterwards. A bit unexpected for me, as this is not how one would usually treat an invited guest.

A major Norwegian newspaper, *Aftenposten*, reported that the leader of the Norwegian screening programme, Steinar Thoresen, had presented very derogatory remarks about our work during the meeting to such a degree that many attendants had perceived it as unprofessional.[59] Thoresen replied that he had quoted a number of internationally renowned epidemiologists and acknowledged – without any regrets – that it had created a bad atmosphere.

Two weeks later, Steinar Thoresen and Rolf Kåresen, medical director and breast surgeon at Ullevål Hospital, published a long article in *Aftenposten* where they attacked our research,[60] and I replied a week later.[61] Thoresen and Kåresen characterised my criticism of the trials as being totally one-sided and based on my own definitions of negative aspects of screening. I was also criticised for having excluded a study from the Netherlands that had shown a clear relation between use of mammography and mortality from breast cancer. This was ridiculous, as it was a case-control study, and we only included randomised trials. Furthermore, such studies are notoriously unreliable and screening experts have agreed that they cannot evaluate the effect of screening.[62]

Thoresen and Kåresen remarked that it was a particularly erroneous and serious claim that more women will lose a breast when there is screening and said that when one of them asked at the meeting whether I had literature that could document this, he received no answer. This was not true. I have a habit of retaining copies of my slides, and I showed at the meeting that my data came from the trials and that there was a 20% increase in mastectomies. I also explained why it necessarily must be so and showed on a slide that carcinoma *in situ* may be treated by mastectomy.

Thoresen and Kåresen made other grave errors. They claimed that new studies had shown that radiotherapy no longer increased mortality from heart and lung diseases. Such studies do not exist. Yet the fact that I had mentioned this adverse effect made Thoresen and Kåresen doubt my 'academic honesty'.[60]

They ended with the seemingly irresistible 'you are killing my patients' argument, saying that it was serious that a few researchers in a groundless and demagogic way can influence women to not attend mammography and thus reduce the effect of the programme.

The Norwegian Cancer Registry had declared that screening would reduce breast cancer mortality by 50%,[58] and Thoresen came up with this remarkable estimate already in 1998, based on preliminary results after screening for only 2 years in four counties in Norway.[63] Thirteen years on, we still haven't seen *any* reduction occur.[64]

In 2006, Thoresen went on leave, as he wished 'to seek new challenges' when journalists helped by a whistle-blower revealed that he had received a large sum of money from the drug-maker Merck in his personal bank account. He had failed to declare this, although the director of the Cancer Registry had repeatedly warned at meetings where Thoresen was present that such money should be declared.[65] Thoresen had single-handedly negotiated a deal for vaccination against cervical cancer with Merck for Norway. The previous Norwegian minister of health remarked that there is a word for such money transactions: corruption.[66]

However, Thoresen continued to publish papers listing his address as the Norwegian Cancer Registry, even as late as 2009,[67] and even though he, in 2008, was described as being research director at GlaxoSmithKline and lectured medical students at the University of Bergen in a professorship position financed by the drug-maker.[68] When this was revealed by a newspaper, he was defended by the director of the Cancer Registry, Frøydis Langmark, who shot the messenger by attacking the journalists who broke the story about corruption 2 years earlier. She also claimed that the education of students would not be influenced by this arrangement.

Her statement goes against overwhelming evidence that conflicts of interest in relation to the drug industry are unhealthy. It doesn't seem likely that Thoresen will tell his students, for example, that the New York State attorney general in 2004 accused GlaxoSmithKline of repeated and persistent fraud by hiding from the public the results of several negative trials about the company's best-selling antidepressant drug, Paxil (paroxetine).[69] Or that the company concealed that the drug causes suicidal thoughts in adolescents by relabelling them 'emotional lability' before the trial reports were submitted to the US Food and Drug Administration. Or that GlaxoSmithKline agreed to pay US$87 million for settlement of accusations of kickbacks.[68] Or that the frauds in research and marketing committed by his previous benefactor, Merck, caused the unnecessary deaths of thousands of patients because the company concealed for many years that Vioxx (rofecoxib) causes heart attacks.[70,71]

No wonder some people become religious and dream of a better world than this one. The amount and scope of dishonesty was amazing. But what we had experienced in 1999 and 2000 was just the beginning. It would become much worse.

Continued troubles in Denmark

Our troubles in Denmark were more civilised at that time. Kristensen from the HTA agency worried about interviews we had given to the *Ugeskrift for Læger*, a national newspaper and a television station. He argued that it was hardly compatible with a good health technology assessment strategy to let a single article be the basis for advising politicians on the very day it was published. He also suggested that our press policy should be discussed at the next meeting of our advisory board.

This seemed a bit weird to us. We don't advise politicians unless being asked and it is in agreement with the press policy of our hospital to make research results widely known. Furthermore, if we had declined to comment on our research, the journalists would likely have sensed a good story and created even more publicity than if we had collaborated with them.

I replied to Kristensen that we would try to avoid statements of a political character, but that we couldn't be evasive about our *Lancet* paper that concluded that screening for breast cancer is unjustified. That might be seen as a political statement, but it was our scientific conclusion.

In March 2000, Kristensen questioned, with reference to the *Cochrane Handbook*,[72] why we hadn't included people with content area expertise in our upcoming Cochrane review. He asked whether we intended to include specialists in breast cancer and screening and referred to the analysis and interpretation of our findings, particularly the obligatory finishing sections of Cochrane reviews, 'Implications for practice' and 'Implications for research'.

We felt this was an inappropriate intrusion in an ongoing research process from a funding agency. We also explained we had contacted the trialists and Nyström, who had all agreed to collaborate with us, apart from Tabár, who had also declined to collaborate with the other Swedish trialists. It would have been a serious impediment if we had included content area experts in our work, as virtually all of them believed so strongly in screening that it would have distorted our results and interpretation. I ended my letter – a bit unkindly, perhaps – by suggesting that our centre should be viewed as the free press, and that our healthcare system needed a free research institute that was independent from political opportunism.

We were under pressure all the time for arriving at similar results as those the Swedish trialists and the Danish National Board of Health had published, particularly at two board meetings where several of the participants were involved with breast screening. It was not said explicitly, of course, but we were strongly recommended to collaborate with certain people and to be 'humble towards judgments made by breast cancer experts' and include their judgements in our analysis. How such judgements should affect a statistical analysis wasn't clear, and Olsen remarked – not so humbly – that it could be 'dangerous' to involve content area experts, as such people are often very biased.

These meetings were dreadful, as our academic freedom was constantly under attack. At the last meeting, we were asked which experts we collaborated with. We corresponded extensively with the trialists and other experts but declined to give this information, as it would have led to renewed pressures about whether those people were the 'right' ones.

I have no doubt that those on the other side of the table found us stubborn and irritating. But it was not a consensus report or a political document we had embarked on. It was science. Pure, unadulterated science.

References

1 Narod SA. On being the right size: a reappraisal of mammography trials in Canada and Sweden. *Lancet*. 1997; **349**(9068): 1846.

2 Atterstam I. [Influential cancer study dismissed, dishonest working practices erodes mammography result] [Swedish]. *Svenska Dagbladet*. 1999 Jul 21: 1, 6.

3 Gøtzsche PC, Nielsen M. Screening for breast cancer with mammography. *Cochrane Database Syst Rev*. 2006; (4): CD001877.

4 Tabár L, Fagerberg CJG, Day NE. The results of periodic one-view mammographic screening in Sweden: Part 2. Evaluation of the results. In: Day NE, Miller AB, editors. *Screening for Breast Cancer*. Toronto: Hans Huber; 1988. pp. 39–44.

5 Andersson I, Aspegren K, Janzon L, *et al*. Mammographic screening and mortality from breast cancer: the Malmo mammographic screening trial. *BMJ*. 1988; **297**(6654): 943–8.

6 Westerholm B. [Shocking view on the worth of middle-aged women] [Swedish]. *Läkartidningen*. 1988; **85**: 4056–7.

7 Gøtzsche PC, Olsen O. Is screening for breast cancer with mammography justifiable? *Lancet*. 2000; **355**(9198): 129–34.
8 Bosely S. Breast screening is a waste of time, says study. *Guardian*. 2000 Jan 7.
9 Schulz KF, Chalmers I, Hayes RJ, *et al*. Empirical evidence of bias: dimensions of methodological quality associated with estimates of treatment effects in controlled trials. *JAMA*. 1995; **273**(5): 408–12.
10 Moher D, Pham B, Jones A, *et al*. Does quality of reports of randomised trials affect estimates of intervention efficacy reported in meta-analyses? *Lancet*. 1998; **352**(9128): 609–13.
11 Kösters JP, Gøtzsche PC. Regular self-examination or clinical examination for early detection of breast cancer. *Cochrane Database Syst Rev*. 2003; (2): CD003373.
12 Baines CJ. The Canadian National Breast Screening Study: science meets controversy. In: Temple NJ, Thompson A, editors. *Exce$$ive Medical $pending*. Oxford: Radcliffe Publishing; 2007. Chapter 12. Available at: www.radcliffe-oxford.com/medicalspending (accessed 22 May 2011).
13 Letters. *J Natl Cancer Inst*. 1992; **84**(17): 1365–71.
14 Letters. *Lancet*. 1991; **338**(8759): 113–14.
15 Letters. The breast cancer screening controversy continues. *Ann Intern Med*. 1993; **118**(9): 746–9.
16 Letters. *J Natl Cancer Inst*. 1993; **85**(21): 1771–6.
17 Baines C. Critiquing the National Breast Screening Study: creative misinformation builds barriers to the dissemination of research findings. *British Columbia Office of Health Technology Assessment*. 1993; **4**: 2–4.
18 Baines C. Screening mammography in women 40–49 years of age: no. In: DeVita V, Hellman S, Rosenberg S, editors. *Important Advances in Oncology*. Philadelphia: Lippincott; 1995. pp. 243–51.
19 Breast cancer screening in women under 50. *Lancet*. 1991; **337**(8757): 1575–6.
20 Lane R, Lemoine N, Hall C, *et al*. Oncology and the media. *Lancet Oncol*. 2000; **1**: 246–9.
21 Holmes-Rovner M, Charles S. The mammography screening controversy: who and what is heard in the press? *Patient Educ Couns*. 2003; **51**(1): 75–81.
22 De Koning HJ. Assessment of nationwide cancer-screening programmes. *Lancet*. 2000; **355**(9198): 80–1.
23 Blanks RG, Moss SM, McGahan CE, *et al*. Effect of NHS Breast Screening Programme on mortality from breast cancer in England and Wales, 1990–98: comparison of observed with predicted mortality. *BMJ*. 2000; **321**(7262): 665–9.
24 Jørgensen KJ, Zahl PH, Gøtzsche PC. Breast cancer mortality in organised mammography screening in Denmark: comparative study. *BMJ*. 2010; **340**: c1241.
25 Gray JA Muir. Reflections and comments on journal article. *Nordic Evidence-Based Health Care Newsletter*. 2001; **5**. Available at: www.folkehelsa.no/dok/rapporter/ebhc.html (accessed 15 January 2002).
26 Wise J. Breast cancer screening may not save lives, study finds. *BMJ*. 2000; **320**(7228): 139.
27 Lerner BH. *The Breast Cancer Wars*. Oxford: Oxford University Press; 2001.
28 Ferraro S. Mammogram blast stirs medical storm. *Daily News*. 2000 Jan 9.
29 DeNoon DJ. Report calls mammography screening 'unjustified'. *WebMD Medical News*. 2000 Jan 6.
30 Jungersen D. [Sensitive research] [Danish]. *Ugeskr Læger*. 2000; **162**: 381–3.

31 Barraud P. [Is it necessary to give up mammography?] [French]. *L'Hebdo*. 2000 Jan 20: 70–1.
32 [Voices in the debate] [Danish]. *Dagens Medicin*. 2000 Jan 13: 3.
33 Bäsén A. [Danish researchers repeat their criticism of mammography] [Swedish]. *Dagens Medicin*. 2000 Jan 25: 17.
34 Rosén M, Lundin A, Nyström L, *et al*. [Incidence and mortality of breast cancer during a 25-year period: international and regional comparisons] [Swedish]. *Läkartidningen*. 2000; **97**(4): 294–9.
35 Rosén M, Nyström L, Stenbeck M. [The National Board of Health and Welfare: stronger evidence basis for the benefits of mammography] [Swedish]. *Läkartidningen*. 2000; **97**(7): 739–40.
36 Raffle A, Gray M. *Screening: evidence and practice*. Oxford: Oxford University Press; 2007.
37 Goldberg KB. Experts raise questions about influential Swedish trial of mammography screening. *Cancer Lett*. 2007; **33**: 1–7.
38 Nyström L. *Assessment of Population Screening: the case of mammography* [dissertation]. Umeå, Sweden: Umeå University Medical Dissertations; 2000.
39 Haran C. Mammography on trial. *MAMM Magazine*. 2002 June.
40 Letters. Screening mammography re-evaluated. *Lancet*. 2000; **355**(9205): 747–52.
41 Gøtzsche PC. On the benefits and harms of screening for breast cancer. *Int J Epidemiol*. 2004; **33**(1): 56–64.
42 Gøtzsche PC, Nielsen M. Screening for breast cancer with mammography. *Cochrane Database Syst Rev*. 2009; (4): CD001877.
43 Duffy SW. Interpretation of the breast screening trials: a commentary on the recent paper by Gøtzsche and Olsen. *Breast*. 2001; **10**(3): 209–12.
44 Levi F, Lucchini F, Negri E, *et al*. Cancer mortality in Europe, 1990–1994, and an overview of trends from 1955 to 1994. *Eur J Cancer*. 1999; **35**(10): 1477–516.
45 Levi F, Lucchini F, Negri E, *et al*. The fall in breast cancer mortality in Europe. *Eur J Cancer*. 2001; **37**(11): 1409–12.
46 Levi F, Bosetti C, Lucchini F, *et al*. Monitoring the decrease in breast cancer mortality in Europe. *Eur J Cancer Prev*. 2005; **14**(6): 497–502.
47 La Vecchia C, Bosetti C, Lucchini F, *et al*. Cancer mortality in Europe, 2000–2004, and an overview of trends since 1975. *Ann Oncol*. 2010; **21**(6): 1323–60.
48 Olsen O, Gøtzsche PC. [There is something wrong in the studies of mammography! No support for the conclusions on benefits of breast cancer screening] [Danish]. *Läkartidningen*. 2000; **97**(4): 286–7.
49 Broeders MJ, Peer PG, Straatman H, *et al*. Diverging breast cancer mortality rates in relation to screening? A comparison of Nijmegen to Arnhem and the Netherlands, 1969–1997. *Int J Cancer*. 2001; **92**(2): 303–8.
50 Ståhle L, Sjönell G. [No evidence that routine mammography screening is effective] [Swedish]. *Läkartidningen*. 2000; **97**(7): 742–3.
51 Rosén M, Stenbeck M. [Unambiguous results in expected direction] [Swedish]. *Läkartidningen*. 2000; **97**(8): 859–60.
52 Mills JL. Data torturing. *N Engl J Med*. 1993; **329**(16): 1196–9.
53 Dean P. The Swedish mammography screening trials: check up on your sources. *Läkartidningen*. 2000; **97**(25): 3105–6.
54 Gøtzsche PC, Olsen O. Openness about the Swedish breast cancer screening trials is needed. *Läkartidningen*. 2000; **97**(25): 3105–6.

55 Dean P. Final comment: the articles by Gøtzsche and Olsen are not official Cochrane reviews and lack scientific merit. *Läkartidningen*. 2000; **97**(25): 3106.
56 Wald N. Populist instead of professional. *J Med Screen*. 2000; **7**(1): 1.
57 Schindele E, Stollorz V. [Be careful, care!] [German]. *Die Woche*. 2000 Mar 3: 28–9.
58 Atterstam I. [Measures should improve mammography] [Swedish]. *Svenska Dagbladet*. 2000 Jan 7.
59 Skogstrøm L. [Scepticism towards breast cancer screening] [Norwegian]. *Aftenposten*. 2000 Nov 23: 1, 3.
60 Kåresen R, Thoresen S. [Breast cancer screening – happiness or misfortune for Norwegian women?] [Norwegian]. *Aftenposten*. 2000 Dec 6.
61 Gøtzsche PC. [Misleading information about breast cancer screening] [Danish]. *Aftenposten*. 2000 Dec 13: 14.
62 Vainio H, Bianchini F. *Breast Cancer Screening*. IARC Handbooks of Cancer Prevention, Vol 7. Lyon, France: IARC Press; 2002.
63 [Can save 120 lives annually] [Norwegian]. *Aftenposten*. 1998 Sep 20: 7.
64 Kalager M, Zelen M, Langmark F, *et al*. Effect of screening mammography on breast-cancer mortality in Norway. *N Engl J Med*. 2010; **363**(13): 1203–10.
65 Gjerding ML, Lia K. [Cancer registry boss received 233 900 kr] [Norwegian]. *Verdens Gang*. 2006 Dec 27.
66 Høybråten: – [Honorarium to research boss is corruption] [Norwegian]. *NRK Dagsnytt*. 2006 Dec 27. Available at: http://web3.aftenbladet.no/innenriks/article390798.ece (accessed 15 April 2008).
67 Kalager M, Haldorsen T, Bretthauer M, *et al*. Improved breast cancer survival following introduction of an organized mammography screening program among both screened and unscreened women: a population-based cohort study. *Breast Cancer Res*. 2009; **11**(4): R44.
68 Langmark F. – [Wrong focus – again!] [Norwegian]. *Verdens Gang*. 2008 Sep 6.
69 Bass A. *Side Effects: a prosecutor, a whistleblower, and a bestselling antidepressant on trial*. Chapel Hill: Algonquin Books; 2008.
70 Topol EJ. Failing the public health: rofecoxib, Merck, and the FDA. *N Engl J Med*. 2004; **351**(17): 1707–9.
71 Nesi T. *Poison Pills: the untold story of the Vioxx drug scandal*. New York: St. Martin's Press; 2008.
72 Higgins JPT, Green S, editors. *Cochrane Handbook for Systematic Reviews of Interventions, Version 5.0.1 [updated September 2008]*. The Cochrane Collaboration; 2008. Available at: www.cochrane-handbook.org (accessed 22 May 2011).

6

Harms dismissed by the Cochrane Breast Cancer Group

We owe almost all our knowledge not to those who have agreed, but to those who have differed.

Charles Caleb Colton (1780–1832)

DOCTORS DON'T LIKE TO FACE THE HARMS THEY ARE CAUSING, AND the storm we had experienced in 2000 when we published our first *Lancet* review turned out to have been a mild breeze compared with what awaited us next. We ended up publishing two versions of our Cochrane review on 20 October 2001. What we published in *The Cochrane Library*, and which was therefore by definition the Cochrane review on mammography screening,[1] was a stymied version of our scientific work, as the data on the most important harms of screening, overdiagnosis and overtreatment had been removed by the editors of the Cochrane Breast Cancer Group. Therefore, we also published a research letter in the *Lancet* that summarised our review and included the harms, and this letter referred the readers to the full review on the *Lancet* website.[2,3]

Cochrane reviews include data on both benefits and harms of interventions, and it was therefore highly unusual that we were not allowed to publish our data on overdiagnosis and overtreatment, which were derived from the same trials as those that provided the estimate of the benefit.

After the events, an Australian colleague, Keith Woollard, past president of the Australian Medical Association, sent the quote at the beginning of this chapter to me in appreciation of the work I was doing against so much opposition.

I also received a nice letter from Ellen Leopold, a non-medical author of a book that examined the unquestioned dominance of Halstead's radical mastectomy for over a century as the gold standard of treatment for breast cancer in the United States, even though no studies ever determined that it reduced the mortality rate. She wrote that the doctors who reviewed her book were scornful and defensive and dismissed her as a wrong-headed radical feminist. Interestingly, it was thanks to courageous women like Rose Kushner, who refused to have the devastating operation, and also to one doctor, George Crile, who didn't neglect the terrible harms, as everyone else did, but pioneered less extensive surgery, that randomised trials ultimately became acceptable. They were carried out by Bernard Fisher and showed that radical mastectomy carried no survival advantage, only tremendous harm.[4]

Alongside our review, the *Lancet*'s editor-in-chief, Richard Horton, published a scathing editorial where he described what had happened.[5] He called our review controversial but acknowledged the problems we had elucidated and concluded that there is no reliable evidence from large randomised trials to support screening mammography programmes. He also noted that the implications for women and policymakers were substantial and required careful reflection and discussion.

Horton praised The Cochrane Collaboration in general, but he noted that the process of collaboration within the Cochrane Breast Cancer Group had broken down badly in the case of our review. He explained that even in the best organisations, raw evidence alone is sometimes insufficient to influence opinion and that our conclusions had been unwelcome. Rather than supporting us in the publication of our research, the Cochrane Breast Cancer Group editors had insisted that changes we disagreed with be made to the review if it was to be published in *The Cochrane Library*. These changes appeared in the Cochrane review against our wishes, but not in the version posted on the *Lancet* website. The Cochrane editors had added statements in the main results section of the abstract, which lent support to arguments in favour of screening, and had excluded data about the effects of screening on subsequent treatment (rates of mastectomy, lumpectomy and radiotherapy) 3 days before the deadline for publication, despite the fact that inclusion of these data was envisaged in the published protocol of the review.

Horton also noted that, according to its 10 key principles, The Cochrane Collaboration bases its scientific reputation on minimising bias and ensuring quality. And that interference by Cochrane editors to insert what the authors of the review believe to be invalid analyses erodes the academic freedom of these investigators. He added that editors make recommendations to authors all the time, but that editors who insist on inappropriate analyses that seem to support a particular point of view hurt not only themselves and the institution they represent but also the credibility of the science they claim to value.

That really said a mouthful, and our actions carried high costs. We made enemies, and some of our colleagues felt we had hurt the collaboration. However, others commended us for our courage, including the founder of the collaboration, Iain Chalmers. Iain told me in no uncertain terms that this should be seen as a learning process for the Cochrane Breast Cancer Group.

I hadn't doubted for a moment that what we did was the right thing to do. In 1993, I was one of 84 people who met in Oxford at the newly established Cochrane Centre and agreed that we should start The Cochrane Collaboration. Iain Chalmers had assembled a remarkable group of researchers for that meeting who were disappointed that the medical research literature generally is so poor and biased. We shared a wish to do better, to work critically with the published papers and synthesise them, in order to get closer to the truth than the original researchers might have intended. Censorship of unwelcome findings about harms was clearly unacceptable. Our loyalties should not be with those people who might have vested interests, or who do not want to have their world view of things disturbed, but with those who are affected by our findings – in this particular case, the women and their families. By displaying the data openly, women and policymakers can judge for themselves.

The process with the Cochrane review

Apart from the harms caused by overdiagnosis, we agreed with the Cochrane Breast Cancer Group on the key points. For example, we agreed that the Two-County trial is flawed and that the Canadian trials and the Malmö trial are reliable. This was in sharp contrast to what people in the pro-screening lobby had agreed to believe.

It was a strong belief that the harms are trivial and nothing to worry about. As a result of our 2000 *Lancet* review, the Cochrane Breast Cancer Group had come under great pressure and criticism, individuals resigned from advisory committees and the editors received letters of complaint and were subjected to pressures requesting that we should be prevented from completing our review.[6] The editors withstood these pressures, but we were unable to convince them that it would be wrong for them to delete our data on the major harms. We found out that there was internal disagreement among the editors, but, unfortunately, the censoring side won the battle.

Whether conflicts of interest were also an issue, we cannot know. The coordinating editor of the group, John Simes, stated at a meeting with us in June 2001 that the editors had no conflicts of interest. However, the group is based in Australia, and I noticed that the National Breast Cancer Centre in Australia, which supports screening, funded the group and that this funding had disappeared the year after the Cochrane review was published. Whether this is coincidental or causal is not important, as it is always problematic to be funded by an institution with strong beliefs. It is difficult to remain objective when making difficult decisions that might be seen as antagonistic to a funding institution's mission.

Eight months after publication of our 2000 *Lancet* review, some of the Cochrane editors published a letter alerting readers to the fact that it was not a Cochrane review and had not been reviewed by them.[7] Although nothing in our paper had suggested this, many journalists had written about 'the Cochrane report'. The editors also wrote that they didn't know about our paper before it was published. We had informed the trialists that the paper was forthcoming but forgot to inform the editors, which we regretted in our reply.[8]

We submitted our Cochrane review in October 2000. The next year was very stressful and involved more than 100 email exchanges with the Breast Cancer Group. At first, there were no signs of the trouble ahead. We informed the group that we also intended to publish the review in a print journal. On 2 January 2001, the group's coordinator, Davina Ghersi, sent comments from three peer reviewers and wrote that the final reviewer, a radiologist, had not yet responded but that she hoped to be able to send this comment within the following week. One of the reviewers was a woman with breast cancer who noted that it had been troubling for her to realise that screening didn't reduce breast cancer mortality, whereas it was easier to accept that it led to more aggressive treatment. Her only caveat was that she knew breast cancer patients 'who WERE saved by mammograms' and that systematic reviews therefore could aid, but never replace, sound clinical reasoning. Well, if true, then why did people bother to do randomised trials of half a million women?

We didn't get the fourth comment. Therefore, we revised our review and sent it on 24 January to Ghersi and also to Mike Clarke, whom we had understood was the lead editor on our review. We noted that we hoped the group didn't feel that publication should be delayed because the radiologist hadn't responded, and we added that the data we presented strongly indicated that the quality of the mammograms had nothing to do with the reported effects on breast cancer mortality.

Ghersi had copied her message from 2 January to two of the Australian editors, John Simes and Nicholas Wilcken, and we therefore believed they should have reacted to our resubmission if they had felt additional peer review was needed. As they didn't, it came as a shock for us when Ghersi wrote on 2 March: 'Attached please find feedback from the Editors of the Cochrane Breast Cancer Group on your systematic review of mammographic screening. Please let me know if anything is unclear or you have any queries.'

We certainly had queries. These editors were Simes and Wilcken. It had been easy to respond to the peer reviews and we had therefore expected the review to be published soon after. However, we received a letter that ran to eight pages, of which only two were comments from the editors. The other six were comments from two new peer reviewers. Simes and Wilcken told us that the issues concerning overtreatment and more aggressive treatment were overstated and not supported by evidence. This was not correct. The evidence came from the same trials as those that provided evidence for a beneficial effect and we had provided other evidence that supported our finding that screening leads to more mastectomies.

Simes and Wilcken also argued that they were conscious that our review would receive a great deal of comment and criticism from the readership and that they wished the review to be able to stand up to any criticism by being based on solid evidence.

Of mites and men

The argument that our review should to be able to stand up to any criticism made me very nervous. The perfect study or review doesn't exist, so if perfection is demanded, the research may never be completed. I had heard exactly that argument before. In the mid-1990s, we had finished a large review on chemical and physical interventions against house dust mites and found that they didn't have any effect on patients with asthma.[9,10] We had worked very carefully with the trials, one of us was a specialist in lung diseases who had done more of the trials than anyone else and I had defended a thesis on meta-analysis that addressed many statistical issues and had published several meta-analyses. Quite a strong team of people, one would think, but we were nonetheless told by the editor for the Cochrane Airways Group that he needed to be absolutely certain that our data extraction for the individual trials was correct, and he therefore asked us to go over it all again. We had to go to London to work at the group's office to get it done, in consultation with the editorial staff. All this extra work was a waste of time, as it didn't change anything in our results.

However, the highly unusual manoeuvre delayed publication of our review considerably and I later learned that, in the meantime, an application in the United Kingdom for public funding amounting to £728 678 for yet another trial, similar to many of those we had reviewed although much bigger, had been granted.[11] If our review had been out, it might have been difficult to obtain this funding.

After we had approved the version to be published in 1998, the editor changed our abstract without telling us so that it became misleading in favour of the interventions. We detected this incidentally and complained about it. Some years later, when we updated the review with new trials, the editor changed our abstract again, and again without our permission. This editor is no longer editor of the group, but his departure was not related to what we regarded as editorial misconduct. We published the most recent version of our review in 2008,[12] and there are now 54 included trials and not a trace of an effect of the interventions, just as when we first published the review.

The editor-in-chief of *Allergy* became so tired of the specialists routinely turning a blind eye to the evidence we produced when they wrote guidelines recommending useless interventions against mites that he asked us to publish our Cochrane review in his journal, which we did in 2008.[13] We have also published a paper showing just how misleading narrative review articles on dust mites written by asthma specialists are, which we called 'Of mites and men'.[14]

Confusion over who is in charge

We were not the only ones that were confused by the escalating number of peer reviewers on our screening review. One of the two new reviewers wrote: 'As I am blind to the comments made by those who have formally reviewed the paper, (I assume that there has been already a formal review) . . .' Thus, it seemed to us that the reviews we obtained initially were the true reviews and that we were now being hassled with additional obstacles.

This reviewer did a good job, but he did not understand our rationale for using surgical interventions as an outcome or that overdiagnosis is an inevitable problem. He suggested the excess surgery was a quality assurance problem. We replied that surgery was an outcome in our protocol that was approved by the editorial group and that Cochrane reviews aim to address outcomes that are meaningful to people making decisions about healthcare.

The second reviewer merely repeated the many false and misleading statements about the Canadian trials that are so popular among screening advocates. He also criticised that we had 'ignored the mortality reductions that have been observed in Canada, the US, the UK and The Netherlands'. Thus, he seemed to suggest that we should have included observational studies in our review of the randomised trials, which is inappropriate.

We consulted with the lead editor on our review, Mike Clarke, who suggested that something must have gone wrong within the review group in terms of internal communication. Apparently, our review had led to tensions and disagreements and some editors didn't know what others were doing. We were left with two sets of peer reviews and editorial recommendations that were in disagreement on a number of points and would be impossible to reconcile.

In an attempt to resolve the issues, I visited two European editors, Mike Clarke and Alessandro Liberati. Liberati was ill and couldn't contribute to the meeting, but 2 days later we received a number of comments from him that were incompatible with those of Clarke. I felt the process had started to become Kafkaesque and wrote, after having carefully addressed all Liberati's comments: 'It seems to me that each one of the editors has vetoing right over the review which indicates that it may never be published, since the editors do not agree! I think you need to solve this problem between you.' I was then told by Clarke that these comments were just to be regarded as friendly advice and that the official comments were those from Simes and Wilcken. This wasn't particularly reassuring, but Clarke's support continued unabated and we noted what his view was when we replied to the peer reviewers: 'There is too much wishful thinking and muddled arguments in this area.'

We submitted the third version of our review in April 2001 and received new demands from Simes and Wilcken in mid-June, with additional issues about the trials and our methods. They told us bluntly that they couldn't accept our review for publication and ended their letter on a strange note, telling us that until our review was accepted as a Cochrane review, we shouldn't list our affiliation as The Nordic Cochrane Centre, because 'Our experience following your publication in the *Lancet* last year indicates that this can be misleading.'

This is unheard of. Ole Olsen and I both worked at The Nordic Cochrane Centre, but we were now asked not to reveal our address on our publications. Simes and Wilcken had no right to require this, and omission of our affiliation could have been regarded as scientific misconduct. Furthermore, we couldn't see the problem. When we published our *Lancet* paper in January 2000, the word Cochrane appeared only as our affiliation and in our search strategy, which was impossible to avoid.

As Simes and Wilcken were coming to the UK Cochrane Centre in Oxford later the same month, I hastily arranged a meeting with them there, in which also Ghershi and Clarke participated. During that meeting, we felt the editors had started a process that would never stop, as in Kafka's novel *The Trial*. However, despite the disappointments, I wrote back optimistically:

> I very much appreciate that it was possible to arrange a meeting to discuss the remaining issues in our review on breast cancer screening. I feel the meeting was very productive and that important compromises were reached which should make it possible to finalise the review this summer as we all agreed to work for, so that it can be published in October. I have made changes in the review according to our discussions and think I have complied fully with your wishes.

I ended my letter thus:

> The final major point for us are the overall summary estimates you insisted we should include for the two subgroups, good quality data and poor quality data. I have done that, but to Ole and me, this makes no sense and violates basic scientific principles for systematic reviews. I have therefore made the necessary reservations in the text but hope you will reconsider this approach carefully again.

I sent the fourth version of our review for approval on 29 June. But the worst was yet to come. I enquired about the process on 6 July and Clarke did the same on 11 July. I received an email about our ongoing review on breast self-examination, but nothing about the mammography screening review. People at the Breast Cancer Group had stopped answering email messages, even from their own editor, Clarke. There was dead silence. Soon it was 26 July, and Ole Olsen came back from holidays and requested a phone call with Clarke.

Then, on 7 August, we received the edited version of our review. It appeared now to be more a question of politics than science. We were told that the editors had changed the 'Implications for practice' section in the conclusion, and the discussion section on 'Does screening lead to less aggressive treatment?' We were painfully aware that we had to accept this if our review should ever come out as a Cochrane review, although some of the changes went directly against what we believed was sound science.

Apart from this, the editors had done a good job with the editing and we thanked them for it. We suggested a few changes and sent it back right away, believing it would now be published.

Then came the next shock. We were told, 'The mammographic screening review is currently in the hands of the editors. As mentioned previously, publication will depend on a majority "yes" vote from the editors.' So, our scientific review was now at the mercy of some sort of consensus conference among the editors of a group that received funding from BreastScreen Australia. Not a situation one would wish to bet on.

We were right. On 24 August, we were told that the main section that was still causing concern was the one about aggressive treatment. The editors did not support our conclusion that mammography leads to more aggressive surgery. Clarke had agreed with us, but what could we do? We had discussed at length the biases that could have affected our estimate of overtreatment and had also mentioned that carcinoma *in situ* is often treated by mastectomy.[3] *The editors flatly denied this*, which reminded me of a Danish politician who once in parliament declared: 'If these are the facts, I deny the facts!'

We were given two options: (i) either to continue working on the review as a whole to sort out the issues relating to treatment, which we perceived as a red herring, as the editors had already had almost a year to think about this, or (ii) to publish only those results relating to mortality and continue working on the section relating to subsequent treatments so that it could be incorporated in a future update of the review. The editors hoped we would agree to the second option and attached a stymied review where they had removed all data and all sections relating to treatment.

We accepted the only option we realistically had, because it was important for the credibility of The Cochrane Collaboration that publication was not further delayed. Already a year earlier, one of the co-chairs of the Collaboration had stressed to the Breast Cancer Group that we should be urged to submit our review as soon as possible. And the director of the German Cochrane Centre, Gerd Antes, told me that journalists, politicians and others were constantly sitting on his neck asking when the Cochrane review would come out. He complained that the review process was far too long if the collaboration considered itself an organisation providing evidence for decision-making. Whether or not screening should be introduced was a very hot issue in many countries, and it had arisen also in the German parliament. As The Cochrane Collaboration has a high reputation, our review was eagerly awaited all over the world.

We were very dissatisfied that the editors had required us to lump the results from the poor trials together with those from the good ones in the analysis and to report this misleading result even in the abstract. As late as 26 August, when we sent last-minute typographical corrections, we made a final attempt to have this changed, but to no avail.

The results and conclusions that were published in the abstract of the Cochrane review in October 2001 read as follows:

Main results

Seven completed and eligible trials involving half a million women were identified. The two best trials provided medium-quality data and, when combined, yield a relative risk for overall mortality of 1.00 (95% CI 0.96–1.05) after 13 years. However, the trials are underpowered for all-cause mortality, and confidence intervals include a possible worthwhile effect as well as a possible detrimental effect. If data from all eligible trials (excluding flawed studies) are considered then the relative risk for overall mortality after 13 years is 1.01 (95% CI 0.99–1.03).

The best trials failed to show a significant reduction in breast cancer mortality with a relative risk of 0.97 (95% CI 0.82–1.14). If data from all eligible trials (excluding flawed studies) are considered then the relative risk for breast cancer mortality after 13 years is 0.80 (95% CI 0.71–0.89). However, breast cancer mortality is considered to be an unreliable outcome and biased in favour of screening. Flaws are due to differential exclusion of women with breast cancer from analysis and differential misclassification of cause of death.

Authors' conclusions

The currently available reliable evidence does not show a survival benefit of mass screening for breast cancer (and the evidence is inconclusive for breast cancer mortality). Women, clinicians and policy makers should consider these findings carefully when they decide whether or not to attend or support screening programs.

It could be argued that we went too far, as it was clear from the abstract that the effect of screening was uncertain. But we knew enough of the screening advocates' tactics to be certain that they would misquote our findings and pretend we had shown that screening reduced breast cancer mortality by 20%, which is exactly what they did. Furthermore, the editors deleted the data on the major harms of screening, which is inexcusable.

I am convinced that no one in the world knew these trials and their weaknesses as well as we did. We had been through a huge amount of literature (*see* Figure 6.1), we had read the most important papers again and again, and we had corresponded extensively with the trialists and many other knowledgeable people on the issues.

Therefore, we felt the editors should have respected our in-depth knowledge rather than forcing misleading analyses upon us. We were not insensitive to

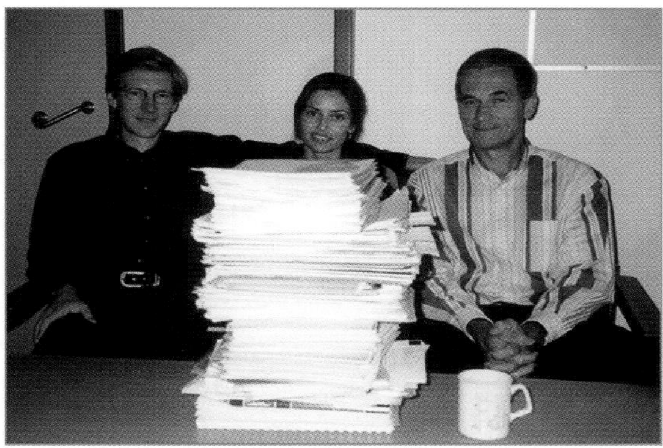

FIGURE 6.1 A peer reviewer once asked: 'What do you mean when you say that you read forty centimeters of literature?' (Ole Olsen, Tine Bjulf and Peter Gøtzsche)

political matters, but science should always trump political concerns, as this principle will have the best consequences for our societies.

The delicacy of the situation and the disagreements among the editors appeared from a comment they published with our review:

> **A Comment from the Editors of the Cochrane Breast Cancer Group**
>
> On this issue of the Cochrane Library appears a systematic review from Ole Olsen and Peter Goetsche on the use of mammographic screening for the early detection of breast cancer. The review has undergone an extensive editorial review process with considerable debate on the conclusions and interpretation of the trial data.
>
> At this stage the editorial group has elected to publish the review of outcomes on mortality and breast-cancer mortality but defer presentation or discussion of results on changes in treatment (mastectomy, radiotherapy, etc) until further editorial review has been completed.
>
> The systematic reviewers have been diligent and conscientious in their efforts and have followed the process they outlined in their protocol. Consequently, it was the majority (but not unanimous) view of the editorial group that the above sections of the review should be published at this time. However, this does not necessarily imply that the editors agree or disagree with each of the interpretations and conclusions reached.
>
> The conclusions of this review will have widespread implications for mammographic screening programmes and the interpretation of the results will be controversial. We would like to invite readers of the review to contribute

comments through the 'Comments and Criticisms' function of the Cochrane Library.

Professor John Simes, Co-Coordinating Editor,
Cochrane Breast Cancer Group
Dr Nicholas Wilcken, Co-Coordinating Editor,
Cochrane Breast Cancer Group
Davina Ghersi, Coordinator, Cochrane Breast
Cancer Group

References

1 Olsen O, Gøtzsche PC. Screening for breast cancer with mammography. *Cochrane Database Syst Rev*. 2001; (4): CD001877.
2 Olsen O, Gøtzsche PC. Cochrane review on screening for breast cancer with mammography. *Lancet*. 2001; **358**(9290): 1340–2.
3 Olsen O, Gøtzsche PC. Systematic review of screening for breast cancer with mammography. *Lancet*. 2001 Oct 20. Available at: http://image.thelancet.com/extras/fullreport.pdf (accessed 5 May 2010).
4 Lerner BH. *The Breast Cancer Wars*. Oxford: Oxford University Press; 2001.
5 Horton R. Screening mammography: an overview revisited. *Lancet*. 2001; **358**(9290): 1284–5.
6 Ghersi D. Comments on The Lancet article on mammography screening from the Cochrane Breast Cancer Group. *Nordic Evidence-Based Health Care Newsletter*. 2001; **5**. Available at: www.folkehelsa.no/dok/rapporter/ebhc.html (accessed 15 January 2002).
7 Wilcken N, Ghersi D, Brunswick C, *et al*. More on mammography. *Lancet*. 2000; **356**(9237): 1275–6.
8 Gøtzsche PC, Olsen O. More on mammography. *Lancet*. 2000; **356**(9237): 1276.
9 Hammarquist C, Burr ML, Gøtzsche PC. House dust mites and control measures in the management of asthma. *Cochrane Database Syst Rev*. 1998; (3): CD001187.
10 Gøtzsche PC, Hammarquist C, Burr M. House dust mite control measures in the management of asthma: meta-analysis. *BMJ*. 1998; **317**(7166): 1105–10.
11 National Research & Development Programme. Asthma management. Commissioned research: ongoing projects. Woodcock A. The effect of mite allergen avoidance by the use of allergen impermeable bedding, on asthma control in adults. Available at: www.asthmar-d.org.uk/FUNDED/ONGOING/Default.htm (accessed 24 June 2010).
12 Gøtzsche PC, Johansen HK. House dust mite control measures for asthma. *Cochrane Database Syst Rev*. 2008; (2): CD001187.
13 Gøtzsche PC, Johansen HK. House dust mite control measures for asthma: systematic review. *Allergy*. 2008; **63**(6): 646–59.
14 Schmidt LM, Gøtzsche PC. Of mites and men: reference bias in narrative review articles; a systematic review. *J Fam Pract*. 2005; **54**(4): 334–8.

7

The *Lancet* publishes the harms of screening

Given the apparent lack of evidence for breast screening programmes, Minerva wonders why women are under such pressure to attend.

BMJ

DEEPLY FRUSTRATED BY THE ACTIONS OF THE COCHRANE BREAST Cancer Group, Ole Olsen and I submitted a research letter to the *Lancet* on 10 September 2001. We asked for rapid assessment and for publication simultaneously with our Cochrane review, if accepted, and we enclosed the full review, including the data on overdiagnosis and overtreatment.

Our research letter was accepted.[1,2] In contrast to the Cochrane review, we didn't pool all the data. We noted that the best trials failed to find an effect of screening on deaths ascribed to breast cancer, relative risk 0.97 (0.82–1.14) after 13 years, whereas the remaining trials with poor-quality data found a marked effect, relative risk 0.68 (0.58–0.78). We explained that, given the strong heterogeneity (the two confidence intervals didn't even overlap), results from the two quality groups should not be combined. About overtreatment, we said:

> We have also confirmed, with additional data (see www.thelancet.com), which the editors of the Cochrane Breast Cancer Group have elected to defer from publication until further editorial review has been completed, our earlier finding[1] that screening leads to more aggressive treatment, increasing the number of mastectomies by about 20% and the number of mastectomies and tumourectomies by about 30%. The greater use of surgery was not merely an

> initial phenomenon caused by the tumours detected at the prevalence screen, but seemed to persist. The increased mastectomy rate in the trials might be higher than in current practice, since there has been a general policy change towards fewer mastectomies. However, screening identifies some slow-growing tumours that would never have developed into cancer in the women's remaining lifetimes, as well as cell changes that are histologically cancer but biologically benign. Furthermore, carcinoma in situ does not always develop into invasive cancer, but since these early lesions are often diffuse, women are sometimes treated by bilateral mastectomy. Therefore, the increase in surgery rates could also be an underestimate, since reoperations and operations in the contralateral breast seemed not to have been included. Furthermore, 'better' diagnostic methods – eg, better mammograms – could lead to additional over-treatment because of detection of even more early or questionable lesions. Quality assurance programmes could possibly reduce the surgical activity to some degree, but the problem cannot be avoided.

The *Lancet*'s editor-in-chief, Richard Horton, reacted very swiftly. We sent a revision on 25 September, responding to the comments of four peer reviewers, and we published the research letter on 20 October 2001, together with the full review on the *Lancet* website, and simultaneously with publication of the Cochrane review.

We later found out from Michael Moss, a journalist from the *New York Times*, who three of the peer reviewers were. Two of them are staunch supporters of screening, and one wrote: 'It strikes me as very strange and disturbing, that the Cochrane Collaboration allowed these two authors to conduct an overview of this topic. It would have served Public Health better had an independent group of authors been commissioned to conduct this review of such an important topic.' The other screening enthusiast was equally blunt: 'To publish this communication would sully the good name of *The Lancet*'; 'it would be imprudent in the extreme to publish further unsubstantiated allegations'; and 'I see nothing publishable here'. These reviewers referred to papers by Nicholas Wald and Stephen Duffy as evidence that there were numerous flaws in our research. As I shall explain later, these two people should not be trusted as judges in such matters. A third reviewer said, 'Gotzsche *et al.* will undermine their own credibility'.

We informed the Cochrane Breast Cancer Group and some other key people in the collaboration about our research letter before it came out and explained the differences between the two reviews in a neutral fashion that could be used when talking to journalists:

> A summary of our findings is published in a research letter in *The Lancet* on 20 Oct 2001 and a full version of our systematic review is freely available on *The Lancet*'s website www.thelancet.com. This version is more comprehensive than the Cochrane review as it contains data on the use of surgery and radiotherapy.

While we were awaiting the publications, we received an email from Mike Clarke, who wanted to see the peer reviews for the *Lancet*'s version, as he felt this might help persuade the editorial team of the Breast Cancer Group to include the results related to treatment in an update of our Cochrane review. Clarke's email led to quite some discussion between Ole Olsen and me, and 5 days later I responded that we could get back to our internal problems after the publications.

I explained to Clarke that our data on surgery had been peer-reviewed extensively; namely, before our *Lancet* paper from 2000; when we submitted the whole Cochrane review to the *Lancet* and to *Annals of Internal Medicine* (the *Lancet* offered us a research letter and *Annals* a shorter version, but we declined, as we felt there would be too little space); when we submitted our research letter to *Lancet*; and three times in the Breast Cancer Group. I also noted that the Cochrane editors had still not responded to our question as to when we could expect to see these data in our Cochrane review.

Clarke replied that the coordinating editors should send us the reasons for their concerns along with suggestions for solutions as soon as possible, so that the data could appear in the issue of *The Cochrane Library* that would come out in January 2002. We asked the group again when we could expect to receive the comments, got no reply, asked again, and again got no reply. It took another 5 years, and required the involvement of the Cochrane publication arbiters and the Cochrane Steering Group (*see* Chapter 12) before these data were included in the Cochrane review.

We seriously considered whether we should make all the peer reviews we had received from the various journals publicly available on our website, but we abandoned the idea, as peer reviews are usually considered confidential, and as some of the comments and phrases we had received were so typical of the person who had written them that we had no doubt who it was. When Clarke asked for the peer reviews again 2 months later, we had still not heard from the Breast Cancer Group. From this I noted that the group was putting the cart in front of the horse, as it was rather obvious that the *Lancet* wanted to publish unbiased research. A final problem with releasing peer reviews to 11 editors is expressed in a maxim by La Rochefoucault, who noted that if you cannot keep a secret yourself, why do you think others can?

Amidst all this, Ole Olsen and I attended a peer-review congress in Barcelona in September 2001. These meetings attract editors and researchers with an interest in the quality and reliability of the scientific literature, and we had hardly arrived before Richard Horton spotted us and came along, carrying our paper. This was a rare opportunity to discuss in depth a hot issue with an editor, and we met several times over a beer, sometimes also with Iain Chalmers. Our conversations were very useful and convinced Horton that he should trust us, rather than the peer reviewers, as we rejected their arguments. On the day our papers came out, Horton described this in an email:

> I can't tell you how pleased I am that we were able to work so closely togther on this paper. The fact that we were all three in Barcleona was a stroke of luck – with Iain there especially. I wish that I could be as involved in all papers as I was with yours! Please keep me updated as news comes in. John Simes is clearly rattled by events. But I think, in the long run, that this will be good for Cochrane. I truly hope so. As Iain said, it is time for Cochrane to grow up, and that can sometimes be painful.

Horton was tremendously helpful in the difficult situation we were in, and also afterwards. Some people have suggested that he was merely interested in creating publicity for his journal, but that is not my perception. He wanted to get as close to the truth as possible in one of the most controversial issues in healthcare. He expressed this in an email: 'Well done, if I may say, for being so brave to stick by the science, and not to be swayed by the desire to confirm what many hoped for.'

As I was a member of the editorial board of the *BMJ*, I knew its editors quite well. When they learned about what was going on, three of them invited us out for dinner in Barcelona to discuss the issues. It was a bit difficult for us to be helpful, as our paper was with another journal, so I suggested the editors contact Horton to get our results. There was a good deal of scepticism about mammography screening among the editors, and Tony Delamothe suggested publishing an editorial with the title: Time to stop screening? That didn't happen, but we made up for our locked position later by publishing several important papers on mammography screening in the *BMJ*. And 10 years later, I actually published an editorial with Delamothe's suggested title (*see* Chapter 26).

On 24 September, just after Barcelona, professor of statistics Nick Day from Cambridge, UK, sent an email to Iain Chalmers, which looked like an attempt at censoring our work:

> I have been asked to approach you by a number of colleagues, here and abroad, as there are rumours that the Cochrane Centre is shortly going to publish

> a review of breast screening by mammography based largely on the Lancet paper by Gotzsche and Olsen. This paper, I'll call it the GO paper, is not simply controversial, it contains a number of serious statistical mistakes which invalidate its conclusions, and uses a selective approach to the studies and data it assesses. It is a worthless piece of work which if it had been produced by one of our masters students, would have been sent back with demands for a complete rewrite. I wrote a review of it for a Danish journal last year which I could send you. Many others have done the same, the mistakes in the GO paper are well publicised. It may be that the Cochrane review is fundamentally different from the GO paper, rendering my concerns unnecessary. However, if the review is largely based on the GO paper, then could I ask you to reconsider it. Publication has the potential not only to damage breast screening, which is beginning to have substantial impact in this country and elsewhere, but also the Cochrane process. The immense benefits brought by the Cochrane Centre [the UK Cochrane Centre that is, not The Nordic Cochrane Centre] will be undermined if its name is associated with incompetent and tendentious reviews such as the GO paper.

Nick Day had co-authored the first publication of the Two-County trial in the *Lancet* in 1985.[3] Anthony Miller has told me that Day visited Tabár in Sweden for a weekend and performed the statistical analyses. If correct, Day cannot have exerted much quality control, but must simply have believed the data Tabár gave him.

Five days later, I received an email from Tabár. He had been unwilling to communicate with us for 2 years, but now he suddenly stepped into the scene, wishing us 'a lovely weekend'.

He referred to the letter by Day, asked whether I had read it and forwarded a comment from an American colleague. Tabár didn't reveal the identity of his colleague, but the style is very typical of radiologist Daniel Kopans, who half a year later was quoted saying something similar in the *Philadelphia Inquirer*: 'If you take all the studies that show the Earth is round and reject them, then the Earth is flat. That's what they have done.'[4] The comment Tabár forwarded contained the familiar 'you are killing my patients' argument:

> What is remarkable to me is that this man (i.e. Dr. G) calls himself a scientist since he obviously and knowingly ignores the scientific method in order to further his own agenda, whatever that may be. I cannot believe he is so intellectually deficient that he cannot grasp the plethora of evidence that so strongly supports the benefit of screening. What then drives him so blindly

> in his crusade to convince us all that the world is flat? To become infamous as a contrarian, standing lonely on the curvature of the earth as he denies it spinning under his feet? Or is it something even more petty? An all-consuming hatred and jealousy of Laszlo Tabar, whose impeccable trial facilitated by meticulous Swedish record keeping and a socialist society provides a setting unparalleled in the world for a scientific trial? what is tragic and makes G's ravings sinister is that I am sure his influence has resulted in women's unnecessary deaths somewhere in the world. The Scandanavians are known for their fair-minded, progressive concern for women, as well as for their intellectual integrity. In this regard, PG is certainly a Nordic contrarian.

Shortly before our paper came out, one of the coordinating Cochrane editors contacted Horton, as he had heard there would be an editorial as well. He was anxious and disputed almost everything Horton told him about the process; he even said that we had not disagreed with the changes he had enforced on us. Therefore, we sent Horton copies of email messages that verified everything we had told him in Barcelona was correct. Impressively, Horton finished his editorial just 2 days before the *Lancet* appeared in print. In May 2002, the other coordinating Cochrane editor repeated the false argument that the editors did not insist on changes.[5]

I was very worried about how The Cochrane Collaboration's leadership would deal with the affair, although we received a lot of support from editors of prestigious journals. Drummond Rennie from the US Cochrane Centre, who is also an editor of *JAMA*, replied to my worries in a characteristically humourous fashion: 'When you are on trial, I shall support you strongly, of course, though, as usual my evidence is for sale to the person who gives me the largest number of free mammograms.'

We were also supported by women with breast cancer who were shocked to learn that the Cochrane editors had deleted all information about carcinoma in situ *from our review.* Apart from these women, no one had anything reasonable to say about our finding that screening leads to more mastectomies. The typical argument, that it couldn't be true because surgeons perform fewer mastectomies today than previously, is a nonsense argument, of course.

Vitriolic mass email from Peter Dean

The same day our paper was published, Peter Dean sent one of his vitriolic mass email messages around. Tabár sent it on to me the same day, after having deleted the recipients, but I received the full email from Finn Børlum Kristensen who had also received it despite his express message to Dean to be taken off his mass-mailing list. There appeared to be 128 recipients:

> Albert Baert, Anders Hemmingsson, Anders Lernevall, Anders Ekbom, Andy Oxman, Anna-Leena Lääperi, Aronen Hannu, Arto Haapanen, Autier Philippe, Beate Wimmer-Puchinger, Bedrich Vitak, Bruce Hillman, C.J.M. de Wolf, Carl Blomqvist, Chris Hyde, Christian Herold, Claudia I. Henschke, Constantine Gatsonis, Daniel Howard, Edward Azavedo, Elisabeth Kutt, Erik Thurfjell, Finn Børlum Kristensen, Folke Lindberg, Danish Radiological Society, Francisco Ruíz Perales, Friedrich Hansen, Gunilla Svane, H Suoranta, Hannu Paajanen, Hans Ringertz, Hans Junkermann, Harry de Koning, Hege Wang, Heikki Joensuu, Hendriks J, Holger Pettersson, Ilmo Parvinen, Inger Gram, Ingvar Andersson, Irma Soini, I Schreer, I Soviita, J Hendriks, J Schouten, Janne Nappi, Jayne Foster, J Jellins, Juha Koskenvuo, Kaija Hartiala, Kaija Holli, Karen Abbe, Karl von Smitten, Kataja Vesa, Kaufman Cary S, Kirsti Karhunen, Koning, Koskinen Seppo, Lars Rutqvist, László Tabár, Lawrence von Karsa, Lennarth Nystrom, Leonard Berlin, Liisa Elovainio, Måns Rosén, Marianne Hjertstrand, Kormano Martti, Mary Codd, Mogens Blichert-Toft, Mary Rickard, NJ Wald, Nicholas E. Day, Nicholas Wilcken, Nick Perry, Nils Bjurstam, Olof Jarlman, Osmo Räsänen, Paajanen Hannu, Päivi Hietanen, Pamilo Martti, Parvinen Ilmo, Parvinen Leena-Maija, Paula Lindholm, Klemi Pekka, Peter Aspelin, Pirkko Kellokumpu-Lehtinen, Pyrhönen Seppo, R Holland, Rainer Otto, Rauni Saaristo, Reichel Margrit, Robert A. Schmidt, Robert B. Dean, Robert Smith, Roberts, Robin Wilson, Roland Holland, Ronald J H Borra, Seppo Soimakallio, Soeto, Standertskjöld-Nordenstam Carl-Gustaf, Steinar Thoresen, Stephen Duffy, Stephen J Golding, Stephen Senn, Stuart Field, Sue Moss, Sulev Ulp, Sullivan Daniel, Sven Tornberg, Sven-Ola Hietala, Sylvia Heywang, Söderström Ove, Teijo Kuopio, Tibor Tot, Timo Ihamäki, U-Bick, Uffe Dyreborg, UK Lammi, Vannier Michael, Vanninen Ritva, Walter Schwartz, Werner Kaiser, Wolf Georg, Y Grumbach, Yrjö Collan, Yoshito, Magnus Stenbeck.

Dean misinformed the recipients and misquoted our research. He said that our *Lancet* paper was not the peer-reviewed Cochrane review, which gives the impression that the *Lancet* paper was not peer-reviewed. Then he seized upon the statement the Cochrane editors had inserted, despite our protests, that the relative risk for breast cancer mortality after 13 years was 0.80, without adding that this estimate was unreliable, although the Cochrane abstract stated that 'the evidence is inconclusive for breast cancer mortality'.

Horton was not one of the recepients of Dean's mail, but I sent it to him and he replied that although editors are used to such things, they usually appear as whispers and rumours, and that he had rarely seen something so personal in print. He added:

> Val Beral was quoted in a newspaper last week as questioning your 'motivations' for doing this review. What I see happenning is direct ad hominem assaults on anybody who dissents from the pro-mammography line, irrespective of the data offered. Jack Cuzick said to me last Friday that your review was an example of context-free statistics. I replied that you had spent a good part of the last 2 years deep in these data – you probably knew the trials better than anybody. But what he seemed to be saying was that one only has the right to comment on screening if one takes a pro-screening line.

Dean claimed that we had turned an exercise in meta-analysis into a personal crusade; that we had been unable to accept the peer-review process of The Cochrane Collaboration; and that we had twice ignored this 'outside control' when publishing in the *Lancet*, while still misleading people into believing that it was a true Cochrane review. We hadn't done that, either in 2000 or now. I admit that we gave our research letter a journalistic title, an appetizer, as people had been awaiting our Cochrane review for so long: 'Cochrane review on screening for breast cancer with mammography',[1] but this was followed by a small summary that made it clear that the research letter was not the Cochrane review:

> In 2000, we reported that there is no reliable evidence that screening for breast cancer reduces mortality. As we discuss here, a Cochrane review has now confirmed and strengthened our previous findings. The review also shows that breast-cancer mortality is a misleading outcome measure. Finally, we use data supplemental to those in the Cochrane review to show that screening leads to more aggressive treatment.

Dean said that we had been supported by the *Lancet*'s editor (what's wrong with that?) and guessed Horton would lose his job as a result. Finally, he spread the lie that our paper was not peer-reviewed and said that he didn't know whether Horton had expertise in evaluating the mammography screening studies, or had knowledge of breast cancer biology, to say nothing of radiology, or even if he was a physician.

Wanting to control science and arguing 'you're not one of us' exactly parallels the Inquisition, when people like Horton and me would have been sentenced to be burned at the stake. Screening had become a religious belief and was fanatically defended.

Beating about the bush in the United Kingdom

The BBC reported on 18 October 2001 that 'as many as 300 lives are saved a year by breast screening'.[6] Although these 300 were described as 'many', that number had risen to 1250 the next day, according to Julietta Patnick, national coordinator of the Breast Screening Programme.[7]

The UK Imperial Cancer Research Fund issued a press release where Stephen Duffy, presented as a breast screening expert at the fund, said that it was rather surprising that we believed screening leads to more radical treatment.[8] This was not our belief; it was our scientific result.

Duffy stated that our suggestion to use deaths from all causes rather than deaths from breast cancer was 'certainly not justified as mammographic screening is aimed at preventing breast cancer deaths, not deaths from things like heart disease or road accidents'. That was a disingenuous remark, as we had written that screening increases deaths from other causes because of the harms related to overdiagnosis and overtreatment, and, indeed, radiotherapy actually causes heart disease. Furthermore, one could argue in a similarly nonsensical fashion that deaths due to bleeding or postoperative infection should not count if a study's purpose is to examine whether cancer surgery saves lives. Duffy also referred to a fatally flawed study he had co-authored with Tabár claiming a 63% benefit (*see* Chapter 14).

Three weeks later, Richard Smith, the editor-in-chief of the *BMJ*, wrote about the agonies of evidence.[9] He quoted John Maynard Keynes arguing that politicians don't like evidence, as it ties their hands. Smith noted that the arrival of a Cochrane review suggesting that mammography did not save lives but simply increased mastectomies must have been painful for those who had invested heavily in screening programmes. He also referred to a letter where I had criticised the NHS Cancer Screening Programme for inaccurate, unscientific and anonymous criticisms of the Cochrane review.

I wrote this letter in response to a *BMJ* news story by Susan Mayor, who described the disagreements between us and the Cochrane Breast Cancer Group.[10] In her article, there were anonymous quotes from the office of the NHS Cancer Screening Programme that misrepresented our research entirely.[11] The office said that our findings on mortality and of more aggressive treatment were based on only two studies. It also claimed that we had not investigated whether more aggressive treatment was beneficial. Perhaps most astonishingly, the office noted that many researchers would classify all studies as of similar quality. When the office claimed that there is clear evidence of the benefit for mammography when all studies are combined, it overlooked not only that some studies are flawed but also our finding that mortality from breast cancer is a misleading and biased outcome measure that favours screening. Finally, I noted that anonymous attacks on scientific work are improper and unfair since there is no accountability. Mayor interviewed Alessandro Liberati from the Cochrane Breast Cancer Group, who noted that it is not unusual that information provided by screening programmes presents results in an overly optimistic fashion, and that this should be changed to reflect the reality of the situation.

Half a year later, one of the editors from the Breast Cancer Group took me aside during a meeting and told me it took time for his wound to heal but that it would ultimately heal. I was very grateful for that remark. I had also been wounded.

Other editors from the Breast Cancer Group were less forthcoming. One year later, Alan Rodger from Australia argued in the *Medical Journal of Australia*: 'That breast screening is unlikely to have an impact on overall population mortality gives the lie to the conclusions of Olsen and Gøtzsche's overview, which are based only on overall mortality.'[12]

An Australian colleague informed me that he thought the comment was unprofessional and should not normally be accepted in a reputable journal. I wrote a letter explaining that it is not appropriate for an editor of the Cochrane Breast Cancer Group that had approved and published our Cochrane review to use a term such as 'gives the lie' to our results. Further, I noted that we had carefully analysed also breast cancer mortality and all-cancer mortality, which meant that Rodger's statement was false.

To my surprise, the deputy editor replied that the journal was happy to publish my letter if I felt strongly about it, but argued, 'we feel that the issue here is one of language and local idiom rather than science'. My Australian colleague suspected this interpretation was flavoured by the wisdom of hindsight, and he didn't think Australians viewed the expression 'giving lie to' differently to the British. Therefore, I published the letter.[13]

In his reply, Rodger, who was a professor of radiation oncology and chair of the Board of Breast-Screen Victoria, stated that cancers detected with mammography are smaller than those detected clinically and therefore have a better prognosis.[14] Immediately after this observation – which is correct but ludicrous, as it says nothing about the benefits and harms of screening – he finished with the 'you're not one of us' argument, noting that perhaps I needed to add a clinical oncology perspective to my 'undoubted expertise in the finer details of trial methodology analysis'. I wonder what difference that should have made to our Cochrane review, which plenty of people with all sorts of expertise had commented on, both before and after publication.

In the letters that followed our review,[15] Hazel Thornton, a patient advocate who had been diagnosed with carcinoma *in situ* without being made aware of this possiblity before attending screening, noted that the actions of the Cochrane editors were a 'blatant threat to the over-riding principle of freedom of appointed investigators to place all legitimate findings in the public domain without judgmental interference.'

Stephen Duffy, László Tabár and Robert Smith (from the American Cancer Society) wrote that our review was 'riddled with misrepresentation, inconsistency in the treatment of the randomised trials, and errors of method and fact', and noted that our 'alleged inconsistencies' in numbers in different reports of the Two-County trial would have been understood by a competent meta-analyst. I would say the opposite. Because we were competent, we spotted all these inconsistencies, which just cannot be explained away. There are even examples of fewer deaths from breast cancer with increasing follow-up.[15,16]

In 2002, we were condemned by Duffy, Tabár and Smith in an editorial in *Cancer: A Journal for Clinicians*, where they wrote about the morale of overworked staff for the third time: 'Women who have developed confidence in breast cancer screening should not be intimidated, and overworked staff who go to great lenghts to make screening work should not have their morale damaged by poor quality reviews such as that of OG [Olsen and Gøtzsche].'[17] They even republished this article, in another journal, and I shall discuss their arguments in Chapter 14.

Condemnations in Sweden

The director of the Swedish National Board of Health, Nina Rehnqvist, admitted that 'if mammography was to be introduced today, we would have put other demands on the scientific documentation than we did in the past', and added that the available trials show 'neither this nor that'.[18] In contrast, Måns Rosén, also from the Board of Health, declared that many lives could be lost because of the debate.[19]

Peter Dean gave his opinion in no uncertain terms under the headline 'A scientific scandal' in the *Läkartidningen*.[20] He started with the 'you're not one of us' argument, which has existed at all times. In Dean's own words, those who criticise mammography screening are rarely experts on screening or have professional experience with diagnosing and treating breast diseases. Dean's views open some interesting perspectives in societal life. Does this mean that you are not allowed to criticise poor car repair work unless you are a mechanic? Or poor surgery because you are not a surgeon? Or excessive interest rates because you are not a banker? Or politicians because you are not a politician? Or Peter Dean because you are not an American?

In an interview, Dean called us outsiders and declared that we had determined, after having read some dozens of articles, to become world-famous experts whose views did not need scrutiny by peer review.[21] He claimed that we had persuaded the editor-in-chief of a respected journal to drop peer review, which wasn't true. *Lancet*'s editor-in-chief, Richard Horton, had stated in an interview 1 week earlier that our paper was thoroughly peer-reviewed, both by experts in the field and by a statistician.[22] I have kept these reviews.

Dean also distorted the truth in other matters. He said that according to 'the approved report's summary, screening reduces breast cancer mortality, but according to the *Lancet* version, it is the opposite'.[20] We wrote in both reports – with slightly different wording – that breast cancer mortality is an unreliable outcome and that the evidence for screening is inconclusive.[1,23] Furthermore, our *Lancet* paper was also 'approved' – namely, by the *Lancet*'s editors.

Dean also said that the Cochrane principles we used for our assessments of the trials were 'homemade' and he called upon the women 'who have always understood that small tumours rarely kill, that big tumours often kill, and that very big tumours usually kill'. Dean added that expertise is needed to interpret the trials and remarked that we neither understood epidemiology principles nor the published literature.[24]

As expected, Dean's misquotations escalated after I had proven him wrong.[25] He said that I should have claimed that there was no difference between our Cochrane review and our *Lancet* review,[26] and added that this wasn't true. What I had stated was: 'Thus, there is no difference, in principle, between our conclusions in the two versions of our review.'[25] This is certainly true.

I noted it was alarming that screening didn't decrease total cancer mortality and explained that if it were true that the effect of screening was a 30% reduction in breast cancer mortality, one would have expected to find a 5% reduction in cancer mortality (including breast cancer mortality).[25] Dean claimed that my calculation was wrong and provided his own calculation, according to which one would have expected only a 1% reduction in total cancer mortality.[26] He didn't explain where his numbers came from and he got it completely wrong.[27,28] He claimed that only 4% of the cancer deaths in the trials were due to breast cancer, but in the Two-County trial, for example, it was 12%.[16]

Finally, Dean joined ranks with the other screening advocates when he denied that screening leads to more mastectomies.

On 13 January 2002, 24 leading clinicians from all over Sweden, described as doctors and cancer experts and counting several professors, published a long article in a leading newspaper, *Dagens Nyheter*.[29] They argued that it speaks against all experience and is not documented that some women lose a breast unnecessarily and claimed that a clear decline in breast cancer mortality was only seen in those countries in Europe that have screening after the Swedish model, whereas mortality continued to increase in other countries. Both comments were blatantly wrong,[16,30,31] which shows how terribly uninformed leading 'experts' can be, unless they are simply dishonest and make statements that conflict with what they know. These people also wrote that the criticism would lead to more women dying from breast cancer. The 'you are killing my patients' argument never dies, it seems.

Because of our criticisms of the trials, the Swedish National Board of Health and the Swedish Cancer Society arranged an international meeting in Stockholm in February 2002. The attendees consisted almost entirely of screening advocates and the atmosphere wasn't friendly towards those who didn't share their views.

This is the only time I have met with Tabár and I used the opportunity to ask him crucial questions. He refused to reply, and one of the participants who worked at the Board of Health later wrote to me that it was a scandal that Tabár wouldn't contribute to clarifying details in his trial, as the money for it had come from the Board of Health and from the Swedish Cancer Foundation. Stephen Duffy didn't contribute to clarifying the essential issues either.

I heard so many 'funny stories' and curious explanations at the meeting that I sent my own minutes to the director of the Board of Health, Nina Rehnqvist, pointing out the errors. Even the lead investigator for the Malmö trial, Ingvar Andersson, whom I otherwise respect, showed misleading numbers on this occasion. He concluded that screening didn't increase the rate of mastectomies because there were nine fewer mastectomies in the screened group than in the control group in his trial between 1984 and 1988. However, the trial started in 1978, and the total number of mastectomies during the 9 years the trial ran were 424 and 339, respectively, i.e. 25% more mastectomies in the screened group.[16]

After the meeting, Robert Smith sent a letter to Nina Rehnqvist:

> I was disappointed to see that the data presented throughout the day had little to no influence on either Dr. Gøtzsche or Dr. Sjönell, despite the efforts made by the Chairs, both you and Dr. Nilsson, to expose a specific criticism to

> evidence and logic for the purpose of resolution. Indeed, what was most unsettling was that neither Dr. Gøtzsche or Dr. Sjönell was prepared to accept any answer to their critiques of trial methodology specifically, or of mammography in general. There is very little doubt that each of them attempt to cloak their disdain for cancer screening in the credibility of science, no matter how weak, ignorant, or shallow their arguments. It is also clear that they begin with a basic belief that there is no justification for breast cancer screening, and then set out to justify their position with an eclectic list of disclaiming statements, which range from incorrect to irrelevant.

One would think this bombastic condemnation would suffice, but Smith went on: 'In the U.S. the American Cancer Society and other organizations have reviewed the Cochrane Report carefully and found it lacking in credibility.' He also remarked that 'this debate is likely to continue, based more emotion, pseudo-facts, and speculation, and less on science'. I agree with Smith on that one, the only difference being – as I demonstrate abundantly in this book – that those who use emotion, pseudo-facts and speculation belong in the screening advocates' camp.

The end of Smith's letter was particularly startling:

> Some in the media have been misled in this debate, which is all too easy when both scientists and institutional icons are lined up on opposite sides of an issue. I have heard disturbing news that Dr. Sjönell has spoken to the press and asserted that your meeting was a clear victory for those who claim mammography has no value. I have also heard that Dr. Tabár has been criticized in the press and accused of intellectual dishonesty. This truly is appalling, for no single individual in the world has done as much to establish the scientific basis for early breast cancer detection than Dr. Tabár. If these stories are true, then I hope there will be an opportunity for someone with authority to speak out against this devious manipulation of the media, since ultimately it sends a deceitful message to the public.

'Someone with authority to speak out against this devious manipulation of the media'? The Swedish prime minister? The pope? And who should censor the free debate? It wouldn't work. We have freedom of speech in the Nordic countries, just like in Smith's own country.

Contempt of science in Denmark and Norway

In Germany, Sylvia Heywang-Köbrunner, director of breast screening in Munich, played the overused 'you are killing my patients' card: 'Those who now demotivate women to take part, play with the lives of thousands of women each year.'[32]

In Denmark, editorials in two leading newspapers cut through all the hype and expressed serious doubt about screening, with telling titles: 'A sick case'[33] and 'The good will'.[34] A third newspaper expressed surprise that the Danish National Board of Health and the politicians paid no attention to our review, but it offered the explanation that elections to parliament were close.[35] Two spokespeople from the Board of Health and the Ministry of Health both declared there was nothing new in our paper.[36] Funny that no news made so many screening advocates enraged by our findings.

Perhaps the prize for the worst argument – although there were many contenders – should go to Danish breast surgeon Mogens Blichert-Toft from the Danish Breast Cancer Group: 'I have never met a woman who was sorry that we found a small tumour rather than a large one.'[37] What is the take-home message in this?

Another non-argument that was repeated over and over was that more women died from breast cancer in Denmark, where we didn't have general screening, than in Sweden. I can provide many pairs of European countries where the opposite is true: that more women die in countries with screening than in countries without. There was no bottom level for the arguments, and this one was even offered by senior spokespeople from the Danish National Board of Health.[38]

It is interesting to see the various ways in which systems immunise themselves against criticism. I once wrote a regular column on science in a newspaper, and in 2003 I did a piece on cancer screening. This provoked a reaction from chief physician Iben Holten from the Danish Cancer Society.[39] She argued that there was no documentation that the cause-of-death assessment was sometimes erroneous; that it was wrong to state that screening leads to 30% overdiagnosis; and that my piece dealt with opinions and had no scientific basis. She also wondered how a chief physician like me could have such a primitive perception of cancer diseases.

In court, we have something called contempt of court and we have perjury. Should we also have contempt of science and punish those who are found guilty? Holten is a pathologist, and if there is anything pathologists know then it is that determination of cause of death is error prone, and that there is a large reservoir of undetected cancers that can be detected at autopsy when women die from something else.[40,41] Furthermore, the numbers I used were scientifically documented in our review of the trials. Finally, what is vulgar about cancer diseases are simple slogans such as 'cancer that is detected in time can be cured', which has been used by the Danish Cancer Society, although it is a circular, and therefore meaningless argument. If you die, it is because it wasn't detected in time; if you don't die, it was detected in time. Even though screening had no effect, or was harmful, this tautology would still be true.

In Norway, the cancer research community was in uproar and Steinar Thoresen remarked that we were on a crusade against screening, that we didn't know what we were talking about, that the technique used in the trials could not be compared with modern-day techniques, and that *Lancet* had become a 'popular science magazine'.[42] He described our work as 'unadulterated nonsense', 'unlimited naiveté', and added that we were undermining our trustworthiness. He also said, 'by the way, no one in the international research community has any confidence in the movement [The Cochrane Collaboration]'.[43] No understatements here!

Norwegian experts 'burned with rage' and Rolf Kåresen insinuated that our conclusion in the *Lancet* was completely wrong and that we knew it was wrong.[22] In December, the Norwegian Research Ethics Committee wrote to the Minister of Health and noted that the information women received was erroneous and also asked that the planned extension of screening to the whole country should take place as a research project.[44] Unfortunately, nothing happened.

No wonder several doctors declined to participate in the Norwegian debate, as they were afraid of being exposed to strong language from the screening advocates.[45]

References

1 Olsen O, Gøtzsche PC. Cochrane review on screening for breast cancer with mammography. *Lancet*. 2001; **358**(9290): 1340–2.
2 Olsen O, Gøtzsche PC. Systematic review of screening for breast cancer with mammography. *Lancet*. 2001 Oct 20. Available at: http://image.thelancet.com/extras/fullreport.pdf (accessed 5 May 2010).
3 Tabár L, Fagerberg CJ, Gad A, *et al*. Reduction in mortality from breast cancer after mass screening with mammography: randomised trial from the Breast Cancer Screening Working Group of the Swedish National Board of Health and Welfare. *Lancet*. 1985; **1**(8433): 829–32.
4 McCullough M. Medical groups rally to back mammography. *Philadelphia Inquirer*. 2002 Feb 4.
5 Wilcken N. Mammography screening. *Lancet Oncol*. 2002; **3**(5): 268.
6 New concerns over breast screening. *BBC News*. 2001 Oct 18.
7 Pearson H. Breast cancer screens scrutinised. *Nature*. 2001 Oct 19.
8 Imperial Cancer Research Fund. *Imperial Cancer Response to Lancet Paper on the*

Effectiveness of Breast Cancer Screening. Press Release. London: Imperial Cancer Research Fund; 19 Oct 2001.

9 Editor's choice: the agonies of evidence. *BMJ*. 2001 Nov 10; **323**(7321).

10 Mayor S. Row over breast cancer screening shows that scientists bring 'some subjectivity into their work'. *BMJ*. 2001; **323**(7319): 956.

11 Gøtzsche PC. Office of NHS cancer screening programme misrepresents Nordic work in breast screening row. *BMJ*. 2001; **323**(7321): 1131.

12 Rodger A. Screening mammography and mortality. *Med J Aust*. 2002; **177**(6): 333.

13 Gøtzsche PC. Screening mammography and mortality. *Med J Aust*. 2003; **178**(4): 189–90.

14 Rodger A. Screening mammography and mortality. *Med J Aust*. 2003; **178**(4): 190.

15 Letters. Screening for breast cancer with mammography. *Lancet*. 2001; **358**(9299): 2164–8.

16 Gøtzsche PC, Nielsen M. Screening for breast cancer with mammography. *Cochrane Database Syst Rev*. 2009; (4): CD001877.

17 Duffy SW, Tabár L, Smith RA. The mammographic screening trials: commentary on the recent work by Olsen and Gøtzsche. *CA Cancer J Clin*. 2002; **52**(2): 68–71.

18 Haverdahl A-L. [Mammography does not decrease mortality from cancer] [Swedish]. *Svenska Dagbladet*. 2001 Oct 19: 4.

19 Blanksvärd H. [The row about our breasts] [Swedish]. *Aftonbladet*. 2001 Dec 19.

20 Dean PB. [Mammographic screening is a reliable examination method] [Swedish]. *Läkartidningen*. 2001; **98**(51–52): 5924–6.

21 Jensen SE. [Lancet paper creates hateful Nordic debate on mammography] [Swedish]. *Dagens Medicin*. 2001 Nov 1.

22 Eiring Ø. [Accuses Lancet for scamped work – experts go against shock report on mammography] [Norwegian]. *Dagens Medisin*. 2001 Oct 25.

23 Olsen O, Gøtzsche PC. Screening for breast cancer with mammography. Cochrane Database Syst Rev. 2001; (4): CD001877.

24 Dean P. 'References are needed – not unsubstantiated opinions'. *Läkartidningen*. 2003; **100**(30–31): 2469.

25 Gøtzsche PC. [Misleading report concerning our work on mammographic screening] [Danish]. *Läkartidningen*. 2002; **99**(1–2): 75–6.

26 Dean P. [Mammographic screening should not be affected by unfounded arguments] [Swedish]. *Läkartidningen*. 2002; **99**(9): 944–5.

27 Gøtzsche PC. [Alarming that the screening trials do not reduce mortality from cancer] [Swedish]. *Läkartidningen*. 2002; **99**(9): 945.

28 Gøtzsche PC, Nielsen M. Screening for breast cancer with mammography. *Cochrane Database Syst Rev*. 2006; (4): CD001877.

29 Anderson H, Arnesson L-G, Bengtsson N-O, *et al*. [Long survival for cured women] [Swedish]. *Dagens Nyheter*. 2002 Jan 13: A4.

30 Levi F, Lucchini F, Negri E, *et al*. Cancer mortality in Europe, 1990–1994, and an overview of trends from 1955 to 1994. *Eur J Cancer*. 1999; **35**(10): 1477–516.

31 Levi F, Lucchini F, Negri E, *et al*. The fall in breast cancer mortality in Europe. *Eur J Cancer*. 2001; **37**(11): 1409–12.

32 Stockinger G. [Search for the tumours] [German]. *Der Spiegel*. 2007; **5**: 126–7.

33 [A sick cause] [Danish]. *Berlingske Tidende*. 2001 Oct 20.

34 [The good will] [Danish]. *Jyllandsposten*. 2001 Oct 22.

35 Hannerup M. [Weak reaction from the Danish National Board of Health] [Danish]. *Dagens Medicin*. 2001 Oct 25.

36 Gøtzsche PC. [We want a scientifically strong National Board of Health] [Danish]. *Dagens Medicin*. 2001 Nov 1.

37 Hansen CF. [Breast cancer experts denounce Lancet paper] [Danish]. *Dagens Medicin*. 2001 Nov 1.

38 Hansen SW, Andersen JS. [Everybody wants a strong National Board of Health] [Danish]. *Dagens Medicin*. 2001 Nov 8: 27.

39 Holten I. [Scare campaign] [Danish]. *Politiken*. 2003 Jun 6.

40 Nielsen M, Thomsen JL, Primdahl S, *et al*. Breast cancer and atypia among young and middle-aged women: a study of 110 medicolegal autopsies. *Br J Cancer*. 1987; **56**(6): 814–19.

41 Welch HG, Black WC. Using autopsy series to estimate the disease 'reservoir' for ductal carcinoma in situ of the breast. *Ann Intern Med*. 1997; **127**(11): 1023–8.

42 Vold JS. [Intense researcher row about mammography] [Norwegian]. *Bergens Tidende*. 2001 Oct 20.

43 Eiring Ø. [Mammography doesn't work] [Norwegian]. *Dagens Medisin*. 2001 Oct 19.

44 Eiring Ø. [Planned breast screening is not recommended] [Norwegian]. *Dagens Medisin*. 2001 Dec 17.

45 Eiring Ø, Dommerud T. [Dissent about mammography in the Cancer Registry]. *Dagens Medisin*. 2001 Nov 8.

8

Delayed media storm in the United States after our 2001 reviews

AT FIRST, THE RESULTS FROM THE NORDIC COCHRANE CENTRE WERE barely noticed in the United States. It is not uncommon that European research results are overlooked, and the Americans themselves say that NIH (National Institutes of Health) means 'Not Invented Here'.

When we published our reviews in the *Lancet* and in *The Cochrane Library* in October 2001, *Reuters* issued a press release,[1] where Robert Smith used as his main argument for screening a fatally flawed observational study authored by himself, Tabár, Duffy and others that reported a 63% reduction in breast cancer mortality in Sweden among those who attended screening.[2] The dramatic effect was very popular and the message spread immediately to many other countries.[3,4] This study will be critiqued in Chapter 14.

That was all. But 2 months later, the media storm in Europe and Australia arrived on American shores when the *New York Times* published a series of articles critical of mammography screening, beginning on 9 December.[5]

In January 2002, an independent panel of US medical experts writing for the National Cancer Institute's website concluded that there is insufficient evidence to show that mammography screening reduces deaths from breast cancer.[6] One of the panel members was Donald Berry, who said that he was aware of the difficulty in questioning an enormous mammography industry: 'Screening programmes bring in patients'.

This was perceived as so threatening that 10 leading medical organisations published a full-page advertisement in the *New York Times* in support of screening using the 'you are killing my patients' argument:[7]

An Open Letter To Women And Their Physicians

We, the undersigned, representing a broad spectrum of concerned health organizations, are responding to coverage in the media and the resulting public discussion questioning the value of mammography. This discussion has been stimulated by a recent report published in the British medical journal, *The Lancet*, which concluded there was no scientific support for breast cancer screening with mammography.

Women and their healthcare professionals should know that numerous independent expert groups in the U.S. and Europe have repeatedly subjected the world's major clinical studies of mammography to careful scientific scrutiny, and also have carefully evaluated the analysis published in *The Lancet*. While the existing studies of mammography screening have known limitations and even some flaws, the evidence as a whole solidly supports reduced breast cancer mortality rates due to mammography screening. Early breast cancer detection means a greater chance for successful treatment and a greater range of treatment options.

We have grave concerns that these public debates have already begun to erode the confidence in mammography that has been built up over the past two decades. While mammography is not a perfect tool, it is effective and has contributed significantly to the declines in breast cancer mortality since 1990. In fact, there will be many thousands fewer breast cancer deaths among U.S. women this year due to the combined progress we've made in early detection and improved therapy. If women are dissuaded from getting regular mammograms, lives will be lost.

We strongly urge women to continue to follow the advice of their physicians and the leading medical organizations. Our organizations will continue to monitor new scientific research in order to offer the best advice to women and their physicians.

This letter is co-signed by the following organizations:
American Academy of Family Physicians
American Cancer Society
American College of Physicians
American Society of Internal Medicine
American College of Obstetricians and Gynecologists
American College of Preventive Medicine
American Medical Association
Cancer Research Foundation of America
National Medical Association

> *Oncology Nursing Society*
> *Society of Gynecologic Oncologists*
>
> For more information about the early detection of breast cancer, call 1-800-227-2345.

Richard Smith, editor-in-chief of the *BMJ*, mentioned the advertisement and remarked that the organisations vigorously upheld the status quo of continuing screening, eschewing any supportive evidence for their stance.[8] He added: 'Is the fact that mammography is worth $3–4 billion a year relevant here?'

An economist from the US National Cancer Institute confirmed that the annual costs for mammography screening amounted to more than US$3 billion.[9] And the *New Republic* reported that the American Cancer Society expected to spend US$20 million in 2002 promoting mammography.[10] *Twenty million dollars*.

Inger Atterstam from *Svenska Dagbladet* also considered the financial benefits for screening advocates. She noted that László Tabár owns an American company, Mammography Education Inc, Arizona, and that he had already started his commercial activities in 1980, 5 years before the results of his Two-County trial were published.[11] This appears to have been unknown in Sweden, but after her revelation, the Council of Ethics in the Swedish Medical Association declared that it would look into this.[12] I don't know if this was done.

Tabár declared an income of SEK5 million in Sweden in 1999, which is an extraordinary amount of money according to Nordic standards, about seven times more than a chief of a hospital department earns. However, I cannot remember having seen any article by Tabár stating his conflicts of interest, not even in a *Lancet* paper where he claimed that screening reduces breast cancer mortality by 40%–50%: 'Conflict of interest statement: None declared.'[13]

Maryann Napoli from the US Center for Medical Consumers reminded her readers that screening creates customers and that mammography screening is a particularly lucrative industry, which explains why this industry fights 'tooth and nail against researchers who find evidence of harm'.[14] She wondered why our finding that screening increases a woman's risk of losing a breast was omitted in virtually all media reports and ended with a question that just won't go away: 'Are we better off not subjecting ourselves to screening tests and, instead, promptly seeking treatment once a symptom appears?'

There were also congressional hearings, but they didn't start well. Senator Tom Harkin, Iowa Democrat, who wanted to hold them, stated:[15]

> There is considerable controversy surrounding the Danish study and women deserve a clear answer. I am personally convinced that had my two sisters had

> access to mammography they would not have died so young because of this terrible disease.

It is a recipe for disaster when politicians mix science, politics, emotions, case stories and prophetic gifts. I was invited to give testimony at the hearings at a time when I planned to be in Thailand on holiday with my family. My travel expenses would not be reimbursed and I didn't sacrifice my holidays.

One of the weirdest arguments in the fierce US debate came from breast cancer screening advocates who wondered whether we might have an economic or political incentive to downplay the benefits of the expensive screening programmes.[16] We have an expression for this in Danish: thieves think everybody steals.

The comedy continued. The *Philadelphia Inquirer* quoted Nick Day as saying that our review was 'total nonsense, and it is a scandal, first, that it was published and, second, that it has had the impact it has'.[17] The newspaper dutifully noted that Day was author of one of the studies (the Two-County trial) that 'the Danes dismissed'. Daniel Kopans felt that the 63% reduction in breast cancer mortality in the fatally flawed observational study[2] 'corroborates the results of the clinical trials of screening mammography',[18] and another professor of radiology was 'not troubled by these revisionist thinkers who are claiming that hundreds of trials were done incorrectly'.[15] Hundreds?

A writer on health for the *New York Times* who had breast cancer noted that 'some small percentage of breast cancers' will not grow to become a threat to the women's lives and that it 'may be a necessary price to pay for the chance to save the lives of the much larger number whose cancers will be life-threatening'.[18] It's the other way round: the 'much larger number' applies to the overdiagnosed women, not to those who benefit.

Larry Norton, president of the American Society of Clinical Oncology, published a letter in the *New York Times* on 3 February 2002, co-signed by 19 organisations,[19] which said:

> Many analyses, including a new study published in the British medical journal *The Lancet* this week, have found that mammograms are lifesaving. Several other thorough reviews are under way.

The new study was published the previous day and it was misleading to the extreme. It didn't show that screening is lifesaving. It couldn't, as it used a faulty method. The study was a research letter published by epidemiologist Olli Miettinen, radiologist Claudia Henschke and others.[20]

Miettinen and Henschke's cherry-picking in the *Lancet*

The research letter was followed by an equally curious letter by other researchers who quoted it.[20,21] Donald Berry and I responded to both letters,[22,23] quite convincingly in our opinion, but that didn't have any effect on Miettinen and Henschke, who now said: 'So grossly does Gøtzsche misrepresent the principles we adduced that they need to be reasserted', whereafter they repeated their mistakes.[24] Not even 6 months later, when other researchers described their errors again, did they admit they were wrong.[25]

Miettinen and colleagues[20] had performed a remarkable act of hocus-pocus. They rightly pointed out that the effect of screening only appears after some delay. But then they used data from the Malmö trial in the time window 8–11 years after the trial started and they concluded that screening reduced breast cancer mortality by 55%, although in fact there was no effect of screening in this trial. Furthermore, they excluded the Canadian trials for no good reason.

If they had wanted to make a very different conclusion, they could have looked at the interval 3–6 years after randomisation, when there was an *increase* in breast cancer mortality of 58%. Obviously, the only legitimate analyses use all the available data from 0 to 11 years. The women cannot come to the interval 8–11 years without first surviving the interval when their risk of dying was increased.

The second letter was also strange. Benjamin Djulbegovic and Iztok Hozo declared that we had made 'elementary analytical errors' and that it was wrong to pool data at a fixed time point (e.g. to report the cumulated breast cancer mortality after 7 years, which is entirely legitimate, relevant and frequently done).[21] They used Miettinen's faulty method, pooled the Canadian and the Malmö trials, and reported a reduction in breast cancer mortality of 39%. They even suggested that Miettinen's cherry-picking method should be used in other systematic reviews in cancer. We noted that we didn't understand how they could have used data from the Canadian trials for their calculations, as we couldn't find useful data for Miettinen's method in the reference they gave. Anthony Miller wrote to Djulbegovic and informed him that he had never published data in a form that would enable anyone to perform a 'Miettinen-type' analysis. Very odd, indeed.

It is difficult to understand why experienced researchers would publish such nonsense. Unless the idea is to create fictitious support for screening, which Claudia Henschke did in relation to lung cancer screening (*see* Chapter 2).

Additional reactions in the United States

David Dershaw, director of the Breast Imaging Center at Memorial Sloan-Kettering Cancer Center in New York, said that Miettinen's study was sound science,[26] and Harmon Eyre, chief medical officer from the American Cancer Society, reported in the congressional hearings that the Miettinen study showed that screening is very beneficial. Donald Berry reported it was junk.

A professor of radiology in Indiana, Valerie Jackson, remarked about our 2001 *Lancet* review that, 'When one closely reads all the available literature', the review 'is highly inaccurate'.[27] I doubt she has read all the available literature because some of it consists of unpublished reports in Swedish, and it took us many months to assemble and read. Furthermore, it is unconvincing to claim a research paper is 'highly inaccurate' without specifying what the problems are.

An editorial in the *New York Times* took issue with all the hype. It found it disappointing that key organisations and individuals in the cancer establishment had mostly chosen to draw their wagons in a defensive circle and noted – with reference to the full-page advertisement in the journal – that the reaction of the cancer establishment 'had been to call on higher authority – itself'.[28] It couldn't be said any better.

The editorial suggested a serious and open reassessment of the data, conducted by an organisation that can be trusted for its objectivity. But that was exactly what we had done. The Cochrane Collaboration is such an organisation, as Napoli acknowledged.[14]

In February 2002, John Crewdson from the *Chicago Tribune* drew attention to a study from Dartmouth by William Black and colleagues[29] that happened to be published in the middle of the maelstrom of the pros and cons of mammography screening.[30] These researchers had looked at screening trials for colon, breast and lung cancer, and although they acknowledged that their results could be chance findings, they went in the expected direction and provided support for our concerns about biased cause-of-death assessments in the mammography trials. Biostatistician Colin Begg from Sloan-Kettering remarked in an interview that 'the notion of a single "cause" of death in an individual is a nebulous one, since death will often result from various frailties that have been endured by the patient.'

Any doctor who has filled out cause-of-death certificates will know how unreliable such data are. The task is left to the most junior doctors, who often do it at night, while they are on call and while they rush busily between acutely admitted patients who are more important than what one writes on a death certificate. When there are several contributing causes, it can be pretty arbitrary and artificial to state *the* cause of death, as doctors are required to do. I noted in Crewdson's article that 'it's of no benefit to a woman to have another cause of death on her death certificate. That's not what they want. They want to live longer.' Paul Meier from Columbia University, co-inventor of the Kaplan-Meier survival analysis, agreed that death from any cause should be the gold standard in cancer screening trials.

Robert Smith mentioned in an interview that what we had done was to accept 'rather uncritically two studies that have been quite controversial' and that we were 'very critical of the other studies that were actually very carefully done'.[31] Smith turned the facts completely upside down. As far as I know, the Malmö study has never been considered controversial by anyone. We also discussed at length in our review why the Canadian studies (described as one study by Smith) are also reliable and why the studies Smith likes are not so reliable. In the same article, Barnett Kramer, senior scientist at the US National Cancer Institute, had an opposite view: 'They did a particularly meticulous examination of all the trials and every publication of every trial . . . It's the most comprehensive look to date at the available data.'[31]

A lawyer, Nancy Newman, past president of the National Conference of Women's Bar Associations, gave her 'perspective on misdirected advocacy'.[32] She noted that, 'people can argue about cause of death, but whether or not someone is alive or dead is generally not debatable', and added that the lack of a discernible effect on overall mortality means that if mammography prolongs life in some women, it may lead to overtreatment or even shortening of life in just as many. She also noted that mammography was a sacred cow and that those responsible for it didn't provide information that allowed informed consent.

Daniel Kopans is a Harvard professor, which looks good on paper. He is not known for his measured reactions, however, although he has declared that he is 'not a terrorist'.[33] In *Science*, he has been described by Richard Klausner, the then director of the US National Cancer Institute, as a person who employs 'a pattern of inflammatory, accusatory approaches that are antithetical to the requirements of scientific discourse'. Kopans called the National Cancer Institute Panel involved in the 1997 Consensus Development Conference 'fraudulent' when it recommended against regular screening of women in their forties (*see* Chapter 18).[33] Kopans published a piece in the *Boston Globe* where he shot in all directions. The *Lancet* was irresponsible, a front-page article in the *New York Times* that highlighted our review's conclusions was 'unconscionable' and our review was 'Not a scientific study, but the summary of an analysis by two individuals in Denmark.'[34] He also complained that our review 'had not even been published, so when experts were questioned by the media about the significance of the summary, most had no idea as to the review's contents'. This was entirely misleading, as the *Lancet* had simply followed the usual embargo rules for papers prior to the publication date.

Kopans fantasised about our scientific methods, claiming, 'When the Danes reviewed the data, they decided that they didn't like the way five out of seven trials had been done, so they discarded the results from those trials that showed clear benefit', and he propagated the usual erroneous claims about the alleged poor quality of the mammograms in the Canadian trials and imbalanced randomisation. He concluded that, 'the fact that the Danish writers approved of this grossly flawed trial is an example of their lack of understanding of the randomized, controlled trial.' So now we are 'writers' rather than 'individuals' and we are still not recognised as researchers. Finally, Kopans demonstrated he doesn't understand the weaknesses of observational studies of cancer screening, because he quoted Tabár's study once more that reported the miraculous 63% effect. Anthony Miller wrote to me that, 'as Kopans is well aware, we have responded to all his points already in the scientific media, but he chooses to ignore this.'

Kopans also wrote a long article in the *American Journal of Roentgenology* in January 2003 with a subtitle leaving no doubt about his views on those who disagree with him: 'Nonsense and nonscience'.[35] As a testimony for his own sense of science, Kopans mentioned the 63% reduction in breast cancer mortality again. There was also an editorial by the editor-in-chief, Lee Rogers, that was even more hostile.[36]

Kopans remarked that the *New York Times* had attacked the 'cancer establishment' and had shown complete disdain for the truth to the detriment of the public, which could result in lives being lost. *Lancet* had violated the peer-review principles, as it had published our review despite criticisms raised by Peter Boyle of the European Institute of Oncology and two other peer reviewers. As these peer reviews were anonymous and their identities are considered confidential, it was quite a revelation how the 'cancer establishment' seems to cooperate in an attempt to censor unwelcome research.

Kopans's counterpart in Europe, Peter Dean, was even worse. He sent Kopans's paper[35] around in one of his mass-email messages and wrote in the *Scandinavian Journal of Surgery* that a letter from the *Lancet*'s ombudsman was read at the Global Summit on Mammography Screening in Milan in 2002, which revealed that all but one of the five peer reviewers had rejected our manuscript, but that Richard Horton had decided to publish it.[37] Dean also wrote that we had been invited to defend our arguments at the meeting, had accepted the invitation, and then didn't participate. Kopans only noted that we 'declined'.[35] However, both statements are misleading. We could not accept the invitation, as we were running a course in Oxford at the same time we had arranged, and we informed the organiser, Peter Boyle, that we couldn't come.

Donald Berry participated in the summit and was not impressed. He wrote to me:

> It was a screening lovefest. You two [Ole Olsen and me] were chastised, as was I. I was shunned as though I was a leper. And after the meeting Peter Dean sent a message to half the Western world that was a vitriolic attack on me personally. There was no sense in which the meeting was objective. Or even honest. For example, Tabar presented an inane analysis of screening and breast cancer trends in Sweden, and no one said a word.

In his mass email, Dean questioned Berry's scientific objectivity and willingness for a constructive dialogue, saying that he had already damaged his 'reputation in the scientific community nearly beyond retrieval'. Berry replied to Dean, 'I am impressed by the size of your "cc" list. I want to thank you for not including my mother.'

I was also mentioned in Dean's letter to 'half the Western world':

> Your letter and your other comments remind me of Peter Gøtzsche, who has made a considerable number of professional mistakes in his evaluation of a subject beyond his expertise, partly by his ignorance of the subject matter, partly by his defective understanding of basic epidemiology principles, partly by his careless reading of the published literature, and evidently also by his susceptibility to confirmation bias and self-deception. His rather elementary mistakes have been pointed out numerous times in print and in conference, yet he continues to repeat them with each new audience. I believe that he failed to respond to Peter Boyle's invitation because he received such a comprehensive refutation of his many allegations at the workshop in Stockholm on February 15, 2002 from many of the same trialists and other authorities in the field who attended the Milan conference. Yet, even at the Stockholm conference, when asked by Elsebeth Lynge if he had changed his mind after hearing the evidence, his response was a firm 'no.'

Another participant, Cornelia Baines, published her experience from the summit:[38]

> We heard the *Lancet* had caused harm to womankind and that because *Lancet* editor Dr. Richard Horton published the manuscript, disregarding five

> peer-reviewers who had recommended rejection, it proved that *Lancet* is not a peer-reviewed journal. In fact, as one of the reviewers I had recommended 'accept with revisions.'

Baines also noticed that after Tabár presented one of his observational studies at the meeting, no one spoke from the floor, even though it was biased and deserved questioning. By the time Baines caught on, the discussion had been closed. She asked several people why there had been no comments and the answer was: 'No one wants to fight with Laszlo.'[38] As already noted, I shall comment on this study in Chapter 14.

References

1 Norton A. Study recharges debate on the value of mammograms. *Reuters*. 2001 Oct 19.
2 Tabár L, Vitak B, Chen HH, *et al*. Beyond randomized controlled trials: organized mammographic screening substantially reduces breast carcinoma mortality. *Cancer*. 2001; **91**(9): 1724–31.
3 Imperial Cancer Research Fund. *Imperial Cancer Response to Lancet Paper on the Effectiveness of Breast Cancer Screening*. Press Release. London: Imperial Cancer Research Fund; 19 Oct 2001.
4 Thye-Petersen C. [Criticism of screening for breast cancer] [Danish]. *Jyllandsposten*. 2001 Oct 19: 3.
5 Kolata G. Study sets off debate over mammograms' value. *New York Times*. 2001 Dec 9: A1.
6 Charatan F. US panel finds insufficient evidence to support mammography. *BMJ*. 2002; **324**(7332): 255.
7 An open letter to women and their physicians. *New York Times*. 2002 Jan 31: A15.
8 Editor's choice: a modest proposal. *BMJ*. 2002 Feb 16.
9 Kolata G, Moss M. X-ray vision in hindsight: science, politics and the mammogram. *New York Times*. 2002 Feb 11.
10 Napoli M, Schiff H. Survey of U.S. media coverage of the review of mammography trials [poster]. 10th Cochrane Colloquium, 31 Jul–3 Aug 2002; Stavanger, Norway.
11 Atterstam I. [Mammography, a lucrative business] [Swedish] *Svenska Dagbladet*. 2002 Feb 16: 8.
12 Rudbeck K. ['Pure defamation.' Now the mammography doctor Laszlo Tabar threatens to leave the country] [Swedish]. *Falu Kuriren*. 2002 Feb 19: 34.
13 Tabár L, Yen M-F, Vitak B, *et al*. Mammography service screening and mortality in breast cancer patients: 20-year follow-up before and after introduction of screening. *Lancet*. 2003; **361**(9367): 1405–10.
14 Napoli M. Center calls for independent mammography review. Center for Medical Consumers. 2002 Feb 2. Available at: www.medicalconsumers.org/pages/call_for_ind_mamm_review.htm (accessed 7 August 2002).
15 Some of the many views on mammography. *New York Times*. 2002 Feb 5.

16 Gorman C. To test or not to test? The mammogram wars are raging again: the facts aren't all in yet, but don't cancel your appointment. *Time*. 2002 Feb 4.
17 McCullough M. Medical groups rally to back mammography. *Philadelphia Inquirer*. 2002 Feb 4.
18 Brody JE. Mammograms: not perfect, but necessary. *New York Times*. 2002 Feb 5.
19 Norton L. Mammogram alert: advice to women. *New York Times*. 2002 Feb 3: 414.
20 Miettinen OS, Henschke CI, Pasmantier MW, *et al*. Mammographic screening: no reliable supporting evidence? *Lancet*. 2002; **359**(9304): 404–5.
21 Djulbegovic B, Hozo I. Re-analysis of data from the high quality trials. Comment on: Olsen O, Gøtzsche PC. Screening for breast cancer with mammography. *Cochrane Database Syst Rev*. 2002: (3): CD001877.
22 Gøtzsche PC. Mammographic screening: no reliable supporting evidence? *Lancet*. 2002; **359**: 706.
23 Gøtzsche PC, Berry D. Re-analysis of data from the high quality trials. Reply in: Olsen O, Gøtzsche PC. Screening for breast cancer with mammography. *Cochrane Database Syst Rev*. 2002; (3): CD001877.
24 Miettinen OS, Henschke CI. Mammographic screening: no reliable supporting evidence? *Lancet*. 2002; **359**(9307): 706.
25 Letters. Mammographic screening: no reliable supporting evidence? *Lancet*. 2002; **360**(9334): 719–21.
26 Bouchez C. Mammograms do save lives, researchers say. *Chicago Tribune*. 2002 Feb 6.
27 Study rekindles debate over clinical benefit of screening mammography. *Health Tech Trends*. 2002; **14**: 1–5.
28 Circling the mammography wagons. *New York Times*. 2002 Feb 6.
29 Black WC, Haggstrom DA, Welch HG. All-cause mortality in randomized trials of cancer screening. *J Natl Cancer Inst*. 2002; **94**(3): 167–73.
30 Crewdson J. Cancer studies may have bias: some deaths likely attributed to other, noncancer causes. *Chicago Tribune*. 2002 Feb 6.
31 Perry S. Do mammograms save lives? *Today's Health & Wellness*. 2002 March/April.
32 Newman N. Women, lawyers and mammograms: a perspective on misdirected advocacy. *Women Law J*. 2003; **88**(3): 13–17.
33 Taubes G. How one radiologist turns up the heat. *Science*. 1997; **275**(5303): 1057.
34 Kopans DB. Needless confusion over mammograms. *Boston Globe*. 2002 Jan 1: A19.
35 Kopans DB. The most recent breast cancer screening controversy about whether mammographic screening benefits women at any age: nonsense and nonscience. *AJR Am J Roentgenol*. 2003; **180**(1): 21–6.
36 Rogers LF. Screening mammography: target of opportunity for the media. *AJR Am J Roentgenol*. 2003; **180**(1): 1.
37 Dean PB. The rationale and current controversies of mammographic screening for breast cancer. *Scand J Surg*. 2002; **91**(3): 288–92.
38 Baines C. Breast practices. *Medical Post*. 2002 Jun 25: 11.

9

The Danish National Board of Health circles the wagons

> *How to discredit an unwelcome report. Stage Two: Some of the main conclusions have been questioned. (If they haven't, question them yourself; then they have).*
>
> *Yes Minister* (BBC series)

IF YOU ARE NOT DANISH, WHICH YOU PROBABLY AREN'T, AS THERE ARE only 5.4 million of us, you might think this chapter is not for you. Who cares about what happens in a small country? But since you have decided to read this book, there is a good chance that you may not believe everything the authorities tell you about healthcare and about what you should do to reduce your risk of becoming ill or dying. This chapter gives you a rare insight into how health policies are made, which, in the case of mammography screening, has involved a glaring disregard for the scientific evidence in order to arrive at preconceived and politically desirable conclusions.

Shortly after Ole Olsen and I had published our Cochrane and *Lancet* reviews in October 2001, the Association of Danish Counties asked the Danish National Board of Health to reconsider its recommendations on screening, noting that it had not been documented that screening leads to better survival, whereas screened women will experience more operations and more radiotherapy.

The association demanded a written report from the Board of Health on its interpretation of our research, and a spokesperson mentioned difficulties, as the counties usually respected both The Nordic Cochrane Centre and the Board of Health highly. The director of the Board of Health replied that it was not the board's obligation to comment on every publication that is published in the *Lancet*, even though its authors are Danish.[1] That remark was pretty inappropriate, considering that the board had funded our research to learn more about screening.

A week later, the board declared that it would look at data from screening programmes in several countries, as there 'are many other data [than those from randomised trials] that can contribute to the evaluation of screening'.[2] This is like first using a strong lamp, and when it is unclear what you see, you shift to a weak lamp, hoping it will help you to see better. The trials didn't show a life-extending effect of screening with certainty, and the authorities would now look at far less reliable evidence – observational studies – which cannot prove an effect of screening, as the biases are too large compared to the magnitude of the expected effect. But perhaps there was another reason. Politically it had been decided that screening is good for people and finding observational studies in support of this view shouldn't be too difficult.

The Board of Health gave in to the association's demands and we were summoned to yet another expert meeting where the board ignored some of our most important observations. We therefore pointed them out at the meeting, and we also sent written comments after the meeting detailing a number of errors and misleading statements in the board's draft report. However, as I shall explain, the board's 26-page report, which was finalised in February 2002, was still seriously misleading.[3] It was sent to the association with the message that there was no reason to change the recommendations.

The board acknowledged that the most important result is the effect on all-cause mortality but added that it would only be realistic to show an effect on disease-specific mortality. The board argued that 'positive experiences' with the Swedish programme had been communicated in a 1997 report from the Swedish National Board of Health. What this report was about and what was 'positive' wasn't described, and I have been unable to find it on the Swedish National Board of Health's website or locate it by other means.

The board also quoted a UK report for 'positive experience with screening', but no data in that report were provided in support of screening,[4] even though it was written by those responsible for the programme. And as we shall see in later chapters, publications from the UK NHS Breast Screening Programme are generally misleading. A more sobering reference would have been to a paper in the *BMJ* published 2 years earlier that received a lot of attention. It estimated that screening in the United Kingdom had decreased breast cancer mortality by only 6%.[5]

The board also referred to the totally misleading articles in the *Läkartidningen* by Måns Rosén from the Swedish National Board of Health and concluded that the effect of screening in Sweden agreed with what was expected. This was an outrageously false statement (*see* Chapter 5). An effect of screening in Sweden hasn't been visible at any point in time, not even today, so many years after screening started.[6,7] In a way, this is yet another example of what the *New York Times* described as calling on a higher authority – itself.[8] One board of health calls on another board of health, and both boards have the same conflicts of interest related to defending screening.

The board made other serious errors. Although the Malmö trial didn't find an effect of screening, the board alluded to the inexcusably flawed research letter by Miettinen and Henschke (*see* Chapter 8). The board even had the audacity to note in its conclusion that it is noteworthy that we had declared that the Malmö trial showed no effect, when Miettinen's analysis showed an effect. This information was not part of the draft report we had seen in advance of the meeting at the Board of Health. It was inserted later, and the final report was quite different from the draft report.

We didn't get an opportunity to protest against the many errors in the final report because it wasn't sent to us before it was finalised and sent to the Association of Danish Counties.

About radiotherapy, we had written in our *Lancet* review that it is harmful when given to low-risk women, such as those who have their cancer detected at screening,[9] as many of these women are healthy but overdiagnosed. The board acknowledged that radiotherapy increases deaths from heart disease, but added that this had not been observed at Danish departments. The study they quoted for this has 13 deaths in one group and 12 in the other,[10] which is far too few for such a strong statement. It requires hundreds of cardiac deaths in a randomised trial that compares radiotherapy with no radiotherapy before one can say anything reliably about this important issue.

The board denied that screening leads to more mastectomies and suggested the opposite, although the trial evidence showed that the board was wrong (*see* Chapter 7). It also noted that long follow-up is needed to see the full effect of screening, but did not discuss the curious contradiction of this that we reported in our Cochrane review:[11]

> We find it disturbing that the largest effects on breast cancer mortality have been reported in trials that had long intervals between screenings (Two-County trial), that invited a large fraction of the women to only 2 or 3 screenings (Two-County and Stockholm trials), that started systematic screening of the control

group already after 3–5 years (Two-County trial, Göteborg trial and Stockholm trial) and that had poor equipment for mammography (New York trial). This doesn't make sense.

Such observations should ring any researcher's alarm bells.

The board dismissed another of our important findings, which we had discussed at length and documented; namely, that cause-of-death assessments inevitably are biased in favour of screening, even when blinded end-point committees are used.[11,12] One of the reasons for this is that radiotherapy is used more commonly in screened women, and as it reduces the risk of local recurrence, this makes it more likely that women with screen-detected cancers will be misclassified as deaths from other causes.

About overdiagnosis, the board noted that in Copenhagen, the number of diagnoses doubled when screening was introduced and that there were now 20%–25% more diagnoses than in the rest of the country. Despite this unequivocal documentation of considerable overdiagnosis, the report disregarded this finding completely. It also dismissed our finding of overdiagnosis with the inappropriate argument that these particular data were not accepted by the Cochrane Breast Cancer Group in our Cochrane review. These data were censored away by the Cochrane Breast Cancer Group, but they were published in the *Lancet*.[13,14] What's wrong with that?

The bumpy ride from one untenable argument to the next continued. The board noted that the trials were old and that there had been considerable technological and professional quality development since then, which should also be considered. It is not clear what the board exactly meant by this. But if the equipment had improved, overdiagnosis was also likely to have increased.

Most astonishingly, the board now considered the Canadian trials problematic, particularly because they were not population based and because the Canadian healthcare system doesn't resemble the Danish one. So what? The same argument could be made against the New York trial; in fact, the US healthcare system is more remote from the Danish one than the Canadian. The arguments are irrelevant and the board contradicted itself, as it wrote in its 1994 report that the Canadian trials were well done and didn't suffer from the shortcomings of other trials.[15]

In the last paragraph of its report, the board emphasised that very careful information to the women, mentioning 'benefits and drawbacks', should follow the invitation to participate in the screening programme. What is so tragic about this is, as I shall explain in Chapter 19, that the board seemed determined to do almost anything it could to ensure that this did *not* happen.

It is difficult to describe what I feel about this. Perhaps the worst thing was that even though I was invited to comment and did so, the board produced a seriously misleading report that is erroneous on many important counts, often relies on poor science rather than our Cochrane and *Lancet* reviews, and consistently favours screening. It was very saddening to witness this, and I cannot help having uneasy feelings about other interventions the board recommends. In fact, I have often seen that the most reliable evidence is ignored also in other areas of healthcare.

Systems will go to great lengths to protect themselves, and it is clear to me that the board is a political body with little respect for science. To ignore sound science in order to please the political system and committees composed of specialists with vested interests is not a healthy attitude for a guardian of the citizens' health. As far as I can remember, at all the meetings we attended at the Board of Health, only one person was present apart from ourselves whose main interest seemed to be to get as close to the truth as possible. Everyone else seemed preoccupied with protecting the status quo, and almost all had important conflicts of interest.

Two things make me particularly sad. One is that what I experienced is similar to the way the drug industry operates. It doesn't really matter whether the information on drugs is misleading, which it usually is, or whether the drugs do more harm than good, as long as people don't know about it. The other is that the Swedish National Board of Health performed equally poorly, as described in other chapters. Therefore, it seems likely that the problems are universal.

In my judgement, the Danish National Board of Health did not take seriously the important concerns the Association of Danish Counties had raised, and the board effectively fooled the association. It seemed determined to defend screening at any cost and succeeded.

References

1 [Screening programmes to be evaluated] [Danish]. *Dagens Medicin*. 2001 Nov 8: 27.

2 Hansen CF. [The Health Technology Institute will assemble data on screening] [Danish]. *Dagens Medicin*. 2001 Nov 15.

3 Sundhedsstyrelsen (National Board of Health). [*Considerations in relation to the effect of an offer of mammography screening*] [*Danish*]. Copenhagen: Sundhedsstyrelsen; 2001 Feb 11. J.nr. 236-1-1999/jsa (26 pages).

4 Patnick J, editor. *NHS Breast Screening Programme Review 1999; meeting new challenges*. Sheffield: NHS Breast Screening Programme; 1999. Available at: www.cancerscreening.nhs.uk/breastscreen/publications/1999review.html

5 Blanks RG, Moss SM, McGahan CE, *et al*. Effect of NHS Breast Screening Programme

on mortality from breast cancer in England and Wales, 1990–98: comparison of observed with predicted mortality. *BMJ*. 2000; **321**(7262): 665–9.
6 Jørgensen KJ, Zahl PH, Gøtzsche PC. Breast cancer mortality in organised mammography screening in Denmark: comparative study. *BMJ*. 2010; **340**: c1241.
7 Autier P, Boniol M, La Vecchia C, *et al*. Disparities in breast cancer mortality trends between 30 European countries: retrospective trend analysis of WHO mortality database. *BMJ*. 2010; **341**: c3620.
8 Circling the mammography wagons. *New York Times*. 2002 Feb 6.
9 Early Breast Cancer Trialists' Collaborative Group. Favourable and unfavourable effects on long-term survival of radiotherapy for early breast cancer: an overview of the randomised trials. *Lancet*. 2000; **355**(9217): 1757–70.
10 Højris I, Overgaard M, Christensen JJ, *et al*. Morbidity and mortality of ischaemic heart disease in high-risk breast-cancer patients after adjuvant postmastectomy systemic treatment with or without radiotherapy: analysis of DBCG 82b and 82c randomised trials. *Lancet*. 1999; **354**(9188): 1425–30.
11 Olsen O, Gøtzsche PC. Screening for breast cancer with mammography. *Cochrane Database Syst Rev*. 2001; (4): CD001877.
12 Gøtzsche PC, Nielsen M. Screening for breast cancer with mammography. *Cochrane Database Syst Rev*. 2009; (4): CD001877.
13 Olsen O, Gøtzsche PC. Cochrane review on screening for breast cancer with mammography. *Lancet*. 2001; **358**(9290): 1340–2.
14 Olsen O, Gøtzsche PC. Systematic review of screening for breast cancer with mammography. *Lancet*. 2001 Oct 20. 1. Available at: http://image.thelancet.com/extras/fullreport.pdf (accessed 5 May 2010).
15 Sundhedsstyrelsen (National Board of Health). [*Breast cancer: early detection and diagnosis*] [*Danish*]. Copenhagen: Sundhedsstyrelsen; 1994.

10

US and Swedish 2002 meta-analyses

US Preventive Services Task Force's meta-analysis

There are many reviews and meta-analyses of the screening trials other than those by The Nordic Cochrane Centre, but very few of them have taken into account the risk of bias in the individual trials or considered the harms as well as benefits. Unsurprisingly, most of these substandard reviews have been written by screening advocates.

A notable exception is a comprehensive 2002 review in the *Annals of Internal Medicine* performed by the US Preventive Services Task Force.[1] It was prompted by our Cochrane and *Lancet* reviews from 2001 and found many of the same problems with the trials as we did. Curiously, however, it listed under harms only false positive tests, unnecessary anxiety, biopsies and cost.

It is pretty euphemistic to talk about unnecessary 'biopsies' when there is good evidence from the randomised trials that screening leads to an increase in both tumourectomies and mastectomies.[2] In their reply to this criticism, the authors argued that, 'because treatment options, radiation doses, and practice styles have changed substantially since the trials we examined were done, we did not see value in focusing on evidence of overtreatment and overdiagnosis.'[3] This argument is invalid. The authors could have focused on the number of diagnoses or the total number of operations, which have little to do with practice styles. Furthermore, if they truly believed in their argument, then the fact that treatment options, radiation doses and practice styles have changed substantially should also make it irrelevant to summarise the beneficial effect.

I think the real reason the authors did not look at the most important harm of screening was that it was politically unpalatable. The US reluctance to tell the population the truth about cancer screening was also apparent in a practice guideline published by the American College of Physicians in 2007.[4] The guideline claimed to 'present the available evidence and to increase the clinicians' understanding of the benefits and risks of screening mammography', and it cited our 2001 *Lancet* review, but not for its data on overdiagnosis. Instead, a completely flawed observational study from Florence by Duffy and Paci[5] was taken as evidence that screening *decreases* the risk for mastectomy. This study will be discussed in Chapter 16.

Nyström's updated Swedish meta-analysis

In March 2002, Nyström and colleagues[6] published an updated meta-analysis of the Swedish trials in the *Lancet*, which responded to some of the concerns we had raised.

Luc Bonneux noted that our distrust of the data from the Two-County trial had been confirmed and that Nyström hadn't documented the harms of screening we had previously shown.[7] This was an important observation. Systematic reviews that only look at the benefits are bound to be misleading, particularly when the intervention is cancer screening, which always does harm. Bonneux also mentioned that although Nyström had data on other cancer deaths, he didn't report on total cancer mortality. This omission gives pause for thought. One of our most important findings was that screening didn't reduce total cancer mortality (including breast cancer), and as this was expected, it raised doubt about whether screening is effective. Furthermore, Nyström and colleagues had published data on total cancer mortality earlier. In 1996, they reported a 2% increase in total cancer mortality,[8] which became a 2% decrease after they had adjusted their data for the age imbalances across the two randomised groups. However, as I have already noted, statistical adjustments often increase bias rather than reduce it.[9]

Nyström and colleagues did report data on total mortality, i.e. mortality from all causes, and they found a 2% reduction.[6] This was surprising, as they didn't find any reduction in total mortality in their 1993 meta-analysis.[10] They stated that, based on the reduction they found in breast cancer mortality, they would have expected a 2.3% reduction in total mortality. This was wrong. I showed – and published my detailed calculation – that they would have expected to see only a 0.9% reduction in total mortality.[11] Most amazingly, my correct estimate was improperly reversed in Nyström's reply: 'The expected effect on total mortality was 0.94% and not 2.3%, as Gøtzsche states.'[12]

As I am very careful when I do calculations, Nyström's error was very embarrassing. People who read his reply would get a mistaken impression that I had been inaccurate. While I was used to people lying about my research, Nyström's reply in the *Lancet* made me angry. Four days later, Nyström wrote to me and said he was really sorry, and that it was an editing error. He attached a Word document that contained his reply to the *Lancet*, and which was much longer than what was eventually published. This acknowledged that my calculation was correct:

> Regarding the total mortality Dr Gotzsche is correct. The reduction in the breast cancer mortality in the age group 60–69 years at randomisation according to the follow-up model is 27% according to Table 7 in our paper and not 17% as was given in the last paragraph of the discussion on page 918. Further, the expected effect on the total mortality is 0.94% and not 2.3% as was stated in the same paragraph.

I wrote to the handling editor at the *Lancet* the same day, inserted Nyström's original text into the email and noted that it seemed to me that the *Lancet*'s editing had gone astray. I also asked the *Lancet* to publish an erratum explaining this and copied Nyström on my email. As I didn't get a reply from the editor, I sent a reminder a month later. She said that she would publish an erratum and that she had replied to my message, but that it seemed I had not received it. This surprised me, as I had corresponded with this editor previously and had had no problems with missing email messages.

The text in the published erratum was:[13]

> In this Correspondence letter by Nyström and colleagues (July 27, p 339), paragraph nine should have read: 'For total mortality, <u>Gøtzsche is correct that the reduction in the breast-cancer mortality in patients aged 60–69 years at randomisation is 27%</u>, and the expected effect on the total mortality is <u>0.94%, not 2.3% as we stated</u>.'

Thus, although I had urged the journal to explicitly admit having made an error, this didn't happen. In fact, the text suggests that the error was made by Nyström and not by the *Lancet*.

I am still mystified by this. If Nyström didn't have any part in it, it means that a *Lancet* editor would rewrite this sentence to mean the opposite, that Nyström would overlook the error when he checked the edited version of his letter, and that *Lancet* would not acknowledge its error.

I had explained to the editor how important it was to get the number right. At first, she deleted my calculation – which takes up four lines – but I wrote back:

> The reason I would like to show the full calculation is that the authors made two mistakes: a spelling error and a calculation error. If I do not document this, the risk is that they, or other screening advocates, will simply conclude that my calculation was wrong, and not the authors'. Sadly, such false accusations have happened to me before when debating with screening enthusiasts, even in medical journals. I feel it is of pivotal importance to get the percentage right here: what reduction in total mortality corresponds to the alleged reduction in breast cancer mortality?

The editor reintroduced the calculation and faxed me the proofs for approval.

In a way, this incident illustrates beautifully how difficult it is to get the truth out about mammography screening. Even though I was careful, errors were made by others, and I ended up being ridiculed for errors I had not made. Very few people read errata, but very many read letters to the editor. And when there are many letters, as in this case, they may only bother to read the authors' reply.

There were several other problems with Nyström's meta-analysis,[11] but I shall mention only the most important ones. The reported estimate of a 2% reduction in mortality was driven by the Östergötland part of the Two-County trial that contributed half the deaths in the entire meta-analysis. Socio-economic factors are strong mortality predictors, and an imbalance in such factors between the screened group and the control group because of the poor randomisation method in this trial could easily explain a 2% reduction in total mortality, but such data remain unpublished.

There were other problems with numbers and they were serious. The number of randomised women was larger in 2002 than in the 1993 meta-analysis, although both meta-analyses were based on exact age at randomisation and the age range is the same. *This shouldn't be possible.* Further, thousands of women were included in the analysis although their age was below the defined age for inclusion, and groups differed substantially in size, although the randomisation method should have guaranteed groups of the same size. People experienced with randomised trials get highly sceptical when numbers of included participants vary so much from report to report and when women are included in the analyses in violation with the inclusion criteria for age. It is a sign of poor trial conduct and poor attention to detail.

Nyström and colleagues didn't respond to these important criticisms. About the possible differences in socio-economic factors in Östergötland, they explained that no pre-trial background data were collected in the Swedish trials.[12] This cannot be true, unless someone else is lying, as the randomisation in Östergötland was stratified for socio-economic factors.[14] Furthermore, if such data were subsequently lost, one could use the postal code as a proxy for socio-economic status.

Screening cannot benefit women who were diagnosed with breast cancer before randomisation and Nyström therefore excluded such women from the analyses, using the Swedish Cancer Registry to identify them regardless of whether they subsequently had been randomised to screening or to control groups. A researcher noted that this process could introduce bias if an invitation to attend screening enhanced the likelihood of a prior breast cancer being ascertained and registered. He referred to our findings that in the New York trial more women with previous breast cancer were excluded from the invited group than from the control group and asked if similar proportions of exclusions had occurred in the two trial arms in the Swedish trials.[15] Nyström and colleagues replied:[12]

> The main reason we did not present details of prerandomisation diagnosis of breast cancer is that the Swedish Cancer Registry is continuously updated and corrected. Therefore, results could vary from day to day. Inclusion of these numbers in each update could cause confusion.

Such a reply is absurdly evasive. Recruitment into the Swedish trials had ended by 1984 apart from the extension of the Malmö trial that lacked a formal protocol and which ended in 1990.[16] By 2002, 18 years later, revisions of registry data were very unlikely to be occurring 'day to day'.

References

1 Humphrey LL, Helfand M, Chan BK, *et al*. Breast cancer screening: a summary of the evidence for the U.S. Preventive Services Task Force. *Ann Intern Med*. 2002; **137**(5 Pt. 1): 347–60.

2 Gøtzsche PC. Screening for breast cancer. *Ann Intern Med*. 2003; **138**(9): 769–70.

3 Humphrey LL, Helfand M, Chan BKS. Screening for breast cancer. *Ann Intern Med*. 2003; **138**: 770.

4 Qaseem A, Snow V, Sherif K, *et al*. Screening mammography for women 40 to 49 years of age: a clinical practice guideline from the American College of Physicians. *Ann Intern Med*. 2007; **146**(7): 511–15.

5 Paci E, Duffy SW, Giorgi D, *et al*. Are breast cancer screening programmes increasing rates of mastectomy? Observational study. *BMJ*. 2002; **325**(7361): 418.

6 Nyström L, Andersson I, Bjurstam N, *et al*. Long-term effects of mammography screening: updated overview of the Swedish randomised trials. *Lancet*. 2002; **359**(9310): 909–19.
7 Bonneux L. Update on effects of screening mammography. *Lancet*. 2002; **360**(9329): 337–8.
8 Nyström L, Larsson LG, Wall S, *et al*. An overview of the Swedish randomised mammography trials: total mortality pattern and the representivity of the study cohorts. *J Med Screen*. 1996; **3**(2): 85–7.
9 Deeks JJ, Dinnes J, D'Amico R, *et al*. Evaluating non-randomised intervention studies. *Health Technol Assess*. 2003; **7**(27): 1–173.
10 Nyström L, Rutqvist LE, Wall S, *et al*. Breast cancer screening with mammography: overview of Swedish randomised trials. *Lancet*. 1993; **341**(8851): 973–8.
11 Gøtzsche PC. Update on effects of screening mammography. *Lancet*. 2002; **360**(9329): 338–9.
12 Nyström L, Andersson I, Bjurstam N, *et al*. Update on effects of screening mammography. *Lancet*. 2002; **360**(9329): 339–40.
13 Department of error. Update on effects of screening mammography. *Lancet*. 2002; **360**(9340): 1178.
14 Tabár L, Fagerberg CJG, South MC, *et al*. The Swedish Two-County trial of mammographic screening for breast cancer: recent results on mortality and tumour characteristics. In: Miller AB, Chamberlain J, Day NE, *et al*., editors. *Cancer Screening*. Cambridge: Cambridge University Press; 1991. pp. 23–36.
15 Cheng KK. Update on effects of screening mammography. *Lancet*. 2002; **360**(9329): 339.
16 Gøtzsche PC, Nielsen M. Screening for breast cancer with mammography. *Cochrane Database Syst Rev*. 2009; (4): CD001877.

11

Scientific debates in the United States

Everyone is entitled to his own opinion, but not his own facts.
Daniel Moynihan (1927–2003)[1]

Peter Dean is wrong again

The scientific debates had so far mostly taken place in European medical journals. In January 2004, a new US journal, *Journal of the American College of Radiology*, saw the light of day. Its editor seemed determined to have a spectacular launch. The front page of its first issue featured 'Turf wars in radiology', and its maiden article was written by Peter Dean, who fired heavy artillery with the title 'Gøtzsche's quixotic antiscreening campaign: nonscientific and contrary to Cochrane principles'.[2] Perhaps I should have dropped dead or at least surrendered, but I replied with a more academic title: 'The debate on breast cancer screening with mammography is important'.[3]

Personal attacks in the titles of scientific papers are extremely rare. Dean made four mistakes in his short title, but he did get my name right. I have never campaigned against screening but I have published research supporting my argument that women need full information to enable them to decide for themselves. And as my research accords with Cochrane principles and has influenced people's thinking about screening, it is not a quixotic enterprise.

Dean based his article on a lecture I gave in Helsinki a year earlier at a seminar in relation to the 10th anniversary of The Cochrane Collaboration. In it, I addressed many other issues than screening, and only four of my 28 slides were about mammography screening. Furthermore, very few of the 90 participants had any particular interest in mammography screening. Nevertheless, Dean dominated the entire discussion after the lectures, focusing it on mammography screening. He also used the occasion to attack me personally. His attack was so embarrassing that several of the participants told me afterwards that it was deeply shocking to witness.

Immediately after the seminar, Dean sent a long manuscript of 4286 words (including 32 references) to all the participants. Similar to but even worse than the paper he published a year later in the *Journal of the American College of Radiology*, it was so malicious that those who had convened the seminar felt obliged to send an email to the participants explaining that:

> the medical tradition is to present arguments openly, supported by references to published evidence, so that all can follow the discussion . . . However, we feel that Professor Dean has crossed the limits of good conduct by writing, for example, on p. 5 of his attachment: 'At that meeting he (P. Gotzsche) had no arguments to prove his accusations that many prominent Swedish physicians were criminals.' We are sorry he has sent this material in connection to our seminar and wish to point out we have had no role in his decision to do so.

Dean's fantasy about 'criminals' was unrelated to the truth. In his published article, he likewise fantasised that I had made 'multiple factual, procedural, and scientific errors' that I had not mentioned in my talk.

As is so typical of screening advocates, Dean didn't specify what he meant by his allegations. I could therefore not refute them, but I countered Dean's various arguments, statements and quotations, many of which were plainly wrong, one by one.[3] Dean's accusations were very similar to those offered by other screening advocates, and as I have dealt with them elsewhere in this book, I shall not repeat my rebuttals, but only list briefly Dean's accusations.

Dean dismissed bias in relation to determination of cause of death in the trials, arguing that we used 'homemade' criteria for judging the reliability of the trials that are not used by other investigators (although the whole Cochrane Collaboration uses them). He claimed that I had no biological explanation for my arguments (which would have been unimportant if true, but in fact I have – *see* Chapter 24).

Dean also said I ignored or didn't understand a letter from a trialist. The only letter I have received fitting Dean's description was sent by Tabár in June 1999, but it was useless, as Tabár didn't answer our questions. It is unclear to this day how the clusters were randomised in the Kopparberg part of the Two-County study. Tabár noted in his letter that his research group had published all the details regarding the comparability of the group invited to screening and the control group, with special emphasis on age and socio-economic status (which Nyström claims doesn't exist; it's really curious),[4] and gave a number of references we were recommended to read.

However, we already knew there was a difference in age, and none of the references contained any data on comparability of socio-economic status or other factors of major prognostic importance. We asked again about the missing data on socio-economic status and were told that they were in an enclosed reprint, but this paper didn't contain the data either.[5]

Dean also claimed that screening reduces total mortality with reference to one of Tabár's flawed studies[6] that I shall discuss in Chapter 14.

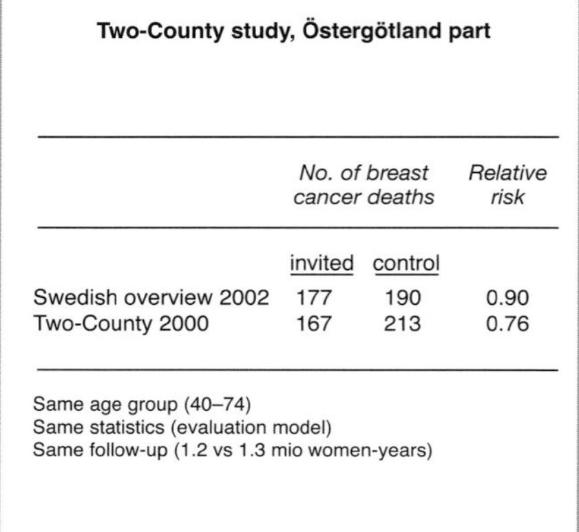

Two-County study, Östergötland part

	No. of breast cancer deaths		*Relative risk*
	invited	control	
Swedish overview 2002	177	190	0.90
Two-County 2000	167	213	0.76

Same age group (40–74)
Same statistics (evaluation model)
Same follow-up (1.2 vs 1.3 mio women-years)

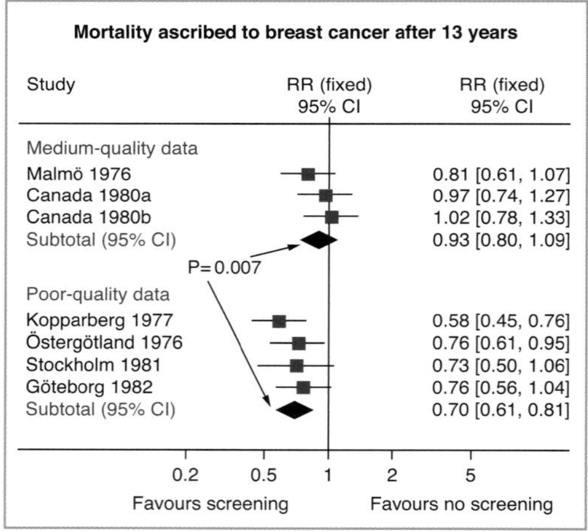

Information on breast screening

The most balanced and comprehensive information on breast cancer screening comes from consumer websites

Websites from cancer charities and governmental agencies are persuasive, not informative

The screening lottery

For every 1000 women screened for 10 years:

1 breast cancer death is avoided (or the woman dies from something else)

5 extra cancer diagnoses

3 extra tumorectomies

2 extra mastectomies

>100 will experience important psychological distress for many months because of false positive findings

FIGURES 11.1–11.4: The four slides presented at a seminar in Helsinki in 2003 celebrating the 10th anniversary of The Cochrane Collaboration

Dean ended by saying that I had harmed The Cochrane Collaboration, which had been powerless to censure my actions. That is quite some comment. True science and censorship cannot coexist. And I believe we had a moral obligation to publish the harms of screening elsewhere when the Cochrane Breast Cancer Group denied us this. I also firmly believe that the outcome for The Cochrane Collaboration was beneficial.

The four slides I presented in Helsinki that triggered Dean's wrath were straightforward and in accordance with the evidence (*see* Figures 11.1–11.4).

Dean criticised the third slide – about more balanced and comprehensive information coming from consumer websites than from cancer charities and governmental agencies – with the argument that I had not referred to a comprehensive analysis of the various organisations. Dean then wrote in his paper that he had previously done his own search of the organisations,[2] but didn't explain how or give a reference to his 'study'. Dean has published very few articles in his career and none of them describes such a study. Yet again, the rules imposed on me by Dean and other screening advocates apparently don't apply to themselves. The irony was intense, as we had in fact done a systematic search of websites, and my coworker, Karsten Juhl Jørgensen, had written a report about our results and had defended it at his exam as a medical student, well in advance of the Helsinki meeting. We published our findings in the *BMJ* in January 2004.[7]

The editor of the *Journal of the American College of Radiology* might have set a record when he accepted my reply to Dean. Fifty-five minutes after I submitted it, I received an email with his minor, very sensible changes and approval.

In February 2003, Mogens Blichert-Toft from the Danish Breast Cancer Group (DBCG) sent a draft version of Dean's quixotic paper to a person who happened to be a senior member of my staff, which he probably didn't know. Blichert-Toft wrote that he should know what thoughts clinicians had about the issues. The draft started by mentioning the 'Peter principle', whereby people are promoted until they reach a position for which they are no longer competent. Obviously, Peter Dean was not thinking of himself, but of me, as Dean asserted, 'Rather than refer to published evidence (from all other workers), he used insinuation, hearsay, and a selective and deliberate misuse of the literature to further his arguments.'

Opinions were divided about the quality of our work. Four months later, I received a letter from the professor of radiology at my own hospital who thanked me for the great work we had done with the Cochrane review and our persistent and always sober way of debating.

Multiple errors in the *International Journal of Epidemiology*

At the same time as my dispute with Dean, a more reasoned debate was started by David Freedman, Diana Petitti and James Robins from the United States in the *International Journal of Epidemiology* in February 2004.[8] They published what they called a qualitative review, which took up 13 pages and had 111 references, and the whole debate, including the contributions of other researchers, ran to 34 pages. As it is difficult to get papers accepted in this journal, the sheer volume suggests that the editors felt the debate was important.

I agree. Good debates move science forwards and I publish many letters. Recently, I even published a study of letters to the editor showing that authors are reluctant to respond to criticisms of their work. This finding made us suggest that journal editors should ensure that authors take relevant criticism seriously and respond adequately to it.[9]

Therefore, I was very positive when I read the paper, but I soon became disappointed. With all its references, I had expected to find new angles on screening I could possibly use when updating the Cochrane review, but the arguments were generally poorly founded and contained many errors and misleading quotations. Freedman and colleagues concluded that our critique of the trials had little merit and that the prior consensus on mammography was correct.[8] They also argued that there was no reason to believe that the Canadian trials were of better quality than the New York trial or the Two-County trial. Few neutral observers would agree to that and even the Cochrane editors had accepted our judgements about the trials.

The title of their paper was 'On the efficacy of screening for breast cancer', as if the benefit was the only thing that mattered. Therefore, I used 'On the benefits and harms of screening for breast cancer' as the title for my response to their article.[10]

The authors didn't discuss the harms of screening. *Not a single word.* They even claimed in their abstract that early detection leads to *less* invasive therapy. They also said in the abstract that our method was to simply discard positive studies as being of poor quality. This echoed Daniel Kopans, who argues in exactly the same way, but we did the opposite. We based our quality assessment on Cochrane criteria,[11] and when we had done that, we found that the effect of screening was much smaller in the better studies than in the poorer studies.

Although Freedman is a statistician, the authors presented an invalid analysis of the data from the New York trial. They used data after 5 years, when there were 39 breast cancer deaths in the study group and 63 in the control group, i.e. a

38% reduction in breast cancer mortality (39/63 = 0.62). Of the 39 deaths in the study group, 16 were among those who were offered screening but declined. They argued that the control group also included 16 women who would have refused screening if they had been invited and who died from breast cancer and therefore subtracted 16 deaths from both groups. With this manoeuvre, they arrived at a 51% reduction in breast cancer mortality (since (39 – 16)/(63 – 16) = 0.49).

They considered their method unbiased, but this is wrong. When the relative risk is not exactly one (i.e. no effect of screening), exclusion of the same number of deaths from both groups leads to biased estimates. If we accept their line of reasoning, we might argue that some of those who died in the screened group couldn't possibly have benefited from screening, as their cancer had already metastasised when it was detected. One might also argue that some only attended by the end of the trial period and therefore couldn't possibly have benefited from screening. We could therefore subtract more deaths than 16 from both groups, and the more deaths we subtract, the bigger the apparent effect of screening. If we subtract 30 deaths, the effect will be 73%, and if we subtract 39 deaths, the effect will be a 100% reduction in breast cancer mortality.

Another analysis was similarly ludicrous. The long-term results from the Canadian trial of women aged 40–49 years showed a 3% reduction in breast cancer mortality,[12] but Freedman and colleagues suggested that the effect would be about 20% if they excluded some advanced cases from the screened group.[8] It is a gross violation of the principles for randomised trials to exclude deaths from one of the groups, and by doing this, the authors demonstrated that my line of reasoning is justified, as they might arrive at almost any result they want by excluding deaths. This absurdity is the most shocking part of their paper.

As 'justification' for the one-sided exclusion of deaths, the authors cited a paper by Anthony Miller, but they ignored Miller's explanation *in the same paper* that the fact that there were more small node-positive cancers in the screened group than in the control group cannot be used to judge the reliability of the randomisation process, as this difference was a result of the screening process. I noted in my reply to Freedman that a similar, spurious 'imbalance' had occurred in the New York trial, where 57% of cancers in the screened group versus 46% in the control group had positive nodes *despite* the fact that many more women with breast cancer were excluded from the study group than from the control group.[10] I also stated that a pathological review found that only 15% of the cancers in the study group were detected solely by mammography and that mammography didn't identify a single cancer smaller than 1 cm. Furthermore, screening had advanced the time of diagnosis by only 3–4 months. These facts don't agree at all with the large reported reduction in breast cancer mortality, 35% after 7 years, but Freedman and colleagues failed to draw the logical consequence of their observations – that it is highly unlikely that the New York trial found a true effect of screening.

They were likely correct on a minor point. We had found several baseline differences between the screened group and the control group, but the papers were very confusing. In one, the text describes all randomised women and refers to a table with percentages and a footnote saying that some of the data are based on 10% and 20% samples. We took account of these reduced sample sizes. However, the table header speaks of women entering the study in a single year, and not of all women as the text does. If the table header is correct, the data presented are subgroups of a subgroup, in which case the resulting samples are too small to study possible baseline differences. This point was immaterial for our Cochrane review, as we excluded the New York trial for other reasons.

Freedman and colleagues also failed when they compared total mortality *among breast cancer* cases in the study group and the control group in the New York trial and considered their comparison fair since numbers of cancers in the two groups were similar. They didn't realise that screening cannot work if it doesn't detect more cancers.[8]

Throughout their paper, the authors quoted the research literature selectively, e.g. when they tried to persuade readers that the discrepancies in numbers in the Swedish trials can be explained. They seemed to have needed considerable help from the investigators to understand the Two-County trial, as they thanked Tabár and Duffy for their patience in answering questions, but the help was not sufficient, as the discrepancies cannot be explained.[10,12,13]

My paper was the middle of a sandwich, with Freedman and colleagues on both sides. In their rejoinder in the same issue,[14] they repeated many of their errors and misleading quotations, and introduced new ones. Therefore, I alerted the readers to these problems in a letter some time later,[15] which Freedman and colleagues also responded to.[16]

I am grateful that Freedman and colleagues – in contrast to most other screening advocates – provided so much detail, as it enabled me to show where they made gross errors, ignored or downplayed evidence that went against their beliefs, or made false statements. They didn't think it was a problem, for example, that the reduction in breast cancer mortality in Östergötland was 24% with one method and 10% with a more reliable method. I shall return to this large discrepancy in Chapter 13.

In their rejoinder, they said I had withdrawn a previous 'near-retraction', but there is no 'near-retraction' in the reference they quoted, where I merely restated my concern that retrospective exclusion of women after 18 years of follow-up in the New York trial may not be reliable.

Cornelia Baines highlighted other grave errors.[17] The radiologists in the Canadian trials had agreed 'only 30–50% of the time' about whether a woman had cancer or not, but Freedman and colleagues didn't reveal that the numbers were kappa statistics,[8] which means that the agreement was much higher. Furthermore, they quoted Baines for something she hadn't written and used it against her, a typical case of the 'if you can't beat them, lie about them' trick.

Shamelessly, in their reply to Baines, they violated the truth once again, saying that she seemed to deny that kappa is a measure of agreement.[16] They were also dishonest when they said that I had repeated 'statistical errors' in my letter. There are no statistical calculations in my letter. Furthermore, the calculations I presented in my paper are correct, and Freedman and colleagues have not shown otherwise.

In our Cochrane review, we stated in the conflicts of interest section that 'we had no a priori opinion on the effect of screening for breast cancer when we were asked in 1999 by the Danish HTA agency, the National Board of Health, to review the randomised trials.' Freedman and colleagues said that our declaration was not supported by the record[13] and quoted a letter in the *Lancet* from 1997, where I discussed two colon cancer screening trials that had just been published:[18]

> The studies also raise a pertinent ethical issue: do we wish to turn the world's healthy citizens into fearful patients-to-be who, in the not too distant future, might be asked to deliver, for example, annual samples of faeces, urine, sputum, vaginal smear, and blood, and undergo X-ray and ultrasound examination with all it entails in terms of psychological morbidity and the potential for harm because of further testing and interventions due to false positive findings?

Peter Dean also cited this *Lancet* letter when he claimed in his quixotic paper that I had a bias against population screening.[2] However, there is genuine reason to worry about the consequences of screening the healthy population for several cancers simultaneously. The harms will increase substantially, compared with screening for only one cancer, whereas the added benefit in terms of living longer could be small or even non-existent. Such a concern cannot be equated with being biased or having a conflict of interest in relation to screening. Furthermore, it is false logic to infer that a concern I raised about multiple cancer screening is incompatible with the fact that we didn't know – and therefore didn't have an opinion about – the effect of breast screening.

The *Lancet* quotation about colorectal cancer screening as Dean used it was also out of context. I suggested that a large, long-term randomised trial in which the experimental group is screened for a number of diseases and the control group for none would be highly relevant. Such a trial is now ongoing – namely, the Prostate, Lung, Colorectal, and Ovarian (PLCO) Cancer Screening Trial – and I welcome it, as it will make us all wiser.

If readers are to be enlightened by an academic debate, it requires that both sides are honest. I believe Freedman and colleagues failed badly in this respect, and they ended their paper by saying that our critique 'is careless at best' and that 'it is time to move on'.[8] Such statements are typical for screening advocates trying to stop intelligent debate.

As always, Dean saw it differently. Freedman and colleagues had posted a report on a website in California a year earlier that was similar to their published paper, and Dean sent a mass email to the participants at the seminar in Helsinki, which he copied to the chair of the steering group of The Cochrane Collaboration. This was an obvious attempt at discrediting me. Dean wrote:

> David Freedman, the senior author, has also written the textbook 'Statistics,' which has been the most popular basic textbook on the subject for the past two decades. The three authors represent the fields of Biostatistics, Public Health, and Epidemiology and have impressive academic credentials, particularly their published output in peer-reviewed journals. The academic credentials of Olsen and Gøtzsche pale by comparison.

Pale by comparison? I have published more than 50 papers in the 'big five', which are the *Lancet*, *BMJ*, *JAMA*, *New England Journal of Medicine* and *Annals of Internal Medicine*. But that isn't the issue. What is important is that Freedman, Petitti and Robins made so many inexcusable errors despite their credentials. I haven't written a textbook on statistics, but I don't make elementary statistical errors.

References

1 Wikiquote. *Daniel Patrick Moynihan*. http://en.wikiquote.org/wiki/Daniel_Patrick_Moynihan (accessed 22 February 2010).
2 Dean PB. Gøtzsche's quixotic antiscreening campaign: nonscientific and contrary to Cochrane principles. *J Am Coll Radiol*. 2004; **1**(1): 3–7.
3 Gøtzsche PC. The debate on breast cancer screening with mammography is important. *J Am Coll Radiol*. 2004; **1**(1): 8–14.
4 Nyström L, Andersson I, Bjurstam N, *et al*. Update on effects of screening mammography. *Lancet*. 2002; **360**(9329): 339–40.
5 Tabár L, Fagerberg G, Duffy SW, *et al*. Update of the Swedish two-county program

of mammographic screening for breast cancer. *Radiol Clin North Am.* 1992; **30**(1): 187–210.
6 Tabár L, Duffy SW, Yen MF, *et al.* All-cause mortality among breast cancer patients in a screening trial: support for breast cancer mortality as an end point. *J Med Screen.* 2002; **9**(4): 159–62.
7 Jørgensen KJ, Gøtzsche PC. Presentation on websites of possible benefits and harms from screening for breast cancer: cross sectional study. *BMJ.* 2004; **328**(7432): 148–51.
8 Freedman DA, Petitti DM, Robins JM. On the efficacy of screening for breast cancer. *Int J Epidemiol.* 2004; **33**(1): 43–55.
9 Gøtzsche PC. On the benefits and harms of screening for breast cancer. *Int J Epidemiol.* 2004; **33**(1): 56–64.
10 Higgins JPT, Green S, editors. *Cochrane Handbook for Systematic Reviews of Interventions: Version 5.0.1 [updated September 2008]*. The Cochrane Collaboration, 2008. Available at: www.cochrane-handbook.org (accessed 22 May 2011).
11 Gøtzsche PC, Nielsen M. Screening for breast cancer with mammography. *Cochrane Database Syst Rev.* 2009; (4): CD001877.
12 Gøtzsche PC. Update on effects of screening mammography. *Lancet.* 2002; **360**(9329): 338–9.
13 Freedman DA, Petitti DM, Robins JM. Rejoinder. *Int J Epidemiol.* 2004; **33**(1): 69–73.
14 Gøtzsche PC. Misleading quotations and other errors persist in rejoinder on breast cancer screening. *Int J Epidemiol.* 2004; **33**(6): 1404.
15 Freedman DA, Petitti DM, Robins JM. Authors' response. *Int J Epidemiol.* 2004; **33**(6): 1405–6.
16 Gøtzsche PC, Delamothe T, Godlee F, *et al.* Adequacy of authors' replies to criticism raised in electronic letters to the editor: cohort study. *BMJ.* 2010; **341**: c3926.
17 Baines CJ. In search of the best available version of the truth. *Int J Epidemiol.* 2004; **33**(6): 1404–5.
18 Gøtzsche PC. Screening for colorectal cancer. *Lancet.* 1997; **349**(9048): 356.

12

Publication of entire Cochrane review obstructed for 5 years

AS ALREADY NOTED, OLE OLSEN AND I WERE NOT ALLOWED TO publish the major harms of screening in our 2001 Cochrane review[1] and therefore we published them in the *Lancet* instead.[2,3] It would take another 5 years before the harms came out also in *The Cochrane Library*, and we didn't get there easily. In fact, the series of events I shall describe here are highly unusual for an academic journal and not something I would wish others to go through.

Our disputes with the Cochrane Breast Cancer Group were discussed in correspondence in the *Lancet* in early 2002,[4] but the editor-in-chief, Richard Horton, alerted readers that much bigger issues were at stake:[4]

> Some senior scientists have said to me that this debate should not be taking place in public. Screening mammography is, they argue, too important for women's health to have its image damaged by questioning the technique's efficacy and safety. Such paternalism assumes that women cannot decide for themselves whether the available evidence supports or refutes the case for mammography. Discouraging a discussion with women about the evidence for and against mammography is more harmful for women's health, not less, if doctors truly believe that patients should be active partners in making decisions about their care.

Horton also noted:

> When Cochrane reviewers [us] produce a review at odds with the opinions

> of Cochrane editors, the normal process of peer review and negotiation will resolve many of the differences. But if a difference remains, let the scientists doing the review publish what they wish to say – it is, after all, their work. The editors can present their own view as a supplementary discussion or comment. That way, the debate proceeds properly, each side is given its voice, accusations of censorship are avoided, and the public sees science as a truly collaborative process, in which differences of opinion are not only respected, but also welcomed.

In his letter in the *Lancet*, the chair of The Cochrane Collaboration Steering Group, Peter Langhorne, alluded to the uniqueness of the Cochrane process when he remarked:

> First, Cochrane editorial groups are committed to try to publish reviews – rejection is very much a last resort. Second, because limited resources must be used responsibly there should only be one Cochrane review addressing a particular question. It therefore needs to be comprehensive and balanced.

I addressed the limitation of this arrangement:

> Should a Cochrane researcher become dissatisfied with the Cochrane editorial group he cannot choose another Cochrane journal for publication to obtain the Cochrane stamp of approval – a quality stamp that, in the case of mammography screening, seems to have been important given that the Cochrane review was eagerly awaited by many policy-makers.

The monopoly situation creates a potential for editorial abuse, and we felt the editors had clearly overstepped their limits. We were willing to negotiate how the harms should be presented and discussed but not to have them deleted.

Langhorne arranged a telephone conference to resolve our dispute with the Breast Cancer Group. He was keen to avoid further damage to the collaboration and therefore asked me to disclose our reply to a letter the Cochrane editors had submitted to the *Lancet* about the dispute. I replied that suppression of academic freedom could be far more damaging to the collaboration and noted that I had already received the Cochrane editors' letter from the *Lancet* and had responded to it. Furthermore, I felt it would be inappropriate for me to circulate my reply to the conference attendees, as Langhorne requested.

When Langhorne insisted, I noted that Horton had made it very clear that in his view, the collaboration 'should not, repeat not' ask me to disclose the contents of my letter. With Horton's permission, I also forwarded his comments to me about this:

> It smacks of censorship and I know of no example where one protagonist has had the right to review the comments of another protagonist pre-publication. That is my public view and I would be happy for you to restate it in full – ie, with the reason behind it rather than just the advice to keep your letter confidential. The way forward, and again I have said this to all parties, is to convene a discussion between you and John Simes. That way, any factual misunderstandings can be ironed out. It is then up to John to revise his letter, and only then for you to amend yours in the light of his changes.

John Simes accepted this.

At my request, Drummond Rennie participated at the meeting in his capacity as an editor of a major medical journal, *JAMA*. Rennie pointed out that majority voting in an editorial group, such as that which had occurred with our review, was not a good way to solve disputes between authors and editors, or between the editors themselves. He agreed with Horton about giving freedom to authors when disputes cannot be resolved, and to let the dissenters have their saying in an accompanying editorial.

Cochrane editors stonewall our Cochrane review

Although the teleconference went well, the process of updating our review was subsequently obstructed by the Australian-based Cochrane Breast Cancer Group. I continued my enquiries about when I would get the Cochrane editors' comments, but to no avail. I gave up after 11 months and contacted Langhorne, who asked the group for a response. Still no reply, even though it was The Collaboration's chair who had asked.

In March 2003, 1½ years after the publication of our curtailed Cochrane review, we had still not heard anything from the Cochrane editors. Therefore, we submitted a revision of our review, which was now out of date, as additional, important data had been published in the Swedish 2002 meta-analysis (*see* Chapter 10). We had reinserted the data on treatments, had expanded our explanations why these data were reliable and had made some compromises in an attempt to accommodate the editors.

The silence continued. In June, I informed the Cochrane editors that it had written about itself that, 'Reviews will not be published in parts (eg reporting on some outcomes in one issue, and other outcomes in the next).' I reminded the editors that it was now almost 2 years since we published our curtailed review. Again I asked when I could expect a response. And asked once more. Dead silence.

In September 2003, I told Langhorne that there were now epidemiological data from the United States and the United Kingdom that clearly confirmed the results the Breast Cancer Group had not allowed us to publish in 2001 – namely, that screening causes about 30% overdiagnosis and overtreatment. I added that the pro-screening lobby had consistently tried to suppress and even ridicule this important information. I also warned that the longer it took, the more the suspicion of censorship would grow, as we had received reports of such worries from many people already in 2001, both in and outside the collaboration.

It was like ringing a bell. I received an email from two of the group's editors, Simes and Wilcken, the next day. But their reply didn't follow standard editorial practice. It mentioned two peer reviews, but they were not enclosed, only a summary of them. Therefore, we couldn't reply to them, and we couldn't tell if they were written recently or some time ago.

We were now convinced that the group was doing what it could to get rid of us. We were told that the two anonymous peer reviewers both strongly recommended against publication and furthermore that our review was not acceptable for publication and that further revision of the review was unlikely to resolve the issues. That was a smart move, leading to a catch-22 situation. By denying us the possibility of updating the review, the group could withdraw our published review at a later stage with the argument that it was outdated. That would be easy to do, as *The Cochrane Library* is an electronic publication that gets regularly updated.

Complete denial of the most important harm of screening continued. The editors talked about 'unsubstantiated claims of harm' and remarked that in the longer run the number of surgical procedures would tend to become the same in the control groups as in the screened groups, which was not only wishful thinking, but plainly wrong.

I informed Langhorne about the permanent roadblock the same day, and he offered to contact the collaboration's newly appointed publication arbiter, David Henderson-Smart, who had a specific remit to address disagreements between authors and editors.

I also asked Drummond Rennie for advice. He replied that the Breast Cancer Group had taken an unbelievable time over all this and furthermore noted that The Cochrane Collaboration is committed to having only one version of a review, which is tantamount to saying that in an area of debatable science there is only one correct answer and one correct version, which is completely anti-science. He suggested that, in exceptional circumstances, there could be two versions of a

Cochrane review, e.g. that of the authors and that of the editors, with an accompanying explanation that it was not possible to agree on the final version. That would be in the fine tradition of science, which acknowledges that information is often hard to interpret, and 'unless Cochrane makes it as a scientific enterprise, it cannot and should not survive'.

Langhorne and I agreed with Rennie. Langhorne added that, in his capacity as editor of the Cochrane Stroke Group, he increasingly found himself disagreeing with the way some reviews had been analysed, but as no one could say which was the more correct approach, the solution was to publish both sets of analyses.

My co-author, Ole Olsen, and I had undertaken a huge piece of work together and had had our happy moments when we found the proof of a suspicion we had shared for a long time. Systematic reviewing has similarities to detective work and faces similar difficulties. It is difficult to detect what is *not* there, when it has been carefully removed from the scene of the crime. This requires experience, and one of the peer reviewers on our Cochrane review actually remarked that, with all its details, it looked like a court case.

But what we had gone through was also very stressful, and Olsen had left our centre, informing the Breast Cancer Group that he didn't want to contribute to the review any longer. The group asked me to find another co-author, as it was its policy to have at least two authors on reviews, which is reasonable, as two detectives see more than one. I promised to do so and asked the group to send their comments on treatments in the meantime but was told I wouldn't get them before I had found an additional author. I informed the group that Donald Berry was the new co-author. However, he pulled out when he realised that the amount of work involved was too much for his busy schedule. The Breast Cancer Group raised concerns about Berry's withdrawal as co-author, and Rennie felt this was a particularly specious reason to turn our review down. I published the updated Cochrane review in 2006 with Margrethe Nielsen from the Danish Consumer Council, who later became a PhD student with me on a different subject, psychotropic drugs.

The letter of rejection from the Breast Cancer Group from September 2003 noted that international working parties had reassessed the evidence and had concluded that screening was of value. I remarked that this was a judgemental and not a scientific statement, and that Cochrane reviews are about presenting the scientific evidence on benefits and harms and letting the readers make up their own minds. They are not policy documents. Therefore, I suggested – to ensure a fair process that distinguished appropriately between science and politics – that we should invite experienced editors from highly respected general medical journals to handle our review.

I met with Langhorne and Henderson-Smart a month later and we agreed that I should ignore the rejection from the editors and submit a revision, with a reply to the comments. We did this in November 2003, with the hope that it could be published in April 2004 (*The Cochrane Library* came out quarterly at that time). However, it took another 3 years.

In January 2004, we submitted yet another version, as advised by the publication arbiter who had also asked the group to find additional peer reviewers. Nothing happened. Four months later, I noted that I believed the group had a serious conflict of interest and that I couldn't understand it could be so difficult, as I could easily suggest dozens of skilled people, both pro- and con- screening, who would agree to peer-review our work within a couple of weeks.

I asked about the peer reviews several times and for a deadline, but after 10 months, no reviews and no deadline. The group's arrogance was unbelievable.

A second publication arbiter, Kay Dickersin, director of the US Cochrane Center, became involved. In December 2004, we discussed breaking the deadlock by moving forwards without waiting for the missing peer reviews. Only a week later, a letter arrived from Wilcken that included three peer reviews. I wondered whether this was merely a coincidence but, again, they were undated, just as those we had received a year earlier. But there was a big difference. The new peer reviews were excellent and remarkably consistent, and it seemed to us that the reviewers' interest this time was to get as close to the truth as possible, rather than to protect screening.

That was certainly a new development. As we agreed with almost all the comments, it would be very easy for us to respond. *But we didn't get the opportunity!* Our update was flatly rejected: 'It is with regret that we inform you that on the basis of this feedback, the CBCG [Cochrane Breast Cancer Group] is unable to accept the review update.'

This appeared to be, in my view, an abuse of a monopoly situation. The rejection at this stage, with no possibility of appeal, was not only entirely inappropriate; it also went against Cochrane principles. What is more, one of the reviewers noted:

> The novel contribution of this review is the information reported on the relative increase in mastectomies and radiation among screened women irrespective of the quality score for a trial. This is important information to be communicated to women who are considering undergoing screening mammography.

The second reviewer stated: 'Overall this is a carefully done review', and the third suggested various changes we could easily make. *Thus, there wasn't the slightest objective reason for rejection.*

I was reminded of Kafka again and I appealed to Dickersin. In my appeal, I mentioned another reply on a related issue we had received from the group just 2 days earlier. Karsten Juhl Jørgensen and I had submitted a protocol to the group for a systematic review on the harms of radiotherapy for breast cancer, as these were very poorly elucidated in randomised trials and were virtually absent in systematic reviews. Interestingly, our proposed review was rejected with the argument that it would not 'offer patients and practitioners an opportunity to balance evidence of harms and benefits within the same review'. What can one say? The same editors had made sure that our published Cochrane review on breast screening *did not allow such a balance*. It seems that the group's rules changed ad hoc, depending on the circumstances; therefore, we abandoned that review.

Stalemate, it seemed. But the publication arbiters now decided to discuss the issues not only with the chairman but also with the whole democratically elected Cochrane Collaboration Steering Group. Five months later, we were asked to reply to the comments and to submit a new version. Most important, the steering group had decided that all benefits and harms should be examined in the review and also that the Breast Cancer Group needed to provide us with an itemised list of what needed to be addressed for the review to be publishable, incorporating the points raised by the peer reviewers and the editorial team.

It was the first time in 3½ years that we received specific suggestions for escaping from the Kafkaesque process. Kay Dickersin offered her assistance with the language, which was very helpful. She had extensive experience with breast cancer and with consumer issues through her active involvement with the US National Breast Cancer Coalition. This evidence-based group consists primarily of women who have been treated for breast cancer, and it has been described as being perhaps the world's most influential medical consumer lobby group.[5]

Three days before we submitted the revised review on 27 November 2005, the Cochrane Breast Cancer Group informed me that our review would be peer-reviewed again. I wrote back that I had understood that it was now up to the editors to look at the paper. Wilcken replied that he would send our paper on 'to reviewers', not to *the* reviewers. That was not a clear reply, and I remained nervous. I enquired again and was then told that it would be sent to the previous reviewers, not new ones (which would have been the fifth time our Cochrane review was getting peer-reviewed).

Again, the delay was grotesque, and repeated requests, both from me and from Dickersin, to get a reply from the group led nowhere. We were told that not all of the three peer reviewers had responded, and I requested a deadline for this but I didn't get one. It took another 7 months before we finally got the message that our updated review was accepted for publication. The updated review was published in October 2006 and was very well received. This was 6 years after we first submitted it. That could be a record for editorial delay, as our revisions took up very little of these 6 years. It is also revealing to compare this with the process at the *Lancet*. We submitted our full review on 10 September 2001 and it was published 40 days later.

On 13 March 2009, we submitted the second update of the Cochrane review, which included a new trial, the UK Age trial in women about 40 years of age. This time, our contacts with the group were fine and uneventful, and the update was accepted without peer review and published in October 2009.[6]

Lessons for the future

At one time, when I was particularly frustrated, one of the two publication arbiters, Henderson-Smart, replied that it would be better to be a tortoise than a hare in this matter. He alluded to Aesop's fable again when he later wrote, 'Slow and steady – sticking to the course (scientific principles) – wins the race.' He was right. The Cochrane review is the most comprehensive scientific evidence there is about mammography screening in one place, and it has benefited from the fact that so many people became involved with it.

What I have described is the most high-profile conflict in The Cochrane Collaboration's history. It concerned one of the most controversial and hugely expensive interventions that have ever been introduced in healthcare. The NHS in the United Kingdom has never invested more in implementing a new type of clinical practice.[7]

The conflict can be analysed from different angles. The overriding perspective for us was ethics. Women should not be denied information about the most important harm of screening. This harm was a well-guarded secret before we stepped into the scene and published our findings in 2000 in the *Lancet*.[8] The screening advocates kept quiet about overdiagnosis, as they were afraid it would deter women from attending screening. Such utilitarian ethics are a form of unsolicited paternalism, which is only acceptable if one deals with incompetent patients, e.g. unconscious patients or children. Women are not children, and the prevailing paternalistic attitude is therefore not acceptable.

The conflict is also interesting from a Cochrane perspective. The Cochrane Collaboration is a charity that aims to help people make evidence-based decisions about healthcare interventions. It builds on volunteerism, and the editorial teams for each of its 52 review groups have been recruited on a somewhat first-come, first-served basis. This means that many editors lack training in issues related to editing, publication ethics and conflicts of interest. Another key value is collaboration, which is helpful, but difficulties are created when hard decisions need to be made that not everybody will agree with.

With a strong leadership, it would have been easy to demand of the Cochrane Breast Cancer Group that it publish the data on harms shortly after our *Lancet* paper with these data came out. On the other hand, it was a strength that the collaboration's steering group wouldn't tolerate that the huge work we had done on the review was thrown in the dustbin by the Breast Cancer Group.

An editor-in-chief was appointed in 2008, but before this happened, the freedom for Cochrane groups to set their own standards sometimes resulted in unusual demands that do not exist in other scientific journals. For example, when performing a review on soft laser therapy for unwanted hair growth with a dermatologist, the Cochrane Skin Group told me that they required a consumer as co-author. It is not clear to me why a woman with too much hair on her upper lip would become a good author of a scientific paper. We found one, but as she didn't contribute in any meaningful way, the group allowed us to publish without her name on the review.

The Cochrane Breast Cancer Group also told us that it was keen to have a consumer as co-author. We had concerns about this, e.g. a woman who had already made up her mind and entered a screening programme might not be a good choice. We replied that we would provide the consumer input ourselves, as Ole Olsen had been a consumer pregnancy and childbirth advocate for many years, and this was accepted.

The Cochrane Anaesthesia Group required that all author teams must have access to a BSc-, MSc-, or PhD-qualified statistician. I argued that I knew an excellent statistician who had never been formally educated in statistics but had worked his whole life as a statistician, and also that I had authored 12 Cochrane reviews without having needed support from statisticians. The group accepted my arguments and now explains that a statistician is someone who has the skills to perform a meta-analysis.

In dealing with a fourth group, the Cochrane Cystic Fibrosis and Genetic Disorders Group, we needed to involve both the publication arbiters and the editor-in-chief, David Tovey. The group refused to send our Cochrane review for peer review before we had found a third author who was a content area expert. We explained that we had plenty of access to such experts, but that they didn't necessarily have to be co-authors, and that it would be impossible to add an author when the work was already done, as such an author would become guest author, a practice uniformly condemned by journal editors. The group provided us with comments from such an expert, who had numerous conflicts of interest in relation to the exceedingly expensive intervention we had studied, which may cost up to US$150 000 annually for each patient in the United States. The group even wrote to us that this expert would be willing to become co-author. In my opinion, this is inappropriate editorial conduct. But as I couldn't persuade the group's editor, I described the case in an anomymised fashion on the email discussion list of the World Association of Medical Editors, of which I am a member. There was no sympathy with the group's attitude. Tovey proceeded cautiously and also involved a person outside The Cochrane Collaboration, Elizabeth Wager, chair of the independent organisation Committee on Publication Ethics, which is a forum for journal editors and publishers, with thousands of members, that handles difficult issues, thereby setting precedents. The deadlock ended when Tovey told the group to send our work out for peer review without demanding a third author. We didn't find convincing evidence that the drug we studied is effective.[9]

It is a big challenge for The Cochrane Collaboration that its editorial teams – in contrast to general medical journals like the *Lancet*, *BMJ* and *JAMA* – to a large extent are based on content area experts. Specialists often share the same opinions, prejudices and biases, and it can be very difficult to get a review accepted that provides evidence challenging their beliefs. Being a Cochrane director, I should perhaps not praise our own organisation, but I think the collaboration has performed exceptionally well for a grass-roots organisation. However, the time has come where impartiality and professionalism – with adoption of the best available standards for journal editing, as expressed in international guidelines and policies for editors – must be the norm for all Cochrane editors. It is the challenging task of the editor-in-chief to ensure that this comes true.

Welcome results in France

In France, our results were much appreciated by the highly respected medical journal *La Revue Préscrire*. This journal aims at providing French doctors unbiased information about interventions, and it also has editions in English.[10] *Préscrire* is a non-profit continuing-education organisation, committed to better patient care; it is wholly financed by its subscribers and accepts no advertising or other outside support. Its editors are healthcare professionals who are specially trained in *Préscrire*'s methods and who are free from conflicts of interest. Thus, it is exactly the type of journal we need to help us decide what is right and what is wrong about healthcare interventions, and I hope we may one day say also about Cochrane editors that none of them have conflicts of interest.

Préscrire published a series of very detailed articles on mammography screening in 2006 and 2007, with numerous references. The editors sent me their drafts to ensure they had not misunderstood anything. I was very impressed by their work; there was virtually nothing I could contribute. The way the editors at *Préscrire* work with the scientific issues offers a startling contrast with how screening supporters and their like-minded editors work. It was such a nice break from the usual screening muddle and wishful thinking to assist the editors of this journal.

I shall mention only one thing from the series. The editors wrote that French women are not being informed in an honest and balanced way, which is in violation of the law; furthermore, they noted that information coming from the French Cancer Institute and other bodies is biased.[11] Déjà vu! Just like in other countries. Why haven't the women protested?

References

1 Olsen O, Gøtzsche PC. Screening for breast cancer with mammography. *Cochrane Database Syst Rev*. 2001; (4): CD001877.
2 Olsen O, Gøtzsche PC. Cochrane review on screening for breast cancer with mammography. *Lancet*. 2001; **358**(9290): 1340–2.
3 Olsen O, Gøtzsche PC. Systematic review of screening for breast cancer with mammography. *Lancet*. 2001 Oct 20. Available at: http://image.thelancet.com/extras/fullreport.pdf (accessed 5 May 2010).
4 Letters. Screening mammography: setting the record straight. *Lancet*. 2002; **359**(9304): 439–42.
5 How consumers can and should improve clinical trials. *Lancet*. 2001; **357**(9270): 1721.
6 Gøtzsche PC, Nielsen M. Screening for breast cancer with mammography. *Cochrane Database Syst Rev*. 2009; (4): CD001877.
7 Gray JA. Breast screening programme. *BMJ*. 1989; **298**(6665): 48.
8 Gøtzsche PC, Olsen O. Is screening for breast cancer with mammography justifiable? *Lancet*. 2000; **355**(9198): 129–34.
9 Gøtzsche PC, Johansen HK. Intravenous alpha-1 antitrypsin augmentation therapy for treating patients with alpha-1 antitrypsin deficiency and lung disease. *Cochrane Database Syst Rev*. 2010; (7): CD007851.
10 Prescrire in English. Available at: http://english.prescrire.org/spip.php?article214 (accessed 3 November 2010).
11 [Mammography screening: honest and balanced information] [French]. *La Revue Préscrire*. 2007; **27**(288): 762.

13

Editorial misconduct in the *European Journal of Cancer*

THE PROBLEMS THE NORDIC COCHRANE CENTRE EXPERIENCED WITH journal editors were not limited to the Cochrane Breast Cancer Group. We were now exposed to editorial misconduct of a very unpleasant nature by the editor of the *European Journal of Cancer*.

This was in 2006. We didn't have the slightest idea that our paper, which was about the Two-County trial, would give us any problems. We thought that our latest revelation about this trial would hardly be noticed, as so many inconsistencies and omissions had already been documented, not only related to numbers but also about how the trial was randomised, when the control group was invited to screening and many other issues. Outside screening advocacy circles, we hadn't met a single researcher who, knowing anything about this trial, wasn't sceptical about it.

Some science journalists were sceptical, too. John Crewdson from the *Chicago Tribune* had already contacted me in November 2000 and asked to have a meeting, which became several meetings. Crewdson won the Pulitzer Prize for a series of articles on US immigration injustices and has a reputation for a Columbo style of information gathering where he feigns confusion and keeps asking questions.[1] He also worked on a case where the evidence strongly suggested that the American Robert Gallo had stolen the credit for the detection of the AIDS virus from the Frenchman Luc Montagnier, who sent specimens of his discovery to Gallo; an affair that was settled at presidential level to save faces.[2] Crewdson reported that Gallo's laboratory was not forthcoming, and that doors closed and the lights went out once the NIH figured out what Crewdson was doing.

Crewdson is not the type of guy one sees on stand-up shows.[1] I have sometimes felt slightly uncomfortable in his company since, like a good police detective, he seems a priori to suspect everybody of wrongdoing until proven innocent. He is the only person I have ever worked with who consistently kept a distance by using my last name when contacting me.

Crewdson has the reasonable view that what people do with taxpayers' money must be open to public scrutiny. He beleaguered Tabár for several days until he got away with data sheets that described causes of death, which he showed to me. These documents were very interesting and Crewdson worked on them for quite a while but never published anything. Several people have informed me that this was because the *Tribune* had been threatened with litigation, but Crewdson has not confirmed this.

Crewdson published other articles. He noted various irregularities in the Two-County trial, e.g. that 750 women disappeared from published reports of the Kopparberg part of the trial after 1989.[3] He also reported that a journalist from a major Swedish newspaper had received anonymous phone calls with death threats and warnings that her articles questioning the value of screening were killing women.[4] This was Inger Atterstam from *Svenska Dagbladet*. Lars Werkö, chair of the Swedish government's health technology agency, noted that although the agency had assessed screening for prostate cancer and found it of no use, it had never been asked to assess mammography screening. It was too controversial, the public believed in it and it was also a political feminist issue.

We had described the various problems with the Two-County trial in some detail already in 2001 and had made it clear that we didn't have much confidence in it. Our scepticism was reinforced when Nyström and colleagues[5] published the updated meta-analysis of the Swedish trials in 2002 in the *Lancet*. Nyström and colleagues could not include the Kopparberg part of the Two-County trial in their meta-analysis, as Tabár withheld his data. Nyström's update was based on official mortality statistics, and the authors reported only a 10% reduction in breast cancer mortality for the Östergötland part of the Two-County trial, whereas Tabár and colleagues[6] reported 24%.

What is so remarkable about these percentages is that Tabár and colleagues[6] reported 10 *fewer* deaths from breast cancer in the screened group despite the fact that the follow-up was slightly *longer* than in the meta-analysis and the age group was identical, and 23 *more* deaths in the control group in Östergötland (Table 13.1).

Thus, the 33 net discrepancies in deaths enhanced the mortality reduction in favour of screening. The probability that this could have happened by chance is extremely unlikely. How could it happen then? The likely reason is that Tabár's

TABLE 13.1 Breast cancer mortality as reported for the Östergötland part of the Two-County trial in two different publications

Publication	Breast cancer deaths		Person-years of follow-up (in 1000s)	Relative risk
	study group	control group		
Nyström *et al.* (2002)	177	190	1161	0.90
Tabár *et al.* (2000)	167	213	1304	0.76

numbers were seriously flawed because the cause-of-death assessments were not performed blindly. A local end-point committee determined the cause of death.[7,8] This has been confirmed by an investigator involved with the trial,[3] other Swedish trialists,[3,5] and *Breast Cancer Screening*, the IARC Handbook of Breast Cancer.[9] When confronted with the large discrepancy in the effect of screening in the two reports, Tabár, Smith and Duffy gave a most peculiar reply in *Lancet*: 'It is asserted in the overview report that the endpoint committees in the Two-County trial were aware of patients' study groups. No evidence is presented for this assertion . . .'[7] No evidence? Surely, there was evidence and Tabár should remember what he and his co-investigators had done.

I have found just one paper, from 2004, where the Tabár/Smith/Duffy trio have declared that cause-of-death assessments were done blindly: 'Cause of death was determined on blind review.'[10] If that was truly the case, then why didn't they say so in their 2002 *Lancet* letter? There was no explanation in their 2004 paper how blinding was achieved and I found out that their statement was false. As is often the case with the Two-County trial, it required detective work to see this. A table shows a 32% reduction in breast cancer mortality, and in a column titled 'Reference' the source of this is given as 'Tabar 2000'. However, although the paper has 55 references, none of them is from 2000 and has Tabár as first author or even as co-author. In two other tables, the mortality is shown by age groups, and the reference is now 'Amy' without a year of publication. There are no publications with Amy as author in the reference list. This was very puzzling, but after a while I got the idea of searching in the PDF file on 'Amy' and discovered that Amy was the fifth author on the paper itself![10] Highly unusual playing hide-and-seek for an academic paper.

The missing reference to 'Tabar 2000' would also have been difficult to find were it not for the fact that I had tabulated all of Tabár's data from all of his publications earlier. The paper I found, which provided the same risk ratio and confidence interval as in Tabár's table,[6] was the paper where Tabár, Duffy and Smith had claimed a 24% reduction in breast cancer mortality in Östergötland

and where the cause-of-death assessments were *not* performed blindly.[3,5,7–9]

There were other curiosities. Nyström and colleagues[5] had explained that the unavailability of the Kopparberg data was because the trialists had declined to collaborate shortly after the publication of the first meta-analysis in 1993, and that they regretted the trialists' decision. In contrast, Tabár, Smith and Duffy[7] claimed that the 'lead investigator of Kopparberg' (which is Tabár) had offered the data to the Swedish collaborative group and that they regretted the group had elected not to include the Kopparberg data. It seems that this statement was misleading. Nyström has described that Tabár tried to stop the 2002 meta-analysis some weeks before it was published, presumably because of its rather frank criticisms of Tabár's trial, and Ingvar Andersson from Malmö responded, 'there is no way that we negotiate in any way like this'.[3] Thus, if an offer was made, it was too late.

The Two-County trial reported a 31% reduction in breast cancer mortality in 1985.[11] This is an implausibly large effect, especially considering that only single-view mammography was used and that women above 50 years of age were only screened every 33 months, on average.[11] Two Norwegian researchers, pathologist Jan Mæhlen and Per-Henrik Zahl, who is both a statistician and a physician, therefore wondered whether some women and deaths could be missing and that this wasn't random, but favoured screening. They initiated a study in collaboration with me in 2005 that used the Swedish population-based registers for cancer and for causes of death. It was relatively easy to do this, as the trial was population based and therefore included all women in the age group 40–74 years. We also used information on the study population and the average study period when estimating the total number of breast cancers and breast cancer deaths in the trial.[12] We found that, compared to official Swedish statistics, 192 breast cancer cases and 43 breast cancer deaths seemed to be missing in the 1985 publication of the trial, and similar discrepancies persisted in two trial updates.

The possibility that some cancers were not included in the trial results is supported by other data. The rate of interval cancers was surprisingly low in the Two-County trial, only 94 per 100 000 based on one publication and 91 per 100 000 based on another, whereas these rates were 158 and 157 per 100 000 in the same age groups in national screening programmes in the United Kingdom and the Netherlands, respectively.[12,13]

We noted in our paper that the difference in the number of breast cancer deaths between the study group and the control group in the Two-County trial is small and that the mortality reduction would therefore no longer be statistically significant if only a few more breast cancer deaths were added to the study group. We also cautioned that we had used a simple and crude method. We submitted our research to the *European Journal of Cancer* and resubmitted it after we had addressed the comments of the peer reviewers.

Editorial misconduct

We published our findings on 9 March 2006 in the articles-in-press section of the *European Journal of Cancer* website.[14]

Twenty days later, Editor-in-Chief John Smyth informed us that his journal had received 'comments from a number of sources regarding some of the claims made in the article' and that our article had been removed from the journal's website pending further discussion and clarification. Smyth also noted that his journal 'believes that science is best served by rigorous debate, which sometimes may even generate controversy, provided of course that the debate and controversy is objective and motivated by the desire to improve science and medical research and practice'. However, by withdrawing our paper, Smyth made sure this couldn't happen.

Smyth didn't forward the comments to us but asked for very minor clarifications and changes. We first asked him to reconsider whether his decision to withdraw our paper was fair, as we hadn't been offered any kind of process, or even a chance of responding to the issues raised. Next, we submitted a slightly revised manuscript in which the most important change was that we had deleted this sentence: 'The numbers of breast cancer deaths in both the study group and in the control group have been changed in favour of screening.'[14] This sentence could be interpreted as suggesting that the trial authors had *deliberately* changed the cause of death in favour of screening, when they reported a 24% effect while it was only 10% using official mortality statistics, which we hadn't intended.

To our great surprise, as our paper had already been published, the revised manuscript was sent out for peer review, and 2 months later the editor informed us that his decision to withdraw our paper was final. He referred to 'the release of new information concerning the randomization process and the trials opening and closing dates' and forwarded selected 'Comments from the peer review process.'

Selected comments? Not again! That was what the Cochrane Breast Cancer Group had also done to us. We were now the victims of another Kafkaesque process where we were only allowed to see selected parts of the evidence raised against us. *And there was now total confusion, as some of this 'new information' contrasted not only with published data but also with randomisation dates we had received in earlier peer reviews.* However, using any of the three different sets of randomisation dates in our analysis, we confirmed our original results. We were

ARTICLE IN PRESS

EUROPEAN JOURNAL OF CANCER XXX (2006) XXX–XXX

available at www.sciencedirect.com

SCIENCE DIRECT

journal homepage: www.ejconline.com

ELSEVIER

EJC

Results of the Two-County trial of mammography screening are not compatible with contemporaneous official Swedish breast cancer statistics

Per-Henrik Zahl[a,*], *Peter C. Gøtzsche*[b], *Jannike Mørch Andersen*[a,c], *Jan Mæhlen*[c]

[a]*Division of Epidemiology, Norwegian Institute of Public Health, P.O. Box 4404, Nydalen, N-0403 Oslo, Norway*
[b]*Nordic Cochrane Centre, H:S Rigshospitalet, DK-2100 København Ø, Denmark*
[c]*Department of Pathology, Ullevål University Hospital, N-0407 Oslo, Norway*

A R T I C L E I N F O

Article history:
Received 6 September 2005
Received in revised form
6 December 2005
Accepted 6 December 2005

Keywords:
Breast cancer
Mammography screening
Randomised trial

A B S T R A C T

National mammography screening programs are based on the results of randomised trials, but the quality of these trials has recently been questioned. The Swedish Two-County trial reported a 31% reduction in breast cancer mortality and was instrumental for the introduction of screening in many countries. In this trial, official Swedish health registries were used to identify breast cancers and breast cancer deaths in the study population. We used data from the registries to estimate the numbers of breast cancer cases and breast cancer deaths among the included women. Our results show substantially higher numbers than those in reports of this trial. Other data show that the mortality results in a recent report were also seriously flawed.

1. Introduction

The Two-County trial of screening mammography in Sweden has been instrumental for the introduction of screening in many countries. It reported a 31% reduction in breast cancer mortality.[1] However, the reliability of the study has later been questioned.[2,3] The mean time of randomisation, as well as the number of women included in the study and the number of breast cancer deaths varied between different papers from the trial, even when the included age groups and follow-up periods were the same.

Another potential problem in the Two-County trial was to identify breast cancers that were not diagnosed during the screening sessions. Such cases included interval cancers in attending women, clinical cancers occurring in invited but non-attending women and all cancers in the control group. Since the researchers used the personal identification number system to link the study population to the Swedish population-based registries for cancer and the causes of death,[1,4] the recorded cancer incidence and mortality in the Two-County trial should be identical to those in the official registers for these women.

We have used official Swedish statistics on breast cancer incidence and breast cancer mortality and compared them with the numbers reported by the researchers. We have combined data from the registries and the information on the study population and the average study period in the Two-County trial to obtain likely estimates of the total number of breast cancers and breast cancer deaths in the trial. As far as we know such a quality control of the Two-County trial has not been done previously.

* *Corresponding author*: Tel.: +47 2340 8150; fax: +47 2340 8101.
E-mail address: per-henrik.zahl@fhi.no (P.-H. Zahl).

0959-8049/$ - see front matter © 2006 Elsevier Ltd. All rights reserved.
doi:10.1016/j.ejca.2005.12.016

FIGURE 13.1 Our paper in the *European Journal of Cancer*, which was later withdrawn by the editor for no good reason and without due process

therefore disappointed when, despite two appeals, Smyth did not offer us the opportunity to document our analyses. I believe a judge behaving like this in a court case would face trouble. But mammography screening somehow always seems to be different.

The peer reviewers complained that we had not responded to 'the letter from the paper's critics', and noted that the letter contained details of the way the randomisation was performed and the screening periods that had never been emphasised before. Kafka again. How could we respond to a letter we hadn't been allowed to see? It was grotesque.

Anyhow, the data in the letter may be of questionable value because one of the peer reviewers noted, 'They are certainly worth reporting, though they should be reported in a far more objective way.' Curiously, like us, this peer reviewer appeared only to have seen selected comments from the other reviewers, as he noted that 'the reference was not provided in the version I received' (although the reviewer, who seemed to have extensive knowledge of the Two-County trial, doubted this reference could be important).

Later, this peer reviewer sent the full review to me. This was revealing. Smyth had deleted only 6% of the whole review before he sent it to us, but the deleted lines were interesting: 'Thus, my conclusion at this time is that it should be pointed out to Zahl *et al.* that they have not adequately responded to the comments received on their paper, and unless they are able to do so, and refute them, the paper will not be accepted.' Thus, we were not supposed to know that this reviewer would recommend publication if we addressed the comments, which we could easily have done.

Four days after Smyth had informed us that he had withdrawn our paper,[14] we observed that our paper was listed as withdrawn in PubMed, in violation of the *European Journal of Cancer*'s own policy. The journal is a member of the International Committee of Medical Journal Editors, which states:[15]

> In no instance should a journal remove an article from its website or archive. If an article needs to be corrected or retracted, the explanation must be labelled appropriately and communicated as soon as possible on a citable page in a subsequent issue of the journal.

The committee goes on to say that it is a serious step to retract a published paper and this should only be done after due process and only if scientific fraud has been established.

Smyth did not only retract our paper but removed it entirely from the journal's website without leaving a trace of it, without sharing essential information with us, without discussing the issues with us and without even notifying us in advance.

The committee's guidelines make it clear that, 'inadequacies exposed by the emergence of new scientific information in the normal course of research . . . require no corrections or withdrawals.' We believe our methods are adequate, our results are reliable and that there was no plausible reason for removing our paper, or for failing to republish it.

Elsevier, the publisher of the journal, is a member of the International Association of Scientific, Technical and Medical Publishers, which states: 'In order to assure the maintenance of the historical record of scholarly publishing, STM supports the principle of favouring "retraction" (erratum) over "removal" in virtually all cases.'[16] The association also notes that 'editors and/or publishers will consult with the authors' and that if an article is removed, 'bibliographic information about the "removed" article should be retained for the scientific record, and an explanation given, however brief, about the circumstances of its removal'. None of this was respected in our case.

We asked Smyth twice, to no avail, to forward all the comments he had received. We also appealed to him to reverse his decision, but we didn't get a reply. We considered appealing to the journal, but we didn't pursue this route as neither the journal nor its editor were members of the World Association of Medical Editors, and because there seemed to be no ombudsman or ethics committee at the journal. Furthermore, we had been informed that the owners of the journal had received complaints from screening advocates, and we therefore felt our chance for a reversal of the editor's decision was remote.

I described our case in an anonymised fashion in June 2006 on the email list of the World Association of Medical Editors and asked for advice. Just an hour later, Richard Horton replied that the *Lancet* would be keen to consider the case for publication, as 'editorial misconduct needs to be as ruthlessly dealt with as any instance of research misconduct', and as it was an important story to make public.

Horton said he would seek the editor's own view, but Smyth didn't accept his invitation. We described the affair in the *Lancet* in November 2006[17] and published our research paper simultaneously in the *Danish Medical Bulletin*.[12] We first considered submitting it to the *International Journal of Epidemiology*, but the lawyers at that journal were worried because we had already assigned our copyright to the *European Journal of Cancer*. This added insult to injury, although it wasn't the lawyers' fault of course. Torben Schroeder, the editor of the *Danish Medical Bulletin*, was bolder and wrote in a note at the end of our paper that he shared our concerns and explained that, 'first, the process that led to removal of the accepted and published paper was unilateral. Second, a withdrawn or removed paper invariably leaves you with an impression of scientific fraud. Therefore, DMB has decided to publish the paper.'

Later, the Committee on Publication Ethics supported the *Lancet* in its decision to bring the case into the public domain. It noted that published work – electronically or otherwise – should not be removed without appropriate correction or retraction and that retraction or removal is a very serious matter for authors and their institutions and should not happen without due process.[18] In a private email to me, the chairman of the committee noted that its members disapproved of the action of the editor of the *European Journal of Cancer* and he wondered what pressures were exerted on Smyth to withdraw the paper.

Threats, intimidation and falsehoods

We also wondered why John Smyth would expose himself to condemnation by editorial colleagues through his actions. A person close to Smyth informed me that Smyth or his journal, or both, were threatened by litigation. If that is correct, the first name that comes to mind is László Tabár. But yet again, Peter Dean led the attack.

Only 11 days after our paper appeared on the *European Journal of Cancer* website, Dean sent two letters by himself and one by Jack Cuzick, associate editor of the journal, to the directors at the National Institute of Public Health in Oslo, where the first author of our paper worked. In his typical fashion, Dean wrote that our paper would hopefully not 'be seen as harmful to your institution, despite the poor scholarship and even poorer ethical standards involved'.

Also typical of Dean, these letters didn't contain any scientific substance or concrete criticism of our work that we could respond to, and this was apparently not the idea either, as we were not copied on the letters. One letter was written to the board of directors of Reed Elsevier, the publisher of the *European Journal of Cancer*. In it, Dean included a letter he had written to John Smyth 2 days earlier, which he had copied to 150 people, including many leaders of screening programmes or outspoken screening advocates and a member of the European parliament:

> Lisa Wood, Autier Philippe, Paola Pisani, International Agency for Research on Cancer, Lawrence von Karsa, Lennarth Nystrom, Les Irwig, Magnus Stenbeck, Martti Pamilo, Marvin Zelen, Mary Codd, Mary Rickard, Matti Hakama, Max Parkin, Michael Linver, Michael Michell, Mike Dixon, Mogens

> Blichert-Toft, Murray Waldren, Måns Rosén, NJ Wald, Nereo Segnan, Nicholas E. Day, CBE, Nicholas Wilcken, Nick Perry, Nils Bjurstam, Olli Miettinen, Olof Jarlman, Osmo Räsänen, Pamilo Martti, Parvinen Ilmo, Klemi Pekka, Peter Boyle, Peter Dawson, Peter Lundsted Hurup, Peter Langhorne, Pyrhönen Seppo, Päivi Hietanen, Rainer Otto, Reichel, Margrit, Rissanen Tarja, Robert A. Schmidt, Robert Smith, Roberts, Robin Wilson, Roger Blanks, N Becker, Europadonna, Claus Blumenroth, Brenner, Cottard MP, Jean-Pierre De-Landtsheer, Jacques Fracheboud, Rhian Gabe, R Holland, K Joens, HakanJonsson, Laura Kotaniemi-Talonen, Lambert, Lucas, C Mahe, Elsebeth Lynge, Nea Malila, Kahan, E Paci, Julietta Patnick, Nick Perry, Niall Phelan, Liga Portuguesa Contra O Cancro, Antonio Ponti, Margrit Reichel, H Rijken, V Rodrigues, M Rosselli, Astrid Scharpantgen, K Joens-assistant, Svobodnik, Laszlo Tabar, Sven Tornberg, CA Wells, Auni Aasmaa, Ahti Anttila, Alfonso Frigerio, Anders Lernevall, Anders Ekbom, Art Elman, Arto Haapanen, Bedrich Vitak, Charlotte McDaniel, Chris de Wolf, Claudia I. Henschke, D. Freedman, Dan Kopans, Dr. Linda Warren Burhenne, Ed Hendrick, Edward A Sickles, Edward Azavedo, Elisabeth Kutt, Erik Thurfjell, Francisco Ruíz Perales, Gunilla Svane, Hannu J Aronen, Harry de Koning, Hilary Dobson, Hirschmann, Jan V, Ilse Vejborg, Inger Torhild Gram, Jaakko Kinnunen, Jack Cuzick, Jan Frisell, Janne Nappi, Kalevi Soila, Karen Abbe, Karl von Smitten, Kaufman, Cary S, Kerstin Moberg, Koskivuo Ilkka, Kronqvist Pauliina, Ronald J H Borra, Samuli Niiranen, Solveig Hofvind, Steinar Thoresen, Stephen Duffy, Stephen Feig, Stergios Prapavesis, Steven Narod, Sue Moss, Sullivan, Daniel, Svedström Erkki, Timo Hakulinen, Timo Ihämaki, Tony Chen, Uffe Dyreborg, Valerie Beral, Walter Schwartz, Wang Hege, Vannier Michael, Werner Kaiser, Wolf Georg, Y Grumbach, Yoshito, Zoltan Péntek, Henderson Craig, Umberto Veronesi, Franceschi.

Dean also copied the chair of the Cochrane Collaboration Steering Group, Peter Langhorne, and Coordinating Editor Nicholas Wilcken from the Cochrane Breast Cancer Group, although our colleagues in The Cochrane Collaboration have nothing to do with what researchers from The Nordic Cochrane Centre elect to publish, with the exception of Cochrane reviews.

Dean's letter to Elsevier was amusing in all its pejorative glory:

- 'patently shoddy scholarship and serious errors'
- our paper claimed that work published by others 'has been fraudulently altered'
- 'the claim amounts to scientific libel and defamation of character'
- 'the claims are preposterous'

- 'since they are now electronically published, they have an air of infallibility on which the authors will use to claim validity'
- 'the accused scientists were never contacted in advance to offer an opportunity to set the record straight.'

The argument that we should have shared our concerns with the trialists was meaningless, as Tabár hadn't provided meaningful answers when asked[19] or he didn't reply at all.

Dean remarked that our paper seriously damaged the reputation of the journal and that he knew that a number of assumptions, estimations and approximations were incorrect and contrary to the published design of the trial. However, as always, he gave himself a free ride, as he offered no concrete evidence in support of his many opinions. Instead, he gave four references to support his views. Three of them were the papers by David Freedman, Diana Petitti and James Robins, which don't contain anything of substance that is correct, as I have explained in Chapter 11, but Dean failed to quote my replies in the same journal.

The fourth reference was to a paper published by Robert Smith of the American Cancer Society in a yearbook quarterly that is not indexed by PubMed.[20] It contains a number of factual errors and untrue statements. For example, our 2000 *Lancet* paper didn't in any way imply that it was a 'Cochrane Collaboration systematic review'; the Cochrane editors weren't caught off guard in 2001, as we had informed them in advance that we had submitted a report to the *Lancet*; and we hadn't omitted mentioning the concerns about the randomisation in the Canadian trials. Worst of all, Smith advised that a comparison of all-cause mortality should not be done for all randomised women but only for those with a breast cancer diagnosis. This approach creates a huge bias in favour of screening because all the overdiagnosed cases in the screened group have an excellent prognosis. It's amazing that a director of cancer screening seems unaware of this elementary flaw or chooses to ignore it.

Dean responded in the *Lancet* to our comment about editorial misconduct with arguments that were all false,[21] which can easily be seen by comparing his letter with our comment and our republished paper.[12,17] Dean ended by stating that he had no conflict of interest, but he had hidden his title as professor of radiology by giving his address as 'Faculty of Medicine'.[22] This is interesting, since a PubMed search showed that Dean and Tabár had collaborated for decades. Since 1979, they had co-authored 16 mammography-related papers and at least three books, including a teaching atlas. Finally, Dean organised the process that led to removal of our paper from the *European Journal of Cancer*.

Tom Jefferson, author of a book about peer review, was very upset.[23] What struck him was not that there might be a debate about our work, but that it was conducted in such a one-sided and occult fashion. Violent letters pressuring Smyth hadn't been published, anonymous referees' reports had been fed in a selective and fragmented fashion to the authors, and the paper was removed without warning.

Dean continued his harassments and informed Schroeder, the editor of the *Danish Medical Bulletin*, that he hoped he would not be liable to litigation. Although Dean considered our paper an 'ephemeral article', he nevertheless offered Schroeder to submit a full-length critique of it, adding that it would reflect poorly on the journal for having published our paper.

Dean also noted that there were several factual errors in the comment we had published in the *Lancet*.[17] It escapes me what Dean alluded to, as there are no errors, but it seems to be Dean's standard behaviour when he harasses people. Dean suggested that Schroeder contact Elsebeth Lynge for her views, as she was 'certainly the most internationally respected investigator from Denmark in the field of breast cancer screening'. I shall discuss Lynge in later chapters.

Finally, Schroeder was told that if he hadn't acted in ways Dean defined for him in his letter, 'this would reflect even more poorly on the *Danish Medical Bulletin*'. Schroeder has a sense of humour and I'm sure he had a good laugh over all this.

Dean copied his letter to Schroeder to an impressive list of people that included the deans for the three Danish medical faculties, the chairman and the director of the Danish Medical Association, the legal editor of the *Ugeskrift for Læger*, the director of the Danish National Board of Health and four other key people working there, the director of the Danish Health Technology Assessment agency, the heads of the Danish screening units, and Elsebeth Lynge, who chaired the working group that wrote the Board of Health's 1997 report that recommended breast screening be introduced in the whole of Denmark.[24] Members of the royal family and our prime minister were not on Dean's list.

Debates in the *Scientist* and the *Cancer Letter*

Journalist Kerry Grens started a debate in the *Scientist* just before Christmas in 2006 by describing the events and interviewing people.[25] Peter Dean used the 'you are killing my patients' argument: 'I get rather upset when people tell lies, especially when it's a matter of life and death for women.' Dean explained that he worked in the hospital where the trial data were collected and that the information was carefully and consistently recorded. I documented in an email to Grens that this wasn't correct, but she paid no attention to this and made no reference to my refutations.

Torben Schroeder said, 'it's very worrisome that a paper is plainly removed from a Web site without further assessment, because it was peer-reviewed and accepted'. Now John Smyth also reacted: 'We at the European Journal of Cancer (published by Elsevier) find it necessary to clarify certain aspects of the article that are incorrect and assure your readers that the editors acted within all legal boundaries and had objective, ethical reasons to support all actions', and added, 'The EJC Editors acted professionally at all times and handled the manuscript fairly and in accordance with the standard editorial policies of the journal.'

Such wording is commonly seen when a drug company has caused the unnecessary deaths of thousands of patients by withholding data on lethal harms from public view. Then we are always told that the company behaved ethically in all possible respects. In his amusing little book *On Bullshit*, moral philosopher Harry Frankfurt starts off by saying that one of the salient features of our culture is that there is so much bullshit.[26] He sees no important difference between humbug and bullshit, but says it's more polite to say 'Humbug!', which he considers short of lying. Smyth's concrete statements were so blatantly untrue[17] that we published a comment explaining this. Other of his comments were misleading, e.g. he noted that our sentence about changing causes of death might be interpreted as potentially libellous, *but Smyth did not mention that this comment was gone when we resubmitted our paper*.

The editor of the *Cancer Letter*, Kirsten Boyd Goldberg, did a better job. She wrote a detailed account of the affair.[27] Cornelia Baines remarked that it was difficult to raise legitimate questions because it undermined core beliefs and noted that her personal experience was that one could get abused for saying things people don't want to be said. She found it unbelievable that a published, peer-reviewed article would be withdrawn because of the protestations of the researchers or the cabal that supports the researchers. Finally, she remarked:

> Although truly libellous things have been said about the Canadian researchers, including committing fraud, we have never attempted to prevent anything being published, because we do have freedom of the press and it's up to people to find out what's true information and what's not true information.

Donald Berry felt we were on shaky ground because of our crude calculations and he would like to see more specifics from Tabár, using actual numbers cited by us. He added that Tabár could clear up questions by submitting his data for an independent audit. John Smyth declined to comment on this occasion, as

'The paper you refer to had to involve legal advice and therefore I would prefer not to comment further.'

Within 3 hours of sending an email to Tabár requesting comment, Goldberg received a phone call from Peter Dean, who introduced himself as a friend and collaborator of Tabár for 30 years and said Tabár's response would be waiting in Goldberg's email inbox. Dean noted that Tabár was brilliant and that we had taken the approach that the best way to advance our criticisms of breast cancer screening was to attack Tabár's personal integrity. Dean's next remark was incredible. He wrote, 'This is effective – attacking any individual, no matter how unjust the accusations, will sow the seeds of doubt in the minds of the reader.' This was exactly what Dean had done to me throughout 7 years.

In an email to the *Cancer Letter*, Tabár described our paper as 'beset by elementary errors and fallacious assumptions'. Tabár very rarely responds to criticism of his trial and I have therefore shown his full comments in Appendix 1, with our replies.[28,29] All of his pivotal statements are either false or misleading.

When Per-Henrik Zahl first contacted me about his suspicion that many cancers and deaths were missing in reports on the Two-County trial and that he wanted to publish his observations, I was rather sceptical, mostly because the information in various reports on the trial on randomisation and other key procedures was inconsistent or absent. I thought it would be a nightmare to try to reconstruct what most likely happened during the conduct of the trial. Furthermore, reported numbers were also inconsistent, and it would therefore be difficult to compare reported cancers and deaths with register data. However, on the other hand, that was exactly the reason to do the study. I therefore agreed to participate and checked very carefully Zahl's calculations and made sure I had understood all the steps involved. This led to a good deal of correspondence between us and also to clarifications in the text.

Some people may feel we went too far, as our study involved assumptions and approximations. But I believe it has merit, particularly after we observed that the comments by the peer reviewers about key feaures of the trial mere mutually incompatible and didn't agree with published information. In addition, no matter what assumptions and which numbers from the various reports on the trial we used, we came to the same result, that cancers and deaths were missing. Unless of course – as we also write in our paper – pivotal information in key papers on the trial was fallacious, which would be equally problematic but less likely, considering the strangely low interval cancer rates in the trial.

References

1 Cohen J. John Crewdson: science journalist as investigator. *Science*. 1991; **254**(5034): 946–9.

2 Marsa M. *Prescription for Profits: how the pharmaceutical industry bankrolled the unholy marriage betwen science and business*. New York: Scribner; 1997.

3 Crewdson J. Swedes doubt mammography trial: disparities found in landmark study. *Chicago Tribune*. 2002 Mar 15.

4 Crewdson J. In Sweden, decades of mammograms barely cut deaths. *Chicago Tribune*. 2002 Mar 18.

5 Nyström L, Andersson I, Bjurstam N, *et al*. Long-term effects of mammography screening: updated overview of the Swedish randomised trials. *Lancet*. 2002; **359**(9310): 909–19.

6 Tabár L, Vitak B, Chen HH, *et al*. The Swedish Two-County trial twenty years later: updated mortality results and new insights from long-term follow-up. *Radiol Clin North Am*. 2000; **38**(4): 625–51.

7 Tabár L, Smith RA, Duffy SW. Update on effects of screening mammography. *Lancet*. 2002; **360**(9329): 337.

8 Nyström L, Andersson I, Bjurstam N, *et al*. Update on effects of screening mammography. *Lancet*. 2002; **360**(9329): 339–40.

9 Vainio H, Bianchini F. *Breast Cancer Screening*. IARC Handbooks of Cancer Prevention, Vol 7. Lyon, France: IARC Press; 2002.

10 Smith RA, Duffy SW, Gabe R, *et al*. The randomized trials of breast cancer screening: what have we learned? *Radiol Clin North Am*. 2004; **42**(5): 793–806.

11 Tabár L, Fagerberg CJ, Gad A, *et al*. Reduction in mortality from breast cancer after mass screening with mammography: randomised trial from the Breast Cancer Screening Working Group of the Swedish National Board of Health and Welfare. *Lancet*. 1985; **1**(8433): 829–32.

12 Zahl PH, Gøtzsche PC, Andersen JM, *et al*. Results of the Two-County trial of mammography screening are not compatible with contemporaneous official Swedish breast cancer statistics. *Dan Med Bull*. 2006; **53**(4): 438–40.

13 Woodman CB, Threlfall AG, Boggis CR, *et al*. Is the three year breast screening interval too long? Occurrence of interval cancers in NHS breast screening programme's north western region. *BMJ*. 1995; **310**(6974): 224–6.

14 Zahl P-H, Gøtzsche PC, Andersen JM, *et al*. WITHDRAWN: Results of the Two-County trial of mammography screening are not compatible with contemporaneous official Swedish breast cancer statistics. *Eur J Cancer*. Epub 2006 Mar 9.

15 International Committee of Medical Journal Editors. *Uniform Requirements for Manuscripts Submitted to Biomedical Journals: writing and editing for biomedical publication*. Available at: www.icmje.org (accessed 22 May 2011).

16 International Association of Scientific, Technical and Medical Publishers. www.stm-assoc.org/home (accessed 22 May 2011).

17 Gøtzsche PC, Mæhlen J, Zahl PH. What is publication? *Lancet*. 2006; **368**(9550): 1854–6.

18 Kleinert S. A withdrawn prepublication. *Lancet*. 2007; **369**(9565): 901.

19 Gøtzsche PC. The debate on breast cancer screening with mammography is important. *J Am Coll Radiol*. 2004; **1**(1): 8–14.

20 Smith RA. Ideology masquerading as evidence-based medicine: the Cochrane review on screening for breast cancer with mammography. *Breast Dis Q*. 2003; **13**(4): 298–307.
21 Dean PB. A withdrawn prepublication. *Lancet*. 2007; **369**(9596): 901.
22 Gøtzsche PC, Mæhlen J, Zahl P-H. Undeclared motives in withdrawing a publication. *Lancet*. 2007; **369**(9574): 1690.
23 Jefferson T. A withdrawn prepublication. *Lancet*. 2007; **369**(9565): 901–2.
24 Sundhedsstyrelsen (National Board of Health). [*Early detection and treatment of breast cancer. Status report*] [*Danish*]. Copenhagen: Sundhedsstyrelsen; 1997.
25 Grens K, with subsequent comments by Gøtzsche PC; Smyth J; Gøtzsche PC, Mæhlen J, Zahl P-H. Mammography article withdrawal sparks dispute: authors of an article critical of mammography believe a scientific opponent forced the retraction. *Scientist*. 2006 Dec 22.
26 Frankfurt H. *On Bullshit*. Princeton, NJ: Princeton University Press; 2005.
27 Goldberg KB. Experts raise questions about influential Swedish trial of mammography screening. *Cancer Lett*. 2007; **33**(18): 1–7.
28 Tabár L. Tabár's reply to the Zahl article. *Cancer Lett*. 2007; **33**(18): 4–6.
29 Gøtzsche PC, Mæhlen J, Zahl P-H. Missing cancers & deaths in the Two-County trial. *Cancer Lett*. 2007; **33**(18): 6–7.

14

Tabár's 'beyond reason' studies

Observational studies based on individual screening history, no matter how well designed and conducted, should not be regarded as providing evidence of an effect of screening.

Harri Vainio and Franca Bianchini[1]

IN MAY 2001, TABÁR, DUFFY, SMITH AND OTHERS REPORTED A historically controlled study in *Cancer*,[2] which illustrates that politically popular messages can beat sound science, at least in the short term.[3] The headline of the paper is 'Beyond randomized controlled trials', but the study is so hopelessly flawed that Donald Berry told Robert Smith that they should have called it 'beyond reason'. *Cancer* is usually regarded as a prestigious journal, but Tabár's article was received on 29 December 2000 and was accepted 6 days later, which suggests that it wasn't peer-reviewed, although this is routine practice for the journal. Perhaps it helped that *Cancer* is published by the American Cancer Society and that Smith was director of cancer screening at the society.

The study was partly based on data from the Two-County trial. Breast cancer mortality during screening was compared with an earlier time period before screening. The authors reported a 63% reduction in breast cancer mortality in those who attended screening, and a 50% reduction in the age group invited to screening. I have already explained in Chapter 2, using data from the Malmö trial, why such an approach is hopeless. The Malmö trial reported a 4% reduction in breast cancer mortality when all women were included in the denominator, but when only women with a breast cancer diagnosis were included in the denominator, there was a 28% reduction. This is spurious of course, and it is the wrong denominator, as all the healthy overdiagnosed women distort the result.

Tabár and colleagues made other serious errors. They had not tried to separate effects of screening from effects of improved treatment, and I showed – based on their data – that the decrease in breast cancer mortality in women below 40 years of age who had not been invited to screening wasn't significantly different from the decrease in the invited age group.[4] This means that what the authors had observed could be explained by improved treatment; in fact, it is entirely implausible that tamoxifen, for example, should be ineffective in Sweden when it is highly effective in the rest of the world.

Elsewhere, Tabár noted, with reference to his own data from the Two-County trial, that adjuvant therapy (such as tamoxifen) didn't seem to reduce mortality in women with tumours that were smaller than 10 mm.[5] Tabár is wrong, and his view was rejected by other Swedish researchers who reminded him of the meta-analyses done by the Oxford group that found that the effect of adjuvant therapy was not related to the size or stage of the cancer.[6] This indicates, once again, that Tabár's data from the Two-County trial are unreliable.

The authors had excluded about half of the breast cancer deaths that had occurred in the two counties. This was because they only included those deaths that resulted from cancers diagnosed during each time interval they compared. This method creates a huge bias in favour of screening since those cancers that were detected in the period before screening were generally more advanced and therefore also more deadly than those detected during screening, which, in addition, included many overdiagnosed cases with an excellent prognosis. Therefore, calculations based on the number of breast cancer deaths in the numerator and the number of detected cancers in the denominator are fatally flawed. Statistical adjustment for this problem cannot solve it, as no one knows by how much the result should be adjusted.[7] The bias in Tabár's study is so large that it can explain reductions in breast cancer mortality of 50% or even more.[8]

In their reply, Tabár, Duffy and Smith introduced new inappropriate comparisons to defend themselves.[9] They compared women who attended screening with women who didn't, although it is clear from their original paper that they were aware that such comparisons are seriously misleading.[2]

An accompanying editorial took up five pages,[10] which, being the size of most reports of original research, is unusually long. Tabár's study was highly praised as seminal, meticulous, a milestone and a final critical test of the effect of screening. This is when the reader must choose between weeping or laughing, as there are no other possibilities (apart from becoming angry by the limitless stupidity demonstrated and allowed to be published by *Cancer*). *The editorialists suggested ways to perform even better, including screening women aged 40–49 years every 6 months, and believed Tabár's estimates were minimum figures.* Pardon me, but this is insane. A 63% reduction in breast cancer mortality is called 'minimum figures'.

The editorial furthermore spoke of a 'marked reduction in the size of invasive cancers' with screening, which is also a perverse statement, as the reduction is so small that large effects of screening are quite impossible (*see* Chapter 24). The authors admitted that there are harms of screening but they didn't mention overdiagnosis and overtreatment, not even when they discussed carcinoma *in situ*, and said that some of the lesions have a lag period of 30 years before they become invasive. They turned the negative into a positive, saying that when such lesions are found, later invasive cancer is prevented.

One would think it couldn't be worse, but it could. The authors believed that the American Cancer Society's goals for the year 2015, to obtain a 50% reduction in cancer mortality and a 25% reduction in cancer incidence, could probably be met for breast cancer. The ignorance demonstrated by this remark is breathtaking. Breast cancer incidence continues to rise dramatically because of overdiagnosis (*see* Chapter 16) and the effect of screening in today's setting is very small, if any (*see* Chapter 25).

Finally, the authors said:

> It is an 'open question whether, with limited resources, a country should focus on expensive and morbid treatments for advanced breast carcinoma and metastatic disease or instead, focus on screening, because finding disease at a much earlier stage means that extensive therapeutic efforts are less necessary, less radical, and less expensive.'

This speaks for itself. I'm sure these authors could sell sand in the Sahara and ice to Greenlandic Eskimos.

The claim that screening reduced deaths from breast cancer by about two-thirds was uncritically repeated elsewhere, e.g. in a news item in the *BMJ*.[11] The *BMJ*'s Minerva section conveyed the strong political message that the case for breast cancer screening programmes was now beyond debate, with reference to a 'meticulous report from Sweden'.[12] And Duffy wasn't modest either: 'The results of this study suggest that we could be underestimating just how many lives mammograms are saving.'[11]

Peter Dean wrote in the *Läkartidningen* that the 'Swedish milestone study' started a new era in the evaluation of breast cancer screening, that others should use the same method and that mammography screening was a large breakthrough for public health.[13] He also noted that the United Kingdom had previously had the largest mortality from breast cancer in Europe but that it had decreased substantially 10 years after screening was introduced, whereas Denmark, where screening had been slowly introduced against considerable resistance, now had the highest breast cancer mortality. As I have already explained in Chapter 15, these statements are deceptive.

But the propaganda worked, of course; the hyperbole was maximal, and the valid and serious criticisms in the letters that followed the 'beyond reason' paper[3] were totally ignored, also by the authors who published a similarly unreliable study in *Cancer* a year later,[14] also based on Swedish women.

It can sometimes be amusing when journalists are too lazy or too busy to do their job properly, or just want to be first. Tabár, Duffy and Smith's second 'beyond reason' study was said in the *Los Angeles Times* to 'effectively refute' the claims that screening wasn't beneficial and to 'confirm beyond any doubt' that reduction in deaths can be obtained in large screening programmes.[15] The person behind this quote was radiologist Stephen Feig. Larry Norton, president of the American Society of Clinical Oncology, added, 'This is a very impressive study' that 'clinches the case for mammography'.

Five days later, I was interviewed for the *Chicago Tribune*:[16]

> Millions of women woke up one day last week to news that the last word had been written in the debate over mammography screening. Newspapers, TV and radio stations reported what many described as the definitive study, proving beyond doubt that getting routine mammograms sharply reduces a woman's chances of dying of breast cancer . . . Too bad it wasn't true. Once again, many in the media fell victim to the well-intentioned authors of a new study without questioning the study's merits or calling an independent expert for a second opinion. Hey, it was published in a scientific journal – it must be right.

The deep irony in all this is that we do randomised trials because this is the most reliable design we have to study the effect of interventions. Then, when the effect is still uncertain after having randomised half a million women and followed them for many years, researchers with vested interests use flawed designs and claim that it has now been proven beyond doubt that mammography screening works. Think of a court case where the judge doesn't find the best available evidence convincing for reaching a verdict and therefore acquits the accused. Would a judge then reopen the case and accept flawed evidence instead and reach a verdict 'beyond doubt'?

Tabár, Duffy and Smith published yet a third 'beyond reason' study in the

Lancet in 2003.[17] I wrote to the *Lancet* that their paper was uninterpretable because of length and lead-time biases.[18] This time, the authors also reported significant decreases in deaths from all causes, and from all cancers, in women with breast cancer, and claimed that this provided support to breast cancer death as a reliable endpoint. Their argument is obviously invalid. When one adds many healthy, overdiagnosed women to the screened group by giving them an unnecessary breast cancer diagnosis, women in this group will of course live longer than women in the control group.

In their reply, Tabár, Duffy and Smith demonstrated an ignorance one would have thought impossible for researchers with so many publications on cancer screening behind them. Furthermore, they blatantly misrepresented their own research.[19] They denied that their results could have been the product of lead-time and length biases, and argued that they had observed a reduction in absolute mortality *in the population invited to screening*.

As they were lying, I sent a second letter to *Lancet* pointing this out. Nowhere in their paper did they report on absolute mortality *in the population invited to screening*. They reported on absolute mortality only *in women with a diagnosis of breast cancer*, which is clear from their abstract, the introduction, the methods section, the results section and the discussion section. This makes a world of a difference.

The editor didn't wish to publish my second letter but sent it to the authors and encouraged me to get an answer directly from Duffy. I wrote to Duffy and asked whether he could inform me where in his paper I could find the data he had described or whether his reply was erroneous. Duffy avoided answering my question and replied, 'We published the absolute mortality reduction from breast tumours diagnosed in the periods studied and this is not affected by lead-time or length bias.' This statement is indisputably false.

I wrote back and noted that I was right that Duffy's reply in the *Lancet* was misleading since he didn't report on 'absolute mortality in the population invited to screening' in his paper. Duffy didn't reply to that email. However, 2 months later, his co-author Tabár wrote a comment about their study in the *Läkartidningen* where he noted that the mortality decrease had been observed *among women with breast cancer*.[20] Thus, Tabár contradicted not only what he wrote in his letter in *Lancet* with Duffy and Smith but also what Duffy wrote to me. The problem with dishonesty is that sooner or later people usually contradict themselves.

Duffy, Tabár and Smith never admitted the fatal flaws in their 'beyond reason' studies, although they are basic knowledge for cancer researchers.[1,8] These flaws were also carefully explained to them on several occasions in correspondences, but this didn't deter them from publishing yet a fourth 'beyond reason' study in 2006, where they claimed that screening had reduced breast cancer mortality by 40%–45%.[21]

Duffy, Tabár, and usually also Smith, have published at least six 'beyond reason' studies,[2,14,17,21–23] and have used them effectively in their screening propaganda.

In 2010, Duffy, Tabár, Nyström and others claimed in *Cancer* that screening in Sweden had reduced breast cancer mortality in women aged 40–49 years by 26%.[23] But they used unclear methods, with complex matching of screened and unscreened areas, and they added and subtracted person-years based on assumed lead times. They were also selective regarding the biases they adjusted for, and if they had adjusted for a prescreening difference in breast cancer mortality of 6%, the effect would have been smaller. *Cancer* rejected our letter to the editor with a curious comment: 'Although it is a possibility to publish letters independent of a response from the authors of the original article, we decline to do so in this case.' We complained to the editor saying that 'whether letters are published should have nothing to do with whether the authors respond to criticism of their work. In fact, it might be even more important to publish letters when the authors refuse to respond, as it suggests there are serious problems with their work, which we believe our letter demonstrate is the case.' We also noted that the American Cancer Society is a political advocacy group and owns the journal *Cancer*, which means that the journal should be very careful to avoid the possibility that conflicts of interest influence editorial decisions. And we drew attention to the fact that the study we criticised provides support to the political agenda of the society, which is to continue to recommend routine breast screening of all women aged 40–49 years.

Our appeal worked, but it took 5 months before our letter was accepted.[24] We noted in it that it is more reliable to count the number of deaths. The breast cancer mortality rate in Sweden in women aged 40–49 years has declined 36% since 1989, although only half were offered screening, whereas the decline was only 16% in women aged 50–69 years who were all offered screening for over 20 years.[25]

Criticism of our work in the *Journal of Surgical Oncology*

In December 2002, Duffy, Tabár and Smith published a criticism of our work in the *Journal of Surgical Oncology*[26] they had published twice before, in another journal[27] and on the homepage of the American Cancer Society. The editor explained that he felt the screening issues had been discussed in such a meaningful way that it would be valuable to reproduce it for his own readership.[28]

I was invited to comment[29] but was not forewarned that I would become the middle of a sandwich, with the Duffy/Tabár/Smith trio on either side, as they responded to my comment in the same issue.[30] The editor seemed determined not to leave any flanks open. He wrote an editorial where he described our *Lancet* review as being selective and remarked that the press coverage seemed committed to exposing what was implied to be another medical hoax, which was why he needed to counter the negative publicity.[28]

Duffy, Tabár and Smith pooled the results from all the trials in a summary estimate, despite the fact that, for example, the Edinburgh trial was so flawed as to be unsalvageable. Furthermore, they preferred, as they said, 'to use the original primary research material where available, rather than figures reported in secondary research',[30] i.e. they used 24% reduction for Östergötland, rather than the 10% reduction that was based on official mortality statistics.[31]

In their paper, they quoted data from their first 'beyond reason' study, without mentioning any of the devastating criticisms that it evoked. They also said that we had dismissed the scientific evidence with 'great confidence, authority, and little detail'. Little detail? Our review is the most comprehensive review of the screening trials that has ever been performed. The main text of our publications in the *Lancet* and *The Cochrane Library* in 2001 took up 11 725 and 10 966 words, respectively, which in both cases correspond to the size of four standard research papers.

There were 'numerous fundamental flaws' in our judgements, they said, but their comments were not relevant and most were misleading or misinterpreted what we had written. In particular, there were no arithmetic inconsistencies, as they claimed. We used the best data we could find, and we can hardly be blamed for the fact that the trialists have often been inconsistent with their numbers. Duffy, Tabár and Smith provided five examples, which were groundless and which I rejected.

To no avail, of course. In the upper part of the sandwich, which is the side people see, my opponents just became even more unreasonable.[30] Although we had adhered to Cochrane principles, we were now told that we had broken fundamental rules of science and that it was absurd to use all-cause mortality or all-cause cancer mortality as end points in a screening trial.

The worst mistake Duffy, Tabár and Smith made was that they considered it especially nonsensical to compare the entire invited and non-invited populations. This is exactly what a randomised trial does in order to avoid bias! They referred to one of their 'beyond reason' papers where they had restricted their analysis of the Two-County trial to *women with a diagnosis of breast cancer*. The paper they quoted reported a 19% reduction in all-cause mortality, or 13% in a more conservative analysis.[22] That paper is perhaps the most unreasonable of all their 'beyond reason' papers. A year later, they repeated their misleading claim of a 13% decrease in all-cause mortality.[32]

Think about it. Duffy, Tabár and Smith apparently wish us to believe that screening leads to a large reduction in all-cause mortality – which it doesn't and which isn't possible – and they arrived at this spurious result by using inappropriate methods.

Duffy, Tabár and Smith seem to be well aware of the biases they have introduced in paper after paper of the 'beyond reason' type, as they have published many papers where they discuss them and claim they have taken them into account in their analyses. This they obviously haven't, at least not fully.

I have rejected their other arguments in other publications, including the Cochrane review, but this is unlikely to impress Duffy, Tabár and Smith, who wrote that many scientists and clinicians have devoted 'hundreds of hours to soberly and carefully refuting the irresponsible and reckless claims of Olsen and Gøtzsche, hours they otherwise might have devoted to their current work'.

From my perspective, it's the other way round. At The Nordic Cochrane Centre, we have used not hundreds of hours but, rather, years to refute 'irresponsible and reckless claims'. I believe that the claim by Duffy, Tabár and Smith that screening reduces all-cause mortality by 13% has ruined their credibility.

References

1 Vainio H, Bianchini F. *Breast Cancer Screening*. IARC Handbooks of Cancer Prevention, Vol 7. Lyon, France: IARC Press; 2002.
2 Tabár L, Vitak B, Chen HH, *et al*. Beyond randomized controlled trials: organized mammographic screening substantially reduces breast carcinoma mortality. *Cancer*. 2001; **91**(9): 1724–31.
3 Letters. Beyond randomized controlled trials. *Cancer*. 2002; **94**: 578–83.
4 Gøtzsche PC. Beyond randomized controlled trials: organized mammographic screening substantially reduces breast carcinoma mortality. *Cancer*. 2002; **94**(2): 578.
5 Tabár L. [The term 'early breast cancer' is misleading] [Swedish]. *Läkartidningen*. 1991; **88**(47): 3996.
6 Rutqvist L, Rydén S. [Reply to the term 'early breast cancer' is misleading] [Swedish]. *Läkartidningen*. 1991; **88**(47): 3996.
7 Zahl P-H, Jørgensen KJ, Mæhlen J, *et al*. Biases in estimates of overdetection due to mammography screening. *Lancet Oncol*. 2008; **9**(3): 199–201.
8 Berry DA. The utility of mammography for women 40 to 50 years of age (Con). In: DeVita

VT, Hellman S, Rosenberg S, editors. *Progress in Oncology*. Sudbury: Jones & Bartlett; 2002. pp. 346–72.

9 Tabár L, Duffy SW, Smith RA. Beyond randomized controlled trials. Authors' reply. *Cancer*. 2002; **94**(2): 581–3.

10 Cady B, Michaelson JS. The life-sparing potential of mammographic screening. *Cancer*. 2001; **91**(9): 1699–703.

11 Mayor S. Study confirms that screening reduces deaths from breast cancer. *BMJ*. 2001; **322**(7295): 1140.

12 Minerva. *BMJ*. 2001; **322**(7296): 1256.

13 Dean P. [Mammographic screening is a reliable examination method] [Swedish]. *Läkartidningen*. 2001; **98**(51–52): 5924–6.

14 Tabár L, Yen MF, Vitak B, *et al*. Mammography service screening and mortality in breast cancer patients: 20-year follow-up before and after introduction of screening. *Lancet*. 2003; **361**(9367): 1405–10.

15 Duffy SW, Tabár L, Chen HH, *et al*. The impact of organized mammography service screening on breast carcinoma mortality in seven Swedish counties: a collaborative evaluation. *Cancer*. 2002; **95**(3): 458–69.

16 Maugh TH. New study validates benefits of mammograms. *Los Angeles Times*. 2002 Aug 1.

17 Women and mammograms. *Chicago Tribune*. 2002 Aug 6.

18 Gøtzsche PC. Mammographic service screening and mortality. *Lancet*. 2003; **362**(9380): 329–30.

19 Duffy SW, Tabár L, Smith RA. Mammographic service screening and mortality. *Lancet*. 2003; **362**: 330.

20 Tabár L. [Screening with mammography contributes substantially to a significant reduction in breast cancer mortality] [Swedish]. *Läkartidningen*. 2003; **100**: 3211.

21 Swedish Organised Service Screening Evaluation Group. Reduction in breast cancer mortality from organized service screening with mammography: 1. Further confirmation with extended data. *Cancer Epidemiol Biomarkers Prev*. 2006; **15**(1): 45–51.

22 Tabár L, Duffy SW, Yen MF, *et al*. All-cause mortality among breast cancer patients in a screening trial: support for breast cancer mortality as an end point. *J Med Screen*. 2002; **9**(4): 159–62.

23 Hellquist BN, Duffy SW, Abdsaleh S, *et al*. Effectiveness of population-based service screening with mammography for women ages 40 to 49 years: evaluation of the Swedish Mammography Screening in Young Women (SCRY) cohort. *Cancer*. 2011; **117**(4): 714–22.

24 Jørgensen KJ, Gøtzsche PC. Unclear methods in estimate of screening effect in women aged 40–49 years. *Cancer*. Epub 2011 Jul 15.

25 Autier P, Boniol M, La Vecchia C, *et al*. Disparities in breast cancer mortality trends between 30 European countries: retrospective trend analysis of WHO mortality database. *BMJ*. 2010; **341**: c3620.

26 Duffy SW, Tabár L, Smith RA. The mammographic screening trials: commentary on the recent work by Olsen and Gøtzsche. *J Surg Oncol*. 2002; **81**(4): 159–62.

27 Duffy SW, Tabár L, Smith RA. The mammographic screening trials: commentary on the recent work by Olsen and Gøtzsche. *CA Cancer J Clin*. 2002; **52**(2): 68–71.

28 Lawrence W Jr. Editorial commentary: screening mammography. *J Surg Oncol*. 2002; **81**(4): 159.

29 Gøtzsche PC. Invited reponse. *J Surg Oncol*. 2002; **81**: 162–3.

30 Smith RA, Duffy S, Tabár L. The authors reply. *J Surg Oncol*. 2002; **81**: 164–6.
31 Nyström L, Andersson I, Bjurstam N, *et al*. Long-term effects of mammography screening: updated overview of the Swedish randomised trials. *Lancet*. 2002; **359**(9310): 909–19.
32 Duffy SW, Tabár L, Vitak B, *et al*. The Swedish Two-County trial of mammographic screening: cluster randomisation and end point evaluation. *Ann Oncol*. 2003; **14**(8): 1196–8.

15

Other observational studies of breast cancer mortality

TABÁR, DUFFY AND SMITH ARE NOT ALONE. THE SCIENTIFIC LITERATURE on breast screening is replete with exaggerated claims based on poor-quality observational studies. The vast majority of these unreliable papers have been written by screening advocates with a vested interest in mammography, particularly radiologists and people involved with screening programmes. Most people who know it is wrong just shrug their shoulders, as they haven't time to 'police' all this. For my part, I have usually only sent letters to the editor when grossly misleading or erroneous papers were published in the *BMJ* or the *Lancet*.

One such paper was published in the *Lancet* in 2003. It described a significant decrease in breast cancer mortality in the Netherlands after screening was introduced.[1] However, a similar decrease had occurred in young women who had not been invited to screening.[2] Furthermore, the authors had cherry-picked countries when they argued that the mortality had declined in some countries that have screening. The same had happened in some countries that didn't have a national screening programme, e.g. in Austria, Germany and Switzerland.[2] I also noted that the age-standardised decrease in breast cancer mortality in Europe was larger in those young age groups that are generally not invited to screening.[3] Other researchers mentioned that the use of adjuvant therapy had increased substantially in the same time period and that it was therefore not possible to separate the possible effect of screening from the effect of better treatment.[4]

It is surprising what slips under the radar of otherwise critical editors and peer reviewers. However, I recently found a rare honest account. Mette Kalager from the Norwegian Cancer Registry and others had looked at breast cancer survival before and after screening was introduced in Norway, just like Tabár, Duffy and Smith had done for Sweden. However, the Norwegians wrote they were unable to adjust for the biases and attributed the increase in survival following the introduction of the mammography screening programmes not to screening but to better management of breast cancer.[5]

Only a year later, in 2010, Kalager and her colleagues published a study in the *New England Journal of Medicine* where they *had* taken the biases into account.[6] They reported a 10% reduction in breast cancer mortality that was not statistically significant ($p = 0.13$) and therefore uncertain. Moreover, they found that most of this little decline was due to better organisation, treatment and breast cancer awareness.

The United States and the United Kingdom

A paper of quite another calibre than Tabár's 'beyond reason' studies was published in the *New England Journal of Medicine* in 2005 by Donald Berry and colleagues.[7] A consortium of investigators had developed seven independent statistical models of breast cancer incidence and mortality based on US data and concluded that screening and adjuvant treatment had contributed about equally to the reduction in breast cancer mortality, and that screening had reduced it by about 15%.

The authors' conclusion was cautious because the increasing use of adjuvant therapy and screening occurred during the same time period; therefore, it is difficult to separate them. A correspondent furthermore noted that because all the models used the same data, any bias would probably appear in all analyses.[8] For example, the statistical models were adjusted for a strong underlying increase in the breast cancer incidence, which was caused by screening and should therefore not have been adjusted for. I pointed out that some countries with national screening programmes (e.g. Sweden) had had little change in breast cancer mortality, whereas others without screening (e.g. Germany and Austria) had had improvements in death rates paralleling those in the United States, and I therefore felt that the estimate of a 15% effect was more likely to be a chance finding than real, particularly because there had been an unusual change in the trend in breast cancer mortality in the United States that coincided with screening becoming more widespread. I suggested that the US study should be replicated in other countries, including those with a reduction in mortality without screening and those without a reduction despite screening, and that such studies should also include young women who are not invited to screening. The authors agreed to this suggestion, but the study hasn't been done. I have already mentioned the large study in the United Kingdom published in the *BMJ* in 2000 that reported a 6% reduction in breast cancer mortality with screening.[9]

Denmark, Lynge's 2005 study

We generally cannot use observational studies to prove that an intervention is beneficial, as the effect is usually too small, compared with the inevitable biases in such studies. We use randomised trials to avoid bias. However, once an effect has been proven, observational studies can be important for evaluating whether the beneficial effect seen in the trials can be reproduced in clinical practice. It is not rare for an intervention that worked well in trials not to work equally well in day-to-day practice.

Denmark is unique in the world for observational studies of the effect of breast screening because there is a concomitant non-screened control group. For 17 years, screening was only offered in about 20% of the country, measured as population size.[10] I will describe first a study from 2005 by Anne Helene Olsen, Elsebeth Lynge and colleagues, and next our own study. Both were published in the *BMJ*.

Lynge and colleagues compared Copenhagen, where screening was introduced in 1991, with non-screened areas in Denmark and reported a 25% reduction in breast cancer mortality that they attributed to screening.[11]

However, there are four major concerns with this result. First, the authors used a statistical model that was unusually complicated: 'We used a Poisson regression model with a study group, a historical control group, a national control group, and a historical national control group.' It doesn't get any easier to follow their methods as one reads on, e.g. 'For all three control groups we constructed five, two year, "pseudo-invitation" rounds and allocated pseudo-invitation dates by using the invitation system from the study group.' The choice of model can have a substantial impact on the results, and 2 years later, Lynge and Olsen reported results from several models, one of which showed an *increase* in breast cancer mortality in Copenhagen compared with non-screened areas.[12] The authors asserted that the model they published originally should be preferred, but didn't explain why. None of the models were validated, and it isn't clear whether the preferred model – which gave the most favourable result for screening – was selected after all the models had been tried first.

Second, the *full* mortality reduction appeared already 3 years after screening started and didn't increase in the remaining observation period. The mechanism of screening is to advance the time of diagnosis, and an effect is therefore not expected to appear in the first years, but is expected to emerge after about 5 years and to increase with further follow-up. When the use of a model gives results that contrast markedly with previous, solid knowledge, the model should be discarded.

Third, the study only included Copenhagen. This was curious, as the county of Funen introduced screening in 1993, has a population of similar size and has a higher proportion of 'faithful users' (76% vs 53%),[10] and also because the head of the Funen screening programme was among the authors.

Fourth, the study didn't describe breast cancer mortality rates in women who were too young or too old to have benefited from screening, although the absence of similar reductions in breast cancer mortality among these women would have strengthened the study's conclusions.

Some of these concerns were raised in letters to the editor.[13–15] Zahl and Mæhlen used an official register and found that in the age group 35–54 years, which can benefit very little from screening, breast cancer mortality declined by 19%. We noted that the authors had not declared any conflicts of interest, although two of them were heads of screening units, and the attendance rate in Copenhagen had dropped to 63%, which is well below the minimum acceptable level of 70% and the desirable level of 75% required for a screening programme, according to the European guidelines for quality assurance in mammography screening.[16] We argued that this conflict of interest could potentially have influenced the authors' interpretation of the data.

The authors replied that we tried to discredit their study 'by use of insinuations, a debate we will not waste time on', but a correspondent noted that this was untrue, as our comment was a statement of fact.[15] A continued low participation rate could lead to the abandonment of the programme.

In their reply to Zahl and Mæhlen, the authors argued that with their model, breast cancer mortality decreased 6% in women aged 40–49 years.[15] However, this was with a wide confidence interval, which went from a 31% decrease to a 27% increase, and it was therefore not a convincing rebuttal. Furthermore, Zahl and Mæhlen followed up on this and noted that, according to Statistics Denmark, there was a 20% drop in breast cancer mortality both in the invited age group 50–69 years and in the uninvited age group 40–49 years.[15]

Then Stephen Duffy joined the debate:[15] 'With respect to criticisms of the Copenhagen mammography study, Dr Lynge's response is measured and correct. With its control for temporal and spatial effects, the Copenhagen study is a model of rigorous evaluation and honest interpretation.' Such undeserved praise – complete empty of scientific arguments – was also heard about Tabár's 'beyond reason' studies that Duffy co-authored. Duffy turned a blind eye to what Zahl and Mæhlen had just demonstrated, arguing that:

> those who believe that the breast cancer mortality reduction observed is due to other factors, have to explain why it did not occur in areas not served by the mammography programme. They have not convincingly done so. Accusations of conflict of interest represent a failure to engage with the scientific issues and are in any case unworthy of debate in the *BMJ*. It is high time this discussion grew up.

As far as I can see, it was Duffy who, in his own words, failed to engage with the scientific issues.

After Duffy's attempt at rescuing the drowning study came a letter from a Danish researcher, Anders Beich, who noted that the question of competing interests was highly relevant, as we all have a tendency to become what we do and defend ourselves tooth and nail, especially if met by criticism of a life's work, the things some even hope to be remembered for. Beich also noted that he had attended meetings on mammography where one of the authors made presentations on the bliss of breast cancer screening in a way that would make Scientologists and used-car salesmen green with envy, and he added that it did not raise the credibility of the paper that this author was now evaluating breast cancer screening in Denmark.

Denmark, our 2010 study

As we had good reason to distrust Lynge's study, and as Denmark is so unique, we decided to do our own study.[10] We used simple and transparent methods and avoided the use of statistical modelling, which is very bias prone.[10] We included the whole country and age groups that couldn't have benefited from screening and also added data from five additional years.

Using Poisson regression analyses, adjusted for temporal changes in age distribution, we found that the decline in breast cancer mortality was 1% per year in women who could benefit from screening (ages 55–74 years) in the screening areas during the 10-year period when screening could have had an effect (1997–2006), whereas it was 2% per year in the non-screening areas. The decline was 5% per year in women who were too young to benefit from screening (ages 35–55 years) in the screened areas, and 6% per year in the non-screened areas in the same time period (*see* Figure 15.1).

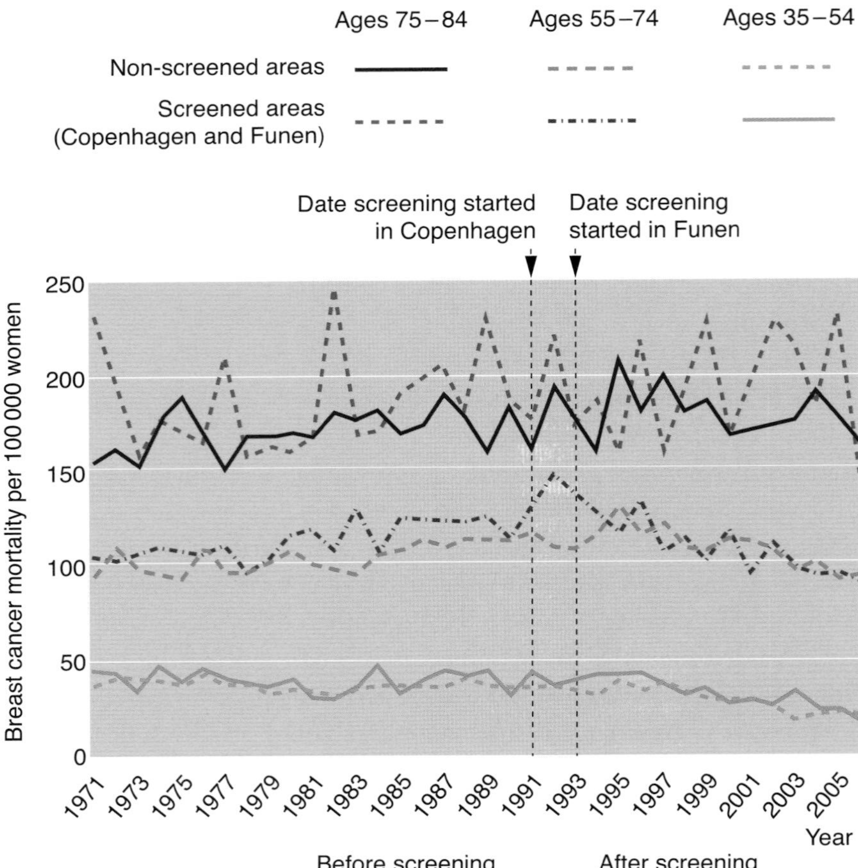

FIGURE 15.1 Unadjusted breast cancer mortality rates for screened and non-screened areas in Denmark

For the older age groups (75–84 years), there was little change over time, both in screened and in non-screened areas.

Thus, we were unable to find an effect of the Danish screening programme on breast cancer mortality. As the reductions in breast cancer mortality were similar or greater in non-screened areas and in younger age groups than in those screened, they are more likely explained by improved treatment, changes in risk factors, and greater breast cancer awareness than by screening mammography.

Since Denmark is the only country with a contemporary unscreened control group and since our results are so clear, our paper was probably the most threatening for the screening advocates of all the papers we had published. Indeed, our research was attacked by the whole choir: Robert Smith, Stephen Duffy, Elsebeth Lynge, Daniel Kopans, Peter Dean, László Tabár and Lennart Nyström. Almost all of the many comments were written by authors that included people with vested interests and they focused on very minor issues that were not important for our results.[17] *This tactic has been called 'weapons of mass distraction'.*

A comment from the Danish Breast Cancer Group (DBCG) was particularly miserable.[17] It stated that, 'DBCG, which represents all the professional expertise of breast cancer diagnosis and treatment in Denmark strongly take exception from the conclusions of the Cochrane Centre.' Well, as just noted, our conclusions were derived from our sound results in a straightforward fashion, and we didn't say anything about whether or not there should be screening in Denmark. We said: 'We believe it is time to question whether screening has delivered the promised effect on breast cancer mortality.'[10] That is a very modest conclusion, as we had just shown screening didn't work.

DBCG furthermore drew the 'you are killing my patients' card: 'It gives rise to considerable professional anxiety that the public attention now leads to womens cancellation from mammography. This may probably lead to unnecessary breast cancer deaths in the future.' We seriously doubt this is true, as we couldn't see any effect. Furthermore, DBCG doesn't consider the harms of screening.

DBCG mentioned an analysis it had made[17] that showed that during the past 30 years, the 5-year mortality had decreased from 'barely 40% to barely 20%', and interpreted this as an effect of better treatment, but also as an effect of earlier diagnosis. Not a word about just how misleading 5-year survival is. Then came an equally misleading argument:

> However, the overall breast cancer mortality is still higher than in our Nordic neighbour-countries, who have had national mammography screening programmes since many years. It is therefore fortunate that eventually we have now nation-wide mammography screening in Denmark. As a result treatment can be introduced at an earlier stage when the tumour is smaller with less frequent positive axillary lymph nodes. As a consequence a larger proportion can be offered breast conserving treatment and modest axillary surgery.

Researchers from the Danish Cancer Society were more truthful when they published a paper comparing Denmark and Sweden and noted that a 10% difference in survival (survival being highest in Sweden) among breast cancer patients had existed for the past 40 years, far longer than the time at which mammographic screening was begun in either country.[18] It is remarkable that Henning Mouridsen co-authored this paper, as he also co-authored the ill-placed criticism of our *BMJ* paper as a member of DBCG, thereby contradicting himself. Furthermore, even in 2010, it hasn't dawned on 'all the professional expertise of breast cancer diagnosis and treatment in Denmark'[17] that screening leads to more mastectomies.

Even more bizarre, DBCG wrote that we raised 'unfounded doubts about the quality of breast cancer treatment in Denmark. The authors must be aware about the nation-wide, internationally adapted guidelines for diagnostic procedures and treatment which are currently quality-controlled.'[17] Yes, we are and we actually mentioned these guidelines in our *BMJ* paper.[10] We noted that national guidelines for breast cancer treatment had been in use in Denmark since 1977 and added that guidelines may not be used to the letter in clinical practice. We gave an example of this: 'In January 2007, for example, several women in one of the non-screened regions were compensated financially for having received treatment that did not live up to "best specialist standards."'[10] Only 4 days before DBCG criticised us in the *BMJ*, an article in a national newspaper described a DBCG report, which showed large differences in the use of breast-conserving surgery between hospitals in Denmark. The Danish Cancer Society stated that it was unacceptable that most women in some hospitals had their whole breast removed. It is blatantly and inexcusably dishonest to try to put the blame on us for describing suboptimal treatment of breast cancer, which the DBCG had just documented themselves.

The DBCG also put the blame on the *BMJ* in a way that is so typical of screening advocates:[17]

> An attempt from The Nordic Cochrane Centre to question the value of the Danish mammography screening programme (1) has been extensively rejected by leading international experts, who also strongly criticize that the distinguished *British Medical Journal (BMJ)* uncritically has published this biased report.

It isn't helpful for science to raise the voice, boast authority and shoot the messenger. As a matter of fact, our paper was peer-reviewed twice and the *BMJ*'s statistician took great care, as the journal wanted to be sure we were right before it published such a provocative finding.

DBCG also wrote a press release, 'Massive international support for the Danish mammography screening examinations', which they sent to the Minister of Health, the Danish regions and the directors at my hospital. Like their letter in the *BMJ*, which it echoed, it was so misleading that we had to issue our own press release explaining the errors.

A newspaper article reported that twice as many women as usual had cancelled their appointments as a consequence of our paper, and the heads of the two major screening units in Denmark, Ilse Vejborg and Walter Schwartz, declared that our paper would lead to loss of lives.[19] Well, if the number cancelling appointments is very small, which I think it is, then double this number is also very small. We were not told what this number was out of the total. Schwartz used the 'everybody agrees' trick by describing us as a 'small group of Danes who had been against screening all the time' and by saying, 'The whole Western world screens for breast cancer. Are we all wrong, and a few people at the Cochrane centre are right?' A leading radiologist was 'very angry' and used the same trick when he talked about a witch-hunt and smear campaign from a small group of people who were outside real life and who were grossly manipulative. I explained that I wasn't worried about the cancellations, as we clearly write in our information leaflet about screening (*see* Chapter 19) that it may be equally reasonable not to attend as to attend screening. I added that our results made it difficult to recommend in favour of screening.

Robert Smith and Stephen Duffy sang the usual refrain about our paper having 'multiple methodological failures' and said that 'to argue that there is no benefit from modern mammography on the basis of such flawed methods means this paper only feeds the medias hunger for controversy, but contributes nothing of substance to the evidence or the on-going debate.'[17] It was easy to dismiss the various criticisms,[17] and our data speak for themselves, unadulterated as they are from massage in statistical models until they confess and give the 'right' answer.[20]

In our 2010 *BMJ* paper on the lack of effect in Denmark, we also noted that, using official mortality statistics, we couldn't see any effect of screening in the United Kingdom or in Sweden.[10] The same applies to the Netherlands, where a larger decline in mortality has been observed in young women than in those invited to screening.[21] Harry de Koning and colleagues[22] suggested otherwise when they wrote in a paper from 2008, 'These results show the profound impact that the implementation of a screening program can have on mortality.' This statement is amazing, as the numbers they presented suggested that screening doesn't work in the Netherlands. The annual decrease in breast cancer mortality was 2.7% in those aged 35–44 years (who cannot benefit from screening) and it was 2.3% and 2.8% in those aged 55–64 and 65–74 years, respectively, who can benefit from it. Thus, their conclusion had no relation whatsoever to their data.

On this background, it is even more amazing that Daniel Kopans in 2009 wrote that studies in Sweden and the Netherlands had shown that at least two-thirds of the decrease in deaths is due to mammography screening.[23] This deserves to be repeated: *at least two-thirds*. Amusingly, the title of Kopan's paper is 'Why the critics of screening mammography are wrong: they distort data, rely on weak science, but refuse to defend when challenged'. This is exactly what Kopans does. To a degree that is beyond belief.

I shall provide some perspective on Kopans's misguided beliefs. In 2010, Philippe Autier and colleagues[24] published breast cancer mortality trends for 30 European countries. These data were so striking that we asked: Where is the effect of mammography screening?[25] Breast cancer mortality had decreased more in women below 50 years of age (median 37% decrease) than in the age range most commonly invited to screening, 50–69 years (median 21% decrease), and *the decreases had consistently started several years before screening could have had an effect*.

Screening advocates both in and outside Denmark have repeatedly claimed that the lower breast cancer mortality in Sweden compared with Denmark is attributable to screening.[26] This argument has also been used by the Danish Cancer Society in its efforts to extend screening to the whole country.[27] However, as already noted, breast cancer mortality has always been lower in Sweden, and it is ironic that it was researchers from the Danish Cancer Society who demolished this argument in a paper from 2004.[18] Perhaps the propaganda department doesn't speak to the research department at the Cancer Society? The new *BMJ* paper showed that this difference between Sweden and Denmark has been present for the past 50 years, and there hasn't been any change in the continuous downward trend in Sweden since 1972, which is long before screening started in the late 1980s.[24] Furthermore, a difference between the two countries has been observed for other cancers, none of which are screened for in either country. The difference is generally attributed to variation in lifestyle, such as alcohol and smoking. Finally, *the decline in breast cancer mortality since 1989 has been markedly greater in Denmark than in Sweden*, 49% versus 36% in women under 50 years of age, and 26% versus 16% in women aged 50–69 years.[24] This has occurred despite the fact that parts of Sweden have offered screening to women in their forties; that Sweden has had nationwide screening for about 15 years with attendance rates of over 90%; and that Denmark has only had screening for about 20% of its population, with very little opportunistic screening of the remaining 80%, and attendance rates of only 60%–70%.[10]

In 2011, Autier published another revealing study.[28] It compared three pairs of very similar neighbouring countries that had introduced screening 10–15 years apart. The country pairs were Northern Ireland and the Republic of Ireland, the Netherlands and Belgium, and Sweden and Norway. There was no relation between start of screening and the reduction in breast cancer mortality. The fall in breast cancer mortality was about the same in all countries. Furthermore, the decline was also about the same as that seen in the United States, where screening started as early as in Sweden.[29] An Australian study found that most, if not all, of the reduction in breast cancer mortality could be attributed to adjuvant hormonal and chemotherapy.[30]

References

1 Otto SJ, Fracheboud J, Looman CWN, *et al*. Initiation of population-based mammography screening in Dutch municipalitites and effect on breast-cancer mortality: a systematic review. *Lancet*. 2003; **361**(9367): 1411–17.
2 Gøtzsche PC. Mortality reduction by breast-cancer screening. *Lancet*. 2003; **362**(9379): 246.
3 Levi F, Lucchini F, Negri E, *et al*. The fall in breast cancer mortality in Europe. *Eur J Cancer*. 2001; **37**(11): 1409–12.
4 Voogd AC, Coebergh JWW. Mortality reduction by breast-cancer screening. *Lancet*. 2003; **362**(9379): 245–6.
5 Kalager M, Haldorsen T, Bretthauer M, *et al*. Improved breast cancer survival following introduction of an organized mammography screening program among both screened and unscreened women: a population-based cohort study. *Breast Cancer Res*. 2009; **11**(4): R44.
6 Kalager M, Zelen M, Langmark F, *et al*. Effect of screening mammography on breast-cancer mortality in Norway. *N Engl J Med*. 2010; **363**(13): 1203–10.
7 Berry DA, Cronin KA, Plevritis SK, *et al*. Effect of screening and adjuvant therapy on mortality from breast cancer. *N Engl J Med*. 2005; **353**(17): 1784–92.
8 Letters. Screening and breast cancer. *N Engl J Med*. 2006; **354**(7): 767–9.
9 Blanks RG, Moss SM, McGahan CE, *et al*. Effect of NHS Breast Screening Programme on mortality from breast cancer in England and Wales, 1990–98: comparison of observed with predicted mortality. *BMJ*. 2000; **321**(7262): 665–9.
10 Jørgensen KJ, Zahl PH, Gøtzsche PC. Breast cancer mortality in organised mammography screening in Denmark: comparative study. *BMJ*. 2010; **340**: c1241.
11 Olsen AH, Njor SH, Vejborg I, *et al*. Breast cancer mortality in Copenhagen after introduction of mammography screening: cohort study. *BMJ*. 2005; **330**(7485): 220–4.
12 Olsen AH, Njor SH, Lynge E. Estimating the benefits of mammography screening: the impact of study design. *Epidemiology*. 2007; **18**(4): 487–92.
13 Gøtzsche PC, Thornton H, Jørgensen KJ. Reduction in mortality from breast cancer: presentation of benefits and harms needs to be balanced. *BMJ*. 2005; **330**(7498): 1024.
14 Zahl P-H, Mæhlen J. Reduction in mortality from breast cancer: decrease with screening was marked in younger age group. *BMJ*. 2005; **330**(7498): 1024.
15 Letters. *BMJ*. 2005. Available at: http://bmj.bmjjournals.com/cgi/eletters/330/7485/220 (accessed 22 May 2011).
16 Perry N, Broeders M, de Wolf C, *et al*, editors. European Commission. *European Guidelines for Quality Assurance in Breast Cancer Screening and Diagnosis*. 4th ed. Luxembourg: Office for Official Publications of the European Communities; 2006.
17 Letters. *BMJ*. 2010. Available at: www.bmj.com/cgi/eletters/340/mar23_1/c1241 (accessed 22 May 2011).
18 Christensen LH, Engholm G, Ceberg J, *et al*. Can the survival difference between

breast cancer patients in Denmark and Sweden 1989 and 1994 be explained by patho-anatomical variables? A population-based study. *Eur J Cancer*. 2004; **40**(8): 1233–43.

19 Albinus N-B. [Women cancel mammography twice as often than usual] [Danish]. *Dagens Medicin*. 2010 April 23.

20 Mills JL. Data torturing. *N Engl J Med*. 1993; **329**(16): 1196–9.

21 Bonneux L. [Advantages and disadvantages of breast cancer screening: time for evidence-based information] [Dutch]. *Ned Tijdschr Geneeskd*. 2009; **153**: A887.

22 Otten JD, Broeders MJ, Fracheboud J, *et al*. Impressive time-related influence of the Dutch screening programme on breast cancer incidence and mortality, 1975–2006. *Int J Cancer*. 2008; **123**(8): 1929–34.

23 Kopans DB. Why the critics of screening mammography are wrong: they distort data, rely on weak science, but refuse to defend when challenged. *Diagnostic Imaging*. 2009; **31**(12): 1–7.

24 Autier P, Boniol M, La Vecchia C, *et al*. Disparities in breast cancer mortality trends between 30 European countries: retrospective trend analysis of WHO mortality database. *BMJ*. 2010; **341**: c3620.

25 Jørgensen KJ, Gøtzsche PC. Where is the effect of mammography screening? *BMJ*. 2010 Aug 16. Available at: www.bmj.com/cgi/eletters/341/aug11_1/c3620 (accessed 22 May 2011).

26 Dean P, Tabár L, Yen M-F. Why does vehement opposition to screening come from Denmark, which has one of Europe's highest breast cancer mortality rates? *BMJ*. 2010 Apr 9. Available at: www.bmj.com/cgi/eletters/340/mar23_1/c1241#234181 (accessed 22 May 2011).

27 Hansen JH. [Denmark has the highest death rate for breast cancer] [Danish] *Information*. 2009 Dec 9.

28 Autier P, Boniol M, Gavin A, *et al*. Breast cancer mortality in neighbouring European countries with different levels of screening but similar access to treatment: trend analysis of WHO mortality database. *BMJ*. 2011; **343**: d4411.

29 Bleyer A. US breast cancer mortality is consistent with European data. *BMJ*. 2011; **343**: d5630.

30 Burton RC, Bell RJ, Thiagarajah G, *et al*. Adjuvant therapy, not mammographic screening, accounts for most of the observed breast cancer specific mortality reductions in Australian women since the national screening program began in 1991. *Breast Cancer Res Treat*. Epub 2011 Sep 29.

16

Overdiagnosis and overtreatment

WHEN WE WERE ASKED TO REVIEW THE BREAST SCREENING TRIALS in 1999, we had no experience with cancer, apart from my 6 months' work at a department of haematology. But haematological cancers, such as leukaemia, are very different from solid cancers and my co-author was a statistician, so we were unfamiliar with cancer screening. Nonetheless, we had no doubt that the worst harm would be overdiagnosis and overtreatment, which is why we looked for the number of operations.

We later discovered that the dishonesty about breast screening hasn't been more consistent, blatant, pronounced and shameless than when its major harms are concerned, overdiagnosis and overtreatment. It is often said that courtrooms are where people lie the most, but screening advocates, cancer charities and representatives of governments supporting screening programmes have massively denied that screening causes substantial harm to healthy people, a deception at least the equivalent of that in the courts.

One would have thought it impossible to conceal overdiagnosis and overtreatment from the public for decades. But that is exactly what has happened. A US survey from 2000 found that only 8% of 479 women were aware that participation in screening can harm healthy women.[1]

The collective denial that overdiagnosis is a problem with breast screening has manifested itself in bizarre ways. For example, some researchers, and particularly clinicians, have argued that since it is not possible to distinguish between an overdiagnosed cancer and a 'usual' cancer such as those found clinically, overdiagnosis is not a problem. This argument is invalid. It is an attempt at preserving the meaningfulness of the clinician's job and the meaningfulness of screening. It is not particularly meaningful for a surgeon to operate on people who don't need it.

As it is not possible to ascertain in the individual case whether a cancer is overdiagnosed or not unless it is followed up without treatment, which rarely happens, the only way overdiagnosis can be defined unambiguously is to do it at a statistical level. The statistical definition is simple and I repeat it from Chapter 2: *overdiagnosis* is the detection of cancers that would not have been identified clinically in someone's remaining lifetime.[2]

Overdiagnosis can be measured precisely in a randomised trial with lifelong follow-up if people are assigned to a screening or a control group for as long as screening would be offered in practice, which in most countries is 20 years for breast screening.[2] Overdiagnosis would then be the difference in number of cancers detected during the lifetime of the two groups, provided the control group and age groups not targeted are not screened.

Overdiagnosis can only be harmful to those who experience it,[3] and currently, all detected breast cancers are treated.[4]

It is well known that most cases of carcinoma *in situ* in the breast do not develop into potentially lethal invasive disease. In contrast, many find it difficult to accept that screening also leads to overdiagnosis of invasive cancer. Harmless invasive cancer is common,[2,4] even with lung cancer, which most people consider uniformly deadly, but after long-term follow-up of patients screened by radiography there was 30% overdiagnosis.[5] Autopsy studies have found many inconsequential breast cancer lesions. In a series of 110 medico-legal autopsies of young women aged 20–54 years, two cancers and 16 cases of ductal carcinoma *in situ* were found, and half of these lesions were visible on radiography.[6]

Cancers that regress spontaneously

Many overdiagnosed cancers are slow growing, and others would have regressed if left alone (*see* Chapter 2). It has been known for decades that many types of cancer can regress spontaneously and a gene has been identified in mice that is so effective in turning cancers on and off that it is almost like turning a light switch on and off.[7]

This knowledge has not been part of the debate on mammography screening. It was as if it didn't exist and had to be rediscovered, although it was clearly laid out in a paper in *JAMA* by Fox[8] in 1979. Fox spoke of regressing cancers and in a series of cases assembled between 1950 and 1973, he identified two subpopulations, one with a relative mortality rate of 25% per year (40% of cases) and one with a mortality rate of only 2.5% per year (60% of cases).[8] Fox wrote that the additional cancers detected at screening were localised and generally harmless.

This agrees well with the data from the Malmö trial I have mentioned earlier that demonstrated 97% 10-year survival for cancers detected at screening.[9] Fox also noted that in women with breast cancer, random biopsies in the other breast had detected cancer in 15%–20% of cases, although disease in the other breast only occurred at a rate of 0.5% per year. This also suggested a large reservoir of inconsequential cancer that might come to light through the use of aggressive diagnostic methods.

The next 25 years were surprisingly quiet about this important issue, although, in 1994, historian and writer Gillian Tindall noted in *Time* magazine that many cancers remit spontaneously.[10] A consultant told her, almost casually: 'Empires have now been constructed. Commitment is on the line. Of course, none of those people employed by the screening programmes can afford to admit that the theories on which they are based have something wrong with them.'

Tindall also wrote that the most discouraging aspect of the whole picture was the lack of general honesty. When a critical article had appeared in *Time* magazine a year earlier, in 1993, a key figure in the NHS Breast Screening Programme said that 'women who come for screening have their risk of dying reduced by 40 per cent'. Tindall asked for details and received a Department of Health Report from 1991 with a note referring her to a particular page. 'What this page turned out to contain was not hard figures but an optimistic, best-scenario projection, a piece of PR that told one nothing about the likely benefits or disbenefits to the individual.'[10] Sounds familiar, doesn't it? A correspondent, with no title attached, drew the 'you are killing my patients' card: 'I can only hope that Ms. Tindall's article will not cost any lives.'

In 2004, Zahl and colleagues[11] wrote in *JAMA* that screening detects so many additional cancers, not only at the prevalence screen but also at subsequent screens, that when all these cancers are accumulated there are many more of them than when women who are somewhat older are being screened. This suggests that many screen-detected cancers undergo spontaneous regression.

Two years later, a study in the *Journal of the National Cancer Institute* by US researchers looked at the breast cancer incidence and mortality rates in the US population during the period 1975–2000 when screening was introduced. In order to explain the observed trends, it was necessary to postulate that approximately 40% of the observed cancers had limited malignant potential and would have regressed if undetected.[12] Thus, these researchers found a large reservoir of exceedingly indolent breast cancers that appeared as a result of screening.

In 2006, Zahl and Mæhlen[13] reported similar results in the *International Journal of Cancer* based on published Swedish data on invasive breast cancers.[14] They concluded that most of the excess cancers would have regressed spontaneously if left untreated.[13] The Swedish researchers agreed with them that cancers regressed.[15]

Zahl, Mæhlen and Welch[16] supported these results in 2008 in an elegant study from Norway with a strong design that involved more than 200 000 women. If cancers regressed spontaneously, one would expect to find more cancers in a group of women who had been screened three times than in a similar group of women at the same ages who had only been screened once. Thus, as an example, a 50-year-old woman in the study group would be invited to screening when she was 50, 52 and 54, whereas a control group woman would only be invited when she turned 54. This was accomplished by selecting control group women who were born in earlier calendar years than the study group women, i.e. the woman had turned 54 before the screening programme was implemented. In both groups, cancers were cumulated over 6 years, whether or not they were detected at screening or clinically. The researchers found 22% more cancers in the group screened three times than in the group screened once, and when they compared four screenings with two screenings, there were 20% more cancers.

This is very convincing evidence that many screen-detected cancers regress if left untreated. Zahl[17] has performed an even stronger study that builds on data from Sweden that confirms this.

The 1986 UK Forrest report

The oldest account of overdiagnosis in the randomised trials that I have found is the 1986 Forrest report,[18] which formed the basis for introducing screening in the United Kingdom. It noted that women might undergo unnecessary procedures for cancer that might not have become invasive. The authors were only thinking of carcinoma *in situ* and failed to realise that invasive cancer could also be overdiagnosed.

Back then, there were only data from two trials. The Forrest report uncritically accepted that overdiagnosis wasn't a problem in the New York trial, as the number of cancers was the same in the screened group as in the control group. The authors also uncritically accepted the results from the Two-County trial. They noted with reference to a workshop report that didn't give the number of cancers[19] that there were 20% more cancers in the screened group than in the control group and advised further follow-up to find out whether this excess persisted for the lifespan of the women. I have carefully tabulated all cancer data from the many publications on the Two-County trial but have been unable to find any data that fit anywhere near 20% more cancers. The closest I got was 22%, but this didn't include carcinoma *in situ*.[20] The idea to follow up the randomised women during their lifespan to see if the excess of cancers persisted is meaningless for the Two-County trial, as the whole control group had been invited to screening. This was mentioned in the 1985 trial report,[21] which the authors of the Forrest report cited, but they paid no attention to this.

The Forrest report speaks volumes about the lack of stringency and reliability of work in committees. Petr Skrabanek participated as an expert and described his experience 2 years later.[22] Dissent was effectively silenced, as those who were invited were bound by secrecy. The Forrest report was a consensus document and it was based on selective evidence, ignoring inconvenient data. Skrabanek had accidentally found data that had only been published in Swedish and which showed increased overall mortality with screening in the Two-County trial. *However, the Forrest report didn't convey these data or the serious criticisms Skrabanek had raised against the trial*, e.g. that cause of death was not assessed by an independent panel, or that age ranges changed all the time in reports of the trial.

Further, the Forrest report claimed it was possible to screen with only 5%–10% interval cancers, which it clearly isn't. In the United Kingdom, the interval cancer rate (as a proportion of the underlying cancer incidence) was 31% in the first 12 months after screening, 52% between 12 and 24 months, and 82% between 24 and 36 months.[23]

The report also downplayed overdiagnosis, although one of the co-authors of the Two-County trial had expressed concern about a 'very serious situation' of 'unacceptable divergence of opinion' among the pathologists who interpreted the breast biopsies.[22] Skrabanek asked who would be blamed if, in 10 years' time, screening had not decreased mortality from breast cancer. Although this is the situation today, the question is still being ignored.

> *It is fair to say that the UK screening programme was based on a report that wasn't evidence-based and on two trials that are unreliable.*

Overdiagnosis in the randomised trials

During the next 15 years, there was virtually nothing in the literature about overdiagnosis. Additional screening trials were reported and many reviews and meta-analyses of the trials were published,[4] but apart from The Nordic Cochrane Centre's own publications in 2000 and 2001, I have found only two reports from this time period, one by Skrabanek[24] from 1989 and one by Swiss epidemiologist Johannes Schmidt[25] from 1990, which analysed the amount of excess cancers and treatments in the trials. People searching for data on overdiagnosis would easily overlook these reports, as the titles and abstracts do not reveal that there are such data in the papers. The report by Schmidt and a subsequent letter[26] described that excess diagnoses were demonstrable in all the trials and he listed rates from three of the four Swedish trials (24%–44%). What is most remarkable is that Schmidt reported exactly the same balance between harm and benefit as we reported 16 years later:[27]

> The occurrence of an excess cancer is almost ten times as likely as the occurrence of a prevented breast cancer death.

Schmidt alerted his readers to another elementary issue that would be actively suppressed by screening advocates; namely, that the question with screening was not one about reducing the mortality from breast cancer, but whether the benefits outweigh the harms. He remarked that the Two-County trial was difficult to evaluate, as the time periods and populations changed from report to report, and as blinding and determination of end points were poorly defined.[25] Finally, he noted that even the 'very optimistic' 40% reduction in breast cancer mortality reported in this trial represented only one case per 10 000 woman-years, which he compared with the traffic mortality risk when driving 14 km daily in England at eight per 10 000.

I believe we were the first to document the extent of overdiagnosis by pooling the results from the trials in 2000 in the *Lancet*, estimating 35% excess surgery.[28] We found additional data for our 2001 *Lancet* review[29,30] and noted that the excess surgery was not only an initial phenomenon, caused by the tumours detected at the prevalence screen, but seemed to persist. We also noted that it was unlikely that a 20% increase in mastectomies had been overestimated since a general policy change towards fewer mastectomies had occurred slowly.[31]

In our 2006 and 2009 Cochrane reviews that included these data, we published a more detailed discussion about whether the randomised trials had over- or underestimated overdiagnosis.[4,27] Our result of 30% overdiagnosis was very robust and was supported by large observational studies. Incidence increases of 40%–60% have been reported for Australia, Finland, Norway, Sweden, the United Kingdom and the United States,[3,14,32–37] without a corresponding decline in incidence after the age of 69 years when the women were no longer screened.[14,37] We also mentioned that opportunistic screening and diagnostic mammography because of a clinical suspicion in the control group would lead to an underestimate of overdiagnosis, e.g. a quarter of the women in the control groups in the trials from Canada and Malmö received mammograms during the trial.[4]

The true increase in surgery is larger than the increase in incidence of breast cancer because many women are operated upon more than once. For example, in New South Wales, one-third of women with carcinoma *in situ* had either mastectomy alone (19%) or after breast-conserving surgery (17%).[38] As we wrote in 2001,[29,30] data on second operations are usually missing from official reports and research papers. They are also missing from the trial reports, as the increase in surgery is very similar to the increase in diagnoses.[4] Therefore, the harm inflicted on women by overdiagnosis is underestimated in the trials.

The Cochrane editors weren't too happy about our description of the excess treatments as harmful and argued that quality assurance could reduce them and that they could also be beneficial. The latter suggestion was difficult to swallow; we couldn't really see how all this unnecessary surgery could be beneficial. But we compromised in a way that looked a bit funny, in our 2006 Cochrane review:[27]

> Quality assurance programs could possibly reduce the surgical activity to some degree, but they could also increase it. In the UK, for example, the surgeons were blamed for not having treated even more women with carcinoma in situ by mastectomy (BASO audit 2000). Not all of the additional operations are necessarily harmful, for example, some cases would represent prophylactic mastectomy in high-risk women.

We succeeded in getting rid of the last sentence about prophylactic mastectomy when we published the 2009 review.[4]

The Canadian trialists reported in 2002 that their trials showed that overdiagnosis is not confined to carcinoma *in situ*, but extends to invasive cancers.[39]

In 2005, statistician Sue Moss, primary author of the most recent screening trial, the UK Age trial, published a review on overdiagnosis and overtreatment based on the trials.[40] The paper was part of a series on overdiagnosis and overtreatment, edited by Nick Day, Stephen Duffy and Eugenio Paci, in *Breast Cancer Research*. I expected the worst, as the whole setup looked like the converted preaching to the converted, and Moss's paper was indeed very poor science. She made virtually all the errors one can possibly make:

- Didn't cite our extensive 2001 Lancet review that provided a meta-analysis of overtreatment and which, in addition, had been extensively peer-reviewed.
- Didn't give any data on overtreatment but stated that its extent was difficult to quantify.
- Included data on diagnoses after the whole control group had been invited to screening, which is an unforgivable error that spuriously removed overdiagnosis.

- Included data from the New York trial, although many cancers in the control group should have been excluded, as the diagnosis was made *before* these women entered the trial.
- Included cancers that were diagnosed many years after the trial ended, which dilutes the estimate of overdiagnosis (see why just below).
- Included the Edinburgh trial, which is hopelessly flawed.
- Didn't pool the data.
- Reported that there were 11%–14% more cancers in the intervention arms in the Canadian trials, but this was long after the trial ended when many women in the control group had been screened.

A persistent criticism of using the randomised trials to estimate overdiagnosis has been that the follow-up was too short. Screening detects cancer earlier and it is therefore only to be expected that there will be more cancers in the screened group than in the control group at the beginning of a trial. Although this is true, I have never been impressed by the argument and will explain why, using the Malmö trial as an example.[4] This trial ran for 9 years, which is longer than for any other trial.

There were 34% more mastectomies and lumpectomies in the screened group than in the control group when the trial ended. After 9 years, most of this excess would seem to be caused by overdiagnosis and not by earlier detection.

In 2006, a long-term follow-up was published in the *BMJ* that purported to have estimated the level of overdiagnosis in the Malmö trial.[41] The number of cancers that had occurred during an additional 15 years after the trial ended were added to those cancers detected during the randomised phase of the trial, and the authors reported 10% overdiagnosis in the age group 55–69 years.

The 10% estimate was seriously biased. During all these extra years, there was very little screening due to the advanced age of the women. Therefore, the estimate of overdiagnosis was considerably diluted, as it was mostly clinically detected cancers that were added to both groups. Moreover, as the incidence of breast cancer increases with age, this dilution becomes even more problematic. Gilbert Welch[42] demonstrated by how much the dilution effect distorted the estimate. It is possible to infer the number of undetected cancers that exist at the end of the trial in the control group because they are subsequently diagnosed as 'catch-up' cancers. This number is simply the difference between number of cancers identified in the screened group and the control group during the 15 years after the trial ended. In this way, it is possible to adjust reliably for the lead-time bias caused by screening, instead of using a complicated model with unverified assumptions that virtually always leads to erroneous results, as I shall describe shortly. The use of real numbers is what is so elegant and yet so simple in Welch's approach. Adding these cancers to the control group, the level of overdiagnosis when the trial ended becomes 18%, rather than the 10% the authors had claimed.

An even more reliable estimate is obtained if we also adjust for the fact that 24% of the women in the control group had undergone screening at least once during the trial.[4] We did just that and found 25% overdiagnosis.[43] This brings me to a conclusion that is so important that I will highlight it:

> *The 25% overdiagnosis in the Malmö trial after very long follow-up suggests that our estimate of 31% overdiagnosis based on the randomised trials is fairly reliable, in fact more reliable than our estimate of a 15% reduction in breast cancer mortality, or any other mortality estimate for that matter.*

The reason that this result is so important is that screening advocates have consistently claimed – just as Sue Moss – that overdiagnosis is difficult to quantify, whereas they have readily accepted implausibly large effects of screening on breast cancer mortality based on the same trials. Even though the harm is better documented than the benefit, the screening advocates have consistently produced estimates of overdiagnosis that are far too low.

Most authors quoting the results from the extended follow-up of the Malmö trial haven't paid any attention to the biasing effects of dilution and the use of mammography in the control group during the trial, although they were described in the *BMJ* after the study was published. Such omissions are the rule in scientific publishing. Even when commentators have demonstrated fatal flaws in a study, it usually continues to be quoted as if its results were true, whereas critical comments are rarely quoted.[44]

Eugenio Paci and San Salvi from Florence didn't even try to conceal that they ignored what we had just demonstrated.[45] They acknowledged that information leaflets directed to women should include correct statements on overdiagnosis, but argued:

> However, these statements should inform women of the conclusions of sound evaluation of research in this field, and not simply of what Gøtzsche or Welch believe is the truth. Our present knowledge, based on several studies, suggests that the problem of over-diagnosis in breast cancer service screening is much less significant than the recent *BMJ* issue has claimed. Quoting Hyppocrates was absolutely correct. The 'first do no harm' rule might also apply to simplistic and superficial conclusions discrediting a current health policy which has been demonstrated to have a major impact on breast cancer mortality.

That came close to the 'you are killing my patients' argument. In my view, the screening advocates lost a good deal of the public's confidence in that issue of the *BMJ* because they displayed their stubbornness and stupidity openly. One can only hope that the public becomes less willing to accept unsolicited paternalism, secrecy, decisions guided by self-interest and political opportunism.

In 2007, Australian researchers published a systematic review on overdiagnosis in the randomised trials.[46] They wrote that it was only 7%–8% in the Malmö trial and only 2% and 7% in the Canadian trials, which disregarded both the dilution and the contamination biases I have just described.[47] Furthermore, they used a model assuming that the incidence of cancer would fall by about 50% immediately after age 69 years. This doesn't happen. The reductions in incidence have been small or non-existent in all the countries we have examined.[48]

To their credit, the researchers learned from their mistakes and published a carefully conducted observational study based on data from New South Wales 2 years later,[49] which showed substantial overdiagnosis (*see* second section below). You might have guessed it already. In this highly contentious area of healthcare, such laudable researchers likely do not have conflicts of interest. Right! They were driven by curiosity, as all good scientists are, and – needless to say – their study wasn't popular with the Australian screening advocates.

Systematic review of overdiagnosis in observational studies

As explained in Chapter 2, we don't randomise people in observational studies but observe what happens, e.g. in a group that is screened and in a group that is not. Observational studies are less reliable than randomised trials, but they are important for estimating overdiagnosis because screening in the real world differs markedly from screening in randomised trials (*see* Chapter 25). Technical developments may improve the performance, and conversely, practising radiologists may be less well trained and less careful than those who participated in the trials. It is difficult to imagine a more boring job for a doctor than to look at mammograms day in and day out throughout a whole career. Further, the increasing demands to extend screening to additional age groups, associated with budget cuts and staffing problems in many hospitals, would be expected to increase the error rate. Fear of litigation increases overdiagnosis, since it is much safer for the radiologist and for the histopathologist to declare cancer when they are confronted with borderline cases.

If overdiagnosis didn't occur, the initial increase in total number of cancers in the screened age groups would be fully balanced by a similar decrease in number of cancers as the group aged and was no longer offered screening, as these cancers would already have been detected.

We compared trends in breast cancer incidence before and after screening in countries with organised screening programmes, taking account of changes in the background incidence and any compensatory drop in incidence of breast cancer among older women.[48]

Our method was simple and transparent, and didn't involve any assumptions about the magnitude of lead-time bias, only concrete data. We included articles with data on breast cancer incidence for at least 7 years before screening and 7 years after screening had been fully implemented in order to estimate the trend in breast cancer incidence, unaffected by the initial peak in prevalence when screening is introduced.

It was the first systematic review of observational studies of overdiagnosis ever performed and it proved to be surprisingly difficult. Numerous papers had published incidence trends, but most data were useless. For example, the data were only shown for the screening years and not for the prescreening years, or data included the elderly that had never been invited to screening and in whom breast cancer is most common. This effectively concealed the incidence increase caused by screening. Another problem was that authors had combined screened and non-screened areas.

Such data are pretty meaningless, and the deficiencies in the presentation of the data were so consistent that it is hard to believe that it wasn't sometimes intentional in order to obscure the evidence from other researchers wanting to estimate overdiagnosis. It was particularly surprising that the data rarely included carcinoma *in situ*, which is virtually always treated as if it were cancer, as most of these cases are overdiagnosed.

Of more than 300 articles we assembled, we could include only five. Three of the authors we contacted provided unpublished data or referred us to Internet resources for additional data. This enabled us to include data from the United Kingdom, Manitoba, New South Wales, Sweden and parts of Norway.

Only from Manitoba did we retrieve the full data set; for the other four areas, we adjusted our estimate of overdiagnosis by assuming that carcinoma *in situ* would contribute 10% of the diagnoses in a population offered screening, in accordance with European data. We couldn't include the United States, as this country doesn't have an organised screening programme and therefore doesn't have well-defined pre- and post-screening periods. Furthermore, comparisons with younger and older age groups is also unreliable, as women are urged to be screened from when they are very young virtually until they die, as there is no upper age limit.

Our findings were remarkably consistent, and I show the results from the United Kingdom as an example (*see* Figure 16.1):

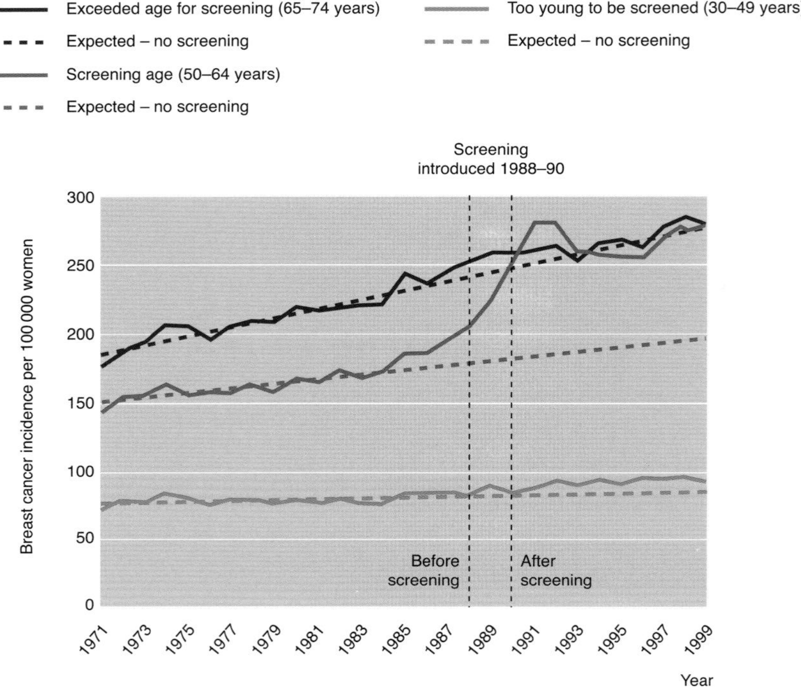

FIGURE 16.1 Incidence of invasive breast cancer per 100 000 women in the UK

It can be seen that introduction of screening during 1988–90 led to a marked increase in the incidence of invasive breast cancer in the screened age groups; in fact, the increase was so large that the incidence became as high as in elderly women, and it stayed at this level. There was no drop in incidence among elderly women, and the incidence in women who were too young to be invited to screening increased slightly over the expected rate, undoubtedly because some opportunistic screening took place.

In some countries, there was a drop in incidence among elderly women, but the reduction in the total number of cancers compared with what was expected if there hadn't been screening was small. We subtracted these cancers before we estimated overdiagnosis, which was 52%, i.e. much higher than that estimated in the randomised trials (*see* Figure 16.2).

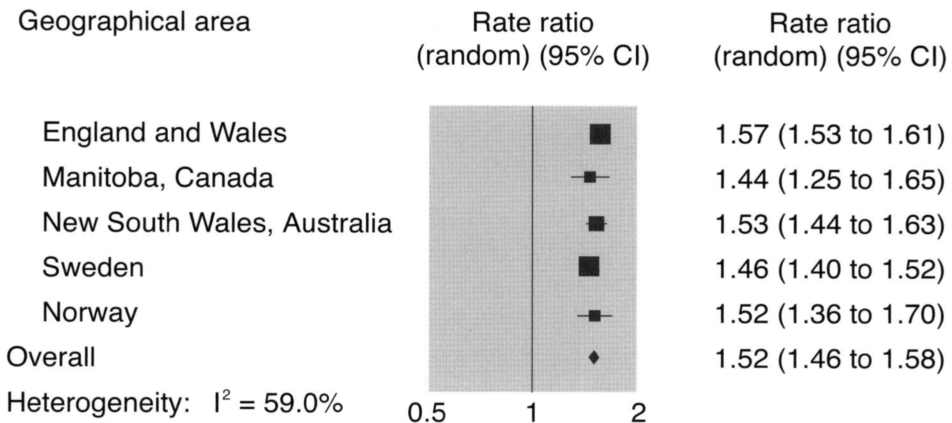

Geographical area
Rate ratio (random) (95% CI)
Rate ratio (random) (95% CI)
England and Wales
1.57 (1.53 to 1.61)
Manitoba, Canada
1.44 (1.25 to 1.65)
New South Wales, Australia
1.53 (1.44 to 1.63)
Sweden
1.46 (1.40 to 1.52)
Norway
1.52 (1.36 to 1.70)
Overall
1.52 (1.46 to 1.58)
Heterogeneity: I² = 59.0%
0.5
1
2

FIGURE 16.2 Meta-analysis of overdiagnosis of breast cancer (including carcinoma *in situ*) in publicly available mammography screening programmes

Since 52% is about one-third of 152% (100% + 52%), this means that *one in three breast cancers detected in a population offered organised screening is overdiagnosed*. A similar result based on registry data from Norway and Sweden was published by Per-Henrik Zahl and colleagues[37] in 2004, although they only included invasive breast cancer.

This result is alarming. Not only because these women will have to live the rest of their lives as cancer patients, fearing that the 'pseudodisease' – which never was a disease and never would have been were it not for screening – would come back and kill them but also because some women die from the unnecessary treatment. It is a new ethical dilemma in healthcare that some people will have to pay with their lives to enable others to live longer. This is what soldiers do, but they at least know about it: most women don't.[1]

Speaking of war, the use of war metaphors in the 'battle' against cancer has a long tradition. US president Richard Nixon declared war against cancer 40 years ago, and it has often been declared under great fanfares that cancer would soon be 'conquered', a misperception actively fostered by cancer charities to their advantage, e.g. 'Make this the decade we win the battle!' (by sending that particular charity more money).[10]

When we published our meta-analysis of overdiagnosis in July 2009 in the *BMJ*,[48] there were many reactions. Michael Baum drew attention to the PR machine that the NHS Breast Screening Programme sets in motion every time screening comes under attack, and to the outdated mindset the pro-screening lobby is locked into.[50] He suggested a risk-adjusted service so that women with a low risk of breast cancer would be advised about lifestyle rather than being advised to have a mammogram, and he further suggested that this approach be tested in a large randomised trial.

A UK cancer patient advocate, Daphne Havercroft, remarked that some experts seem intent on preventing women from exercising their right to decide for themselves by depriving them of full information about the harms and benefits of screening and steering them towards unquestioning acceptance of it. She argued that people who are ill are told of the potential harms of the treatment as well as the benefits, and when offered surgery they must sign a consent form.[51]

Breast surgeon Jayant Vaidya showed interesting data from Scotland.[52] Some regions are attended by a screening van for 1 year every 3 years, with no screening occurring in the interim 2 years. Vaidya found that the population incidence of invasive breast cancer peaks every 3 years when the region is visited by the van, but without any reduction in incidence (compared with the level before screening was introduced) in the 2-year periods between the peaks. Thus, *there was no reduction in symptomatic cancers* despite the peaks in incidence, which continued to be high even after several visits by the van.

In our reply to all the letters, we published more up-to-date statistics from the United Kingdom and drew attention to the remarkable fact that when the women in the age group 65–70 years were included in the programme in 2001–03, their incidence level increased dramatically[53] (*see* Figure 16.3), although they had been

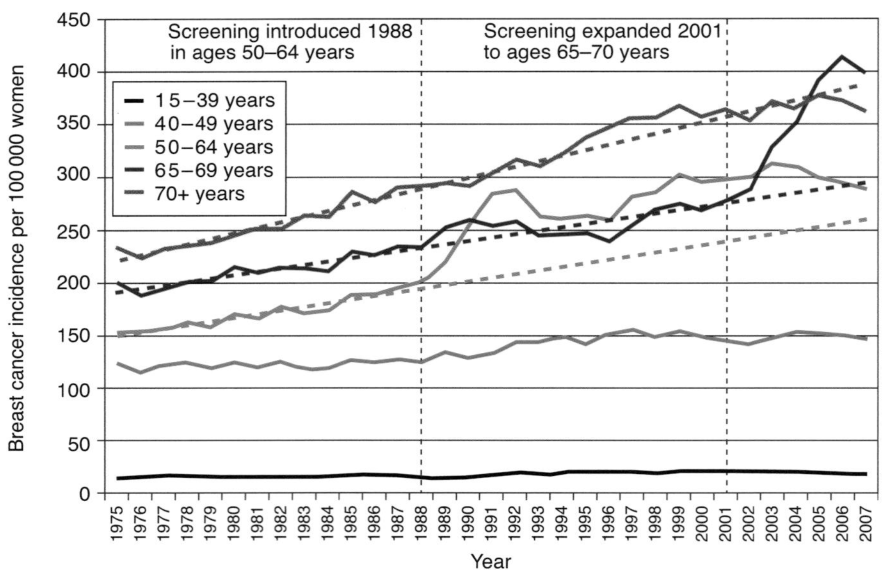

FIGURE 16.3 Incidence of invasive breast cancer per 100 000 women in the UK, by age group. Dashed lines: expected incidence without screening

invited to screening earlier when they were younger! Not only is this evidence of substantial overdiagnosis but also it suggests that many cancers detected by screening would have regressed spontaneously.

We also noted that the debates about overdiagnosis fitted well with Thomas Kuhn's ideas of scientific revolutions. Ever since the 1986 Forrest report stated that 'screening is not likely to lead to a significant increase in the numbers of breast cancers treated', the tacit knowledge, as Kuhn calls it, in the screening community has been that overdiagnosis doesn't occur, and the prevailing paradigm of 'no harm done' has been fiercely protected. As the Kuhnian anomalies (clear demonstrations that more diagnoses occurred in the screened groups) accumulated, screening advocates resorted to wishful thinking based on false theories, or manipulated their data in models so that they appeared to fit with the paradigm, or ignored them. For example, we haven't seen a single screening advocate trying to explain how the New York trial could produce a 35% reduction in breast cancer mortality, apparently without advancing the time of diagnosis, which is a *conditio sine qua non* for cancer screening. The British statistician Sir Richard Peto asked the principal investigator of the trial three times at a meeting in 1983 why the number of breast cancers was about the same in the screened group as in the control group.[54] This discussion is largely unknown and is highly unlikely to be found in a literature search, as only a formal paper, and not the ensuing discussion, is listed in PubMed. The trial is often cited, as it yielded the ideal answer people wanted to hear: a large benefit and no harms.

For the first time ever, we made an impression on power circles in Sweden. The director of the Swedish National Board of Health, Lars-Erik Holm, admitted that the high amount of overdiagnosis should pave the way for a renewed debate on mammography screening.[55] Holm even declared that the Board of Health would look at the information provided to women invited to screening. However, it is easy to appear forthcoming and yet do nothing. The Swedish debate has been hermetically sealed for 25 years and there are no signs that this will change. Swedish women still get no information about overdiagnosis.

Robert Smith of the American Cancer Society dismissed our findings in the same way as he always does, saying they were the result of 'poor methodology'.[56] Smith is very consistent in delivering derogatory remarks with no substance when screening comes under attack. Frankly, we cannot see how our study could have been done better, and there was nothing in the many letters that followed our article that detracts from its credibility.

Psychologists have performed interesting experiments on the tension between belief and fact.[57] Belief is very difficult to overturn, especially when it is held by people with a vested interest in the old message. When people are presented with evidence that their belief was wrong, this doesn't cause them to adjust their erroneous beliefs, but often reinforces them. Considering this formidable psychological handicap for the advancement of science, it is incredible that it has been possible for the naked ape – which is largely steered by emotions rather than logic – to land people on the moon and get them back.

When our *BMJ* paper came out, a journalist asked representatives from the US breast cancer advocacy group Susan G. Komen for the Cure, about our finding that screening needlessly turned many healthy women into cancer patients. The CEO, Hala Moddelmog, replied: '*I don't think there's evidence of overdiagnosis*', and Elizabeth Thompson, vice-president of health sciences, said: 'We're very concerned that insurance companies will stop funding mammograms when these kinds of studies come out.' When the journalist then asked what they were telling women about the risks associated with mammograms, Thompson continued, 'We believe early detection saves lives, and we need to focus on getting out that message.'[57] What an unholy mixture of denial of facts, unsolicited paternalism and financial issues for a patient advocacy group.

The official reaction in Australia was also one of denial. The Australian National Breast and Ovarian Cancer Centre declared, 'The vast majority of breast cancers found through screening would progress if left untreated.'[58] The statement was linked to a position statement from 2008 that said that the estimates of overdiagnosis from the randomised trials ranged from negative values to a high of around 10% of diagnoses, with a midpoint of 2%–3%. Pretty startling, considering that we found about 30% in the same trials.

Three months later, on Sweden's National Breast Cancer Day, the Swedish Cancer Foundation started a month-long campaign about teaching women to examine their breasts every month,[59] although it had been known for more than 6 years that this intervention is harmful.[60] Women who paid SEK1 a month would get an SMS on their mobile phone that reminded them about the examination.

No need to read novels. Real life is much more unexpected.

Observational studies from Denmark and New South Wales

In 2010, we published a study of overdiagnosis in Denmark,[61] comparing areas with screening to areas without. We found 33% overdiagnosis, which is somewhat lower than in other countries, but it was expected. The Danish programme has low recall rates, e.g. only 1.3% per round in one of the regions. Further, a deliberately conservative attitude towards detection of microcalcifications means that only 6% of all breast cancer diagnoses are carcinoma *in situ*. Finally, the uptake is only 63% in Copenhagen.

Stephen Morrell and colleagues[49] estimated overdiagnosis in New South Wales by comparing the observed incidence of invasive breast cancer in the screened age groups (50–69 years) with the expected incidence without screening. The expected incidence was estimated in two ways: from the incidence in unscreened age groups and from the incidence prior to screening. They adjusted their estimates for trends in major risk factors for breast cancer and also for lead-time bias, using two estimates of lead time – 2½ and 5 years. Their approach was deliberately conservative, i.e. provided a minimum estimate of overdiagnosis, but even so, they found 42% and 30% overdiagnosis of invasive breast cancer with the two methods for a lead time of 5 years, and 51% and 36% when the lead time was 2½ years (which is closer to the truth, *see* Chapter 24).

We included New South Wales in our systematic review of overdiagnosis, and although we used very different methods, we obtained similar results, 38% overdiagnosis of invasive breast cancer and 53% when we included carcinoma *in situ*.[48]

The authors published an instructive graph that compared the number of diagnoses per 100 000 women in various age groups in two different time periods (*see* Figure 16.4). This is the sort of graph that shows us that overdiagnosis around zero, or 'a high of around 10%', as declared by the Australian National Breast and Ovarian Cancer Centre,[58] should be distrusted.

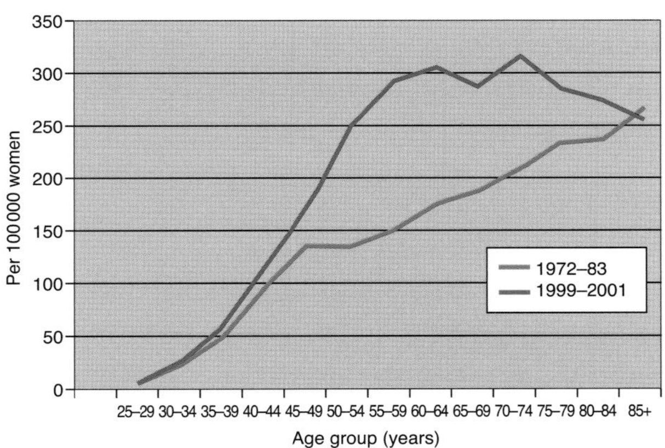

FIGURE 16.4 Mean annual age-specific breast cancer incidence in women prior to universal health insurance (Medicare) (1972–1983) and under established organised mammography screening (1999–2001) in New South Wales (data supplied by author)

There is one more thing about this study, and it is so worrying that I will highlight it:

> The detection rates had increased, not only since the mammography screening trials were conducted in the 1980s, but also within the New South Wales programme itself, where the rates increased from about 28 to 42 per 10 000 women screened. Furthermore, these increased detection rates in Australia have not been accompanied by decreased interval cancer rates, which suggests that the increased detection is harmful, as it simply produces greater overdiagnosis.

However, even overwhelmingly clear data such as these may fall on deaf ears. When cancer epidemiologist David Roder, based at the Cancer Council South Australia in Adelaide, was interviewed, he said the study was 'technically competent', but based on debatable assumptions, and he added: 'I think there are equally rigorous studies that come to different conclusions.'[62]

This is a prime example of the damaging influence that flawed research can have on healthcare. I shall comment below on the studies Roder likely had in mind (Duffy's and Lynge's studies on overdiagnosis). But first, a note on the doubt industry, as flawed studies are routinely used to spread doubt about unwelcome scientific facts.[63]

The doubt industry

> *Most of our so-called reasoning consists in finding arguments for going on believing as we already do.*
>
> James Harvey Robinson (1863–1936)

A tobacco executive once said, 'doubt is our product', and the tactic of knowingly spreading doubt is called the doubt industry.[64] It was easy for the tobacco companies to buy skilled scientists whose job it was to cause confusion by publishing numerous papers that superficially looked like good science. This pollution of the scientific literaure worked; it took much too long before the hazards of smoking were generally accepted. The drug industry also uses hired guns, which has led to the unnecessary deaths of tens of thousands of healthy people who didn't know the drugs they were taking were dangerous.[65,66]

It's a challenge to write about the doubt industry in relation to the denial of overdiagnosis. I don't fancy conspiracy theories, but the denial is so massive and consistent that it looks like collusion. I have selected some publications that have been important for spreading doubt when there was clarity, or which illustrate particular points that are essential for understanding the tricks of the trade.

The most common manoeuvre has been to adjust estimates of overdiagnosis for lead time. I will explain why we have reservations about such adjustments.[47,67] As described in Chapter 2, lead time is the average difference between the time cancers are detected by screening and the time they would have been detected clinically because of symptoms. Such cancers do not contribute to overdiagnosis. Overdiagnosed cancers are those detected by screening that would not have come to the women's attention in their remaining lifetime. The problem is that we cannot separate these two types of cancer. We cannot know how many cancers that would – and how many that would not – have come to the women's attention in their remaining lifetime unless we perform a lifelong randomised trial of screening where all women are followed up until they have all died. As such a trial hasn't been done, lead time hasn't been measured, only approximated, and there is great uncertainty. It is not possible to exclude the overdiagnosed cancers from the calculation of lead time, and the average lead time will therefore be artificially prolonged. This creates a real risk that adjustment for lead time falsely removes true overdiagnosis. Furthermore, several of the assumptions involved in estimates of lead time[68] are wrong. For example, the assumption in a paper by Nick Day[68] that the benefit a woman gains from screening is related directly to her lead time doesn't hold because her cancer might be overdiagnosed, in which case she doesn't benefit but is harmed. And Day's assumption that no tumours regress[68] is also wrong. I shall explain in Chapter 24 why the commonly used estimates for lead time of 2–5 years are far too high.

By adjusting for lead time, screening advocates have successfully spread doubt about the fact that overdiagnosis is an important problem with screening. I believe the collective will to disregard overdiagnosis gathered momentum in 1994 when a correspondence in the *Lancet* claimed that the overdiagnosis in the Dutch breast screening programme was less than 2% over the entire lifetime of the women.[69] One of the authors was Harry de Koning, a major figure in the Dutch screening programme.

The letter is politically correct – telling people that screening does no harm – but scientifically wrong. Correspondences are not peer-reviewed and the letter is so short that it's impossible to judge its methodology. The authors developed a model based on the Malmö trial and predicted overdiagnosis, assuming a lead time of 4.8 years. With such a long lead time, many overdiagnosed cancers will be statistically 'adjusted away', so to speak. To put it simply, many women who had their breast cancer detected at screening would have died before these cancers would ever have given rise to symptoms, which can easily be seen if we compare with the randomised trials in Sweden. In these trials, about 10% of the women had died from causes other than breast cancer after 10 years,[4] and many had therefore died also after 4.8 years.

In their letter, de Koning and colleagues published a figure that showed a huge drop in the expected incidence of breast cancer after age 69 when screening stops (*see* Figure 16.5).[69] However, this is purely wishful thinking. Such a huge drop – or even just a moderate one – hasn't been observed in any country.[48,61]

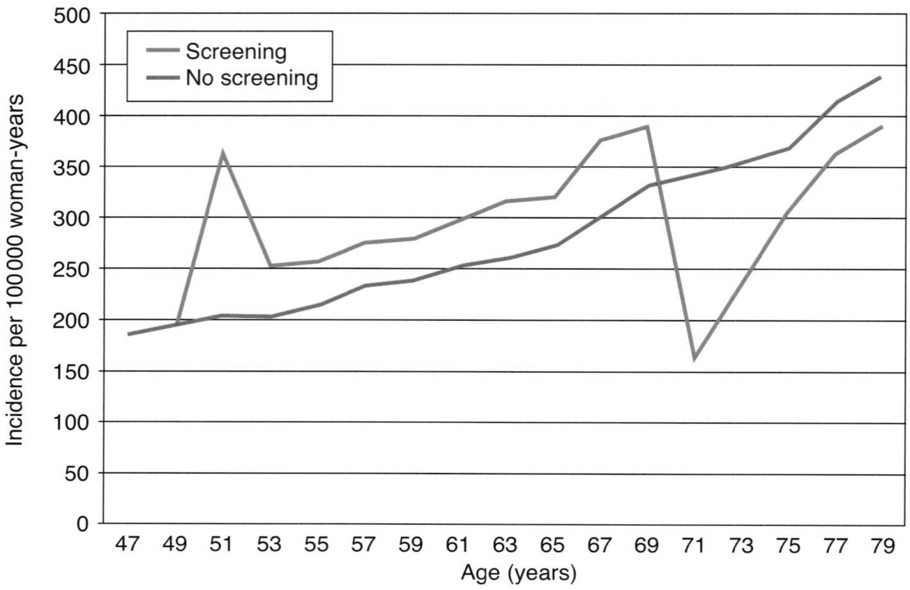

FIGURE 16.5 Expected breast cancer incidence with screening (green line) and without screening (red line). Wishful thinking, as the huge drop in elderly women has never been observed in practice (redrawn)

Such fantasies also pervaded official reports recommending politicians to screen. For example, the report from the Danish National Board of Health from 1997, chaired by Elsebeth Lynge, stated, 'Numbers from Sweden and the Netherlands do not suggest that introduction of screening leads to a persistent increase in the incidence of breast cancer.'[70] Most astonishingly, this report used data from the Malmö area and argued that as the incidence in 1990 didn't seem to be higher than what it would have been without screening, the numbers didn't suggest overdiagnosis. The fact that there was a huge peak in diagnoses between 1976 (when the randomised trial in Malmö started) and 1986 (when it ended) was actually shown in a graph, but that didn't seem to have left any impression on the authors of the Board of Health's report, most of whom had conflicts of interest. Paper is grateful, as we say in Denmark. It doesn't protest, no matter what you write on it.

A report from the Swedish National Board of Health from 1986 noted that there remained a small increase in diagnoses at the second and third screening rounds,[71] but it also stated that screening leads to milder treatment and fewer mastectomies. This early report admitted that most women recalled for further testing are 'deeply anxious'. I cannot recall having seen such honesty anywhere else in reports from supporters of screening. On the other hand, the information was not directed towards the women but towards the surgeons so that they would accept the recalls without delay. And very few non-professionals would ever read a typewritten report located at the Swedish National Board of Health.

In 1998, when screening was in full swing in the whole country, another report from the Swedish National Board of Health noted that a few women received a diagnosis they wouldn't have received without screening,[72] but then added that the diagnosis was treatment-demanding. This shows a poor understanding of overdiagnosis. Such cancers should *not* be treated, if only we could separate them from the dangerous ones. The mistake illustrates how difficult it is for authorities to accept the harms of the interventions they recommend. The report also misrepresented the benefit. It noted that women who were diagnosed during the 1980s had a better 10-year survival than women who were diagnosed during the 1960s and 1970s,[72] ignoring the issues of lead-time and length biases.

The work of the doubt industry is best illustrated by Duffy's and Lynge's papers on overdiagnosis that I shall discuss next.

Duffy's studies on overdiagnosis

Stephen Duffy published five papers on overdiagnosis between 2003 and 2006 that purported to have found virtually no overdiagnosis. He reported that only 4% of the carcinoma *in situ* cases at the incidence screen didn't progress, based on data from the Two-County trial, the United Kingdom, the Netherlands, Australia and the United States;[73] that there was no overdiagnosis in the Two-County trial;[74] around 5% overdiagnosis in Florence;[75] 1% in the Two-County and Gothenburg trials;[76] and 5% in Copenhagen.[77]

Duffy's methods are difficult to follow and even more difficult to swallow. Michael Baum has tried to find out where the estimates Duffy uses, e.g. for lead time, come from and how reliable they are. He went through the reference lists and found that the explanation given in the quoted papers was insufficient. He then retrieved references to the referenced papers and so forth, in backward cycles, but he still wasn't able to make an informed judgement. We have had exactly the same type of experience, not only related to Duffy's studies but also when we tried to find crucial details about the Two-County trial.

There must be grave errors in the assumptions, data, or calculations that are the basis for Duffy's estimates. If not, he would have found considerable overdiagnosis in his studies, which is evident if one looks at published graphs of breast cancer incidence in the countries he has studied.[36,48,49] It is wrong, for example, to imply that only 4% of carcinoma *in situ* cases are overdiagnosed. We know that most cases never progress into invasive cancer,[6,78] i.e. *most* cases are overdiagnosed, not 4%.

In the study where Duffy reported about 1% overdiagnosis in the Two-County and Gothenburg trials,[76] he used Markov chain Monte Carlo methods and a multistate model. Such methods are notoriously unreliable and highly bias prone. It has been said that with these methods, it is possible to get almost any result one had hoped for. In one of Duffy's studies, which had Anne Helene Olsen as first author, the authors actually cautioned themselves against their approach and noted that the estimation might be unstable due to overparameterisation, and they also noted that their assumptions might be incorrect.[77] Indeed.

We have explained what the main problems are with Duffy's approach.[79] Most important, he doesn't review the literature systematically; his models involve assumptions that cannot be correct; he extrapolates far beyond the data at hand; and he does subgroup analyses of attenders at screening.

Like Baum, we fail to understand how Duffy can arrive so consistently at estimates of virtually no overdiagnosis, based on very different data sources from different parts of the world. This doesn't make sense. Duffy adjusts his estimates for lead time, but as we have seen, it didn't really matter for New South Wales whether the authors used small or large estimates of lead time; there was very substantial overdiagnosis in any case.[49]

We have found one paper where Duffy's estimate is considerably higher. However, this study wasn't one of Duffy's own, but was carried out by Håkan Jonsson and two other Swedish researchers who had not been involved with any of the Swedish screening trials. They showed that 7 years after the start of screening in Sweden, the incidence of invasive breast cancer was considerably higher than expected.[14] Even after adjustment for lead time, and even though they had excluded carcinoma *in situ*, there were 54% more diagnoses in the age group 50–59 years and 21% more for 60–69 years. When I pointed out that their results were in good agreement with those from the randomised trials,[80] they replied that it was misleading to include the first round of screening when studying overdiagnosis, as the 'objective of mammography screening is to detect cancer early, which will lead to an increased incidence in the first round'.[15] Thus, they failed to understand that there are many overdiagnosed cases in the prevalence round and argued that overdiagnosis is confined to the incidence rounds (the rounds after the first round).

This error is interesting, as the Duffy/Tabár/Smith trio make the opposite error when they assume that overdiagnosis is confined to the prevalence round,[74] saying that essentially all incidence increase with screening in the Two-County trial represents earlier diagnosis (and therefore not overdiagnosis).[81]

Both groups of researchers cannot be right, and let me be absolutely clear about this. Both groups of researchers are wrong. Screening leads to overdiagnosis at any time, at the prevalence screen and at subsequent screens. It's very simple. We cannot 'forbid' slow-growing or regressing cancers to be detected at the prevalence screen or to be detected at incidence screens in order to comply with wishful thinking on the part of researchers.

Three years later, Duffy published a paper with Jonsson and the excess was now only 39%, after adjustment for a lead time of 2.4 years and also for increased use of hormone replacement therapy.[82] This estimate, which is far more realistic than Duffy's other estimates, may easily be overlooked, however, as *it wasn't mentioned in the abstract of the paper*. We didn't find Duffy's approach reliable this time either.[67]

Lynge's studies on overdiagnosis

In 2003, Elsebeth Lynge, Anne Helene Olsen and colleagues reported a study from Denmark where the last sentence in the abstract was: 'The experiences from Copenhagen and Fyn show that organised mammography screening can operate without overdiagnosis of breast cancer.'[83] The claim is silly; it so obviously *cannot* be true. There are several problems with their approach.

They based their study on a false premise; namely, that the breast cancer incidence in a screened population should decline rapidly after the prevalence peak to the level expected without screening, if there is no overdiagnosis and a closed cohort of women is studied. The error in this reasoning is that they assume there is no overdiagnosis in the prevalence peak. Furthermore, they didn't present a statistical analysis in support of their claim, and as there was very little follow-up, they missed many overdiagnosed cases from subsequent screening rounds.

I was invited to take part in a scientific debate with Nick Day at a European Cancer Meeting shortly after their paper was published. I showed the graph from Olsen's paper (*see* Figure 16.6) and argued that it is impossible to say there is no overdiagnosis when there is a mountain of extra diagnoses and no valley of fewer diagnoses later on to compensate.

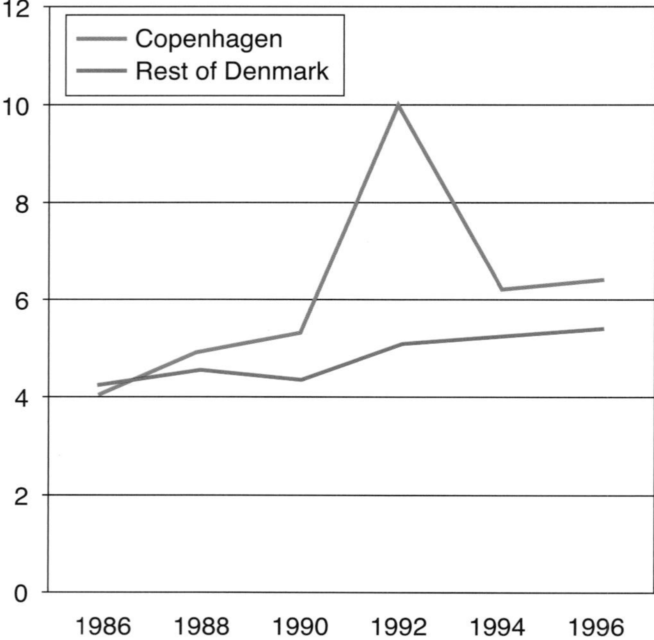

FIGURE 16.6 Graph of breast cancer diagnoses that was supposed to show that '. . . organised mammography screening can operate without overdiagnosis of breast cancer.' Y-axis shows the cumulative risk of invasive breast cancer in per cent (redrawn). The peak in diagnoses corresponds to the prevalence round

My logic led nowhere. Day was very positive towards the Danish study and it was impossible to move him the slightest bit. It was an awkward experience, considering Day's expertise, both in statistics and in screening.

Lynge co-authored a paper in 2006 with longer follow-up that contradicted her 2003 paper, as it showed the incidence in Copenhagen didn't return to the expected level without screening but remained elevated.[84] Curiously, however, although the title of the paper was 'Breast cancer incidence and mortality in the Nordic capitals, 1970–1998: trends related to mammography screening programmes', the authors didn't mention with a single word that the sustained increase in incidence means overdiagnosis.

Lynge, Olsen and colleagues reported yet another Danish study in 2006 and concluded, 'The data from the current study do not provide evidence of overdiagnosis of invasive breast cancer in the 2 Danish screening programs or, if overdiagnosis was found to occur, it was only of limited magnitude.'[85] This study was very similar to the one they had published 3 years earlier,[83] but they broke another academic rule by not quoting their first study, which is required in order to avoid false novelty of subsequent similar studies.

Their 2006 study appeared in *Cancer*, which is notoriously pro-screening, as I have illustrated in relation to Tabár's 'beyond reason' studies. The authors proceeded in a way that made it virtually impossible to detect overdiagnosis. First, they lost power in their analysis by splitting Copenhagen from Funen and analysing the two regions separately, which is meaningless if one wants to study overdiagnosis. Second, they evaluated whether the observed rates for the two regions were within the 95% confidence interval of the expected rate, which they projected from the prescreening rates using regression analysis – instead of testing whether the observed rates were significantly higher than expected, which is how one should analyse such data. Third, their confidence interval is seriously misleading; it is way too broad. When I calculated a confidence interval for a single year based on their numbers, it was much narrower than where it is narrowest in their figure. This suggests that they used a faulty method. Fourth, they left out diagnoses of carcinoma *in situ* from their calculations, although these cell changes contribute substantially to overdiagnosis. Fifth, they made the logical error of concluding 'evidence of absence' from 'absence of evidence'. Sixth, they made all these mistakes despite having a statistician, Anne Helene Olsen, among the authors.

All this contrasts greatly with our findings. We found 33% overdiagnosis, with a 95% confidence interval of 28% to 39%.[61] With such a narrow confidence interval, one would have thought it impossible to *avoid* finding overdiagnosis in Denmark.

Lynge's study in *Cancer*, like her first one, represents a serious violation of basic scientific principles. According to science philosopher Karl Popper, one should subject one's null hypothesis (which in this case is: 'There is no overdiagnosis') to the strongest possible falsification attempts, and one should assemble as much power as possible in the attempt at refuting the null hypothesis. Lynge's study is fatally flawed, and it came as no surprise to us that a recent systematic review of overdiagnosis excluded it.[46] It also contains fallacious arguments, e.g. 'Given the known participation rate and sensitivity, a lead time of approximately 3 years would be compatible with no overdiagnosis occurring during the first screening round.' Pure nonsense, which unfortunately may look convincing for readers knowing little about cancer screening. Try to analyse this sentence. Can you understand it? I think not because it's empty. Screening always leads to overdiagnosis, no matter which fine words – rather than data – have been used to conceal this fact.[3,5]

Carcinoma *in situ* and the increase in mastectomies

I have given many examples that the fact that screening leads to more mastectomies has been flatly and often aggressively denied by the screening advocates. The documented increase in mastectomies contrasts with assertions by trialists,[86] policymakers,[70,87,88] websites supported by governmental institutions and advocacy groups,[89] and invitational letters sent to women invited to screening[90] that early detection spares patients more aggressive treatments – in particular, mastectomy.

Julietta Patnick, director of the NHS cancer screening programmes, perpetuated this error when our updated Cochrane review came out in 2006: 'Women who were screened were also less likely to have a mastectomy than those who were not screened.'[91]

It is easy to see that screening leads to more mastectomies, not only in the trials,[4] but also in practice. Again, Denmark is ideal, as only 20% of the country was screened throughout 17 years (*see* Figure 16.7).

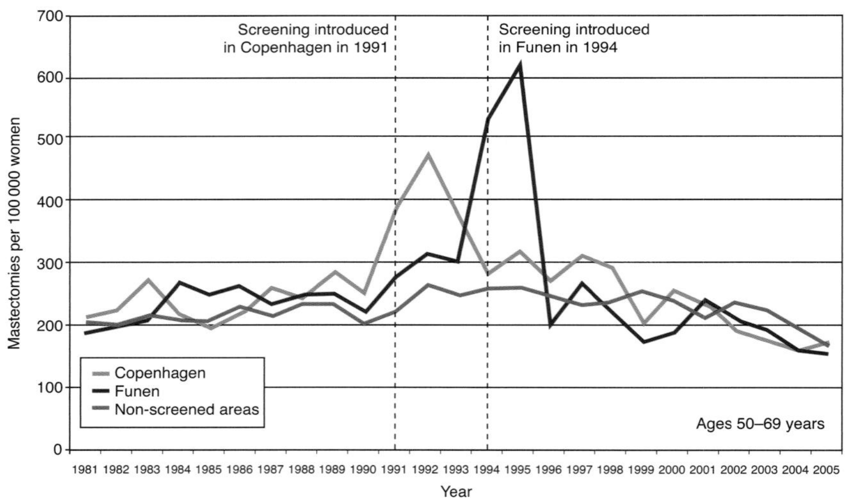

FIGURE 16.7 Mastectomies in Denmark in areas with (Funen and Copenhagen) and without screening. Data from Statistics Denmark

The doubt industry has been surprisingly quiet on this issue, perhaps because it is hard to produce data that suggest that screening doesn't increase mastectomies, and even harder to concoct data that suggest that screening leads to *fewer* mastectomies. But it has been done. And the Tabár/Smith/Duffy trio were again those who did the impossible. They asserted there were *fewer* mastectomies (actually it was about the same, with no significant difference) in the Kopparberg part of the Two-County trial in the group invited to screening compared with the control group.[92] As always, some detective work was needed to demonstrate where they had . . . well, what can I say without being threatened with libel by Tabár (*see* Chapter 21)? I will leave it to the reader to fill in the gaps. *The authors didn't reveal that the numbers they used for the control group were derived after the whole control group had been offered screening.* Such data are totally meaningless. Before the control group was screened, there were 17% more mastectomies with screening in Kopparberg.[4]

The most common manoeuvre is more subtle than adding mastectomies to the control group that don't belong there. Imagine a town with a certain level of crime. You divide the crimes into serious ones and less serious ones. Over a period of time, the rate of serious crime increases by 20% and the rate of less serious crime increases by 40%. This is clearly a development for the worse. But although *more* people are exposed to serious crime and *more* people are exposed to less serious crime as well, a trickster would say that, as there are now *relatively* fewer cases of serious crime, the situation has improved.

The trickster didn't show us the absolute numbers but talked about a proportion. This is highly misleading, but it is precisely what screening advocates often do. It was stated in the Danish report that paved the way for screening that 13% of the patients had a breast-conserving operation before screening was introduced in Copenhagen, and 45% had such an operation after screening was introduced.[70] Such statistics have fooled many people who don't realise that because of overdiagnosis, proportions are bound to be misleading. The number of operations increases with screening, both the breast-conserving ones and the mastectomies.

Duffy co-authored a small study from Florence in 2002 with Eugenio Paci and others[93] that built on a false assumption.[94] They asserted that if screening increased the number of mastectomies, populations in which screening has been introduced should see a subsequent increase. Obviously, since the mastectomy rate has gone down steadily throughout many years, also in countries without screening, it is only to be expected that the authors found a decrease in the mastectomy rate when screening was introduced.

The relevant question is whether the decline is smaller when women are screened than when they are not screened, and the randomised trials show that this is the case.[4] Furthermore, Duffy's findings from Florence are contradicted by a much larger study from the southeast Netherlands, where screening was introduced in the same time period. I calculated that the number of invasive cases increased by 78%, the number of women who underwent breast-conserving surgery increased by 71% and *the number of women who underwent mastectomy increased by 84%*.[95] (Note that this is a legitimate way of using percentages, as we deal here with each operation type separately over a given time period, and not with a proportion of breast-conserving operations out of the total.) What is more, it was an underestimate, as the authors didn't include carcinoma *in situ*, which is rarely detected without screening, but is frequently treated by mastectomy. It is worth noting that breast-conserving surgery with subsequent radiotherapy is also a pretty rough treatment that, in addition, can lead to decreased survival.[96]

When Duffy's flawed study was published in the *BMJ*, it was welcomed by the media and led to hasty endorsements by public figures implying a refutation of the findings that mammographic screening leads to overdiagnosis and overtreatment.[97] A commentator complained that the authors hadn't shown the trend in mastectomies prior to screening and that we therefore didn't know whether the downward trend had preceded screening,[98] but Paci and Duffy did not address this serious criticism in their reply.[99]

The denial of overdiagnosis and the associated increase in mastectomies continued everywhere. In 2007, Anne Helene Olsen and the heads of the two screening centres in Denmark, Ilse Vejborg and Walter Schwartz, published a 'state-of-the-art' article about screening that in the title promised to deal with its advantages and disadvantages.[100] The authors noted that if overdiagnosis of invasive cancer existed, Danish studies suggested it was very limited. They also argued that screening could lead to more opportunities for breast-conserving surgery rather than mastectomy. They didn't cite the Cochrane review.

It has received little attention that the detection and treatment of carcinoma *in situ* leads to a lot of harm in healthy women, including a lot of mastectomies. In Europe, about 10% of all diagnoses in the screened age groups (including interval cancers) are carcinoma *in situ*, and in the United States, the rate is much higher. Between 1991 and 1998, 25% of all findings in the first screening round were carcinoma *in situ*, which increased to 33% in subsequent rounds.[101]

In the United Kingdom, 29% of the women with a diagnosis of carcinoma *in situ* received a mastectomy in 1999–2000,[102] and the number of women who were treated by mastectomy almost *doubled* from 1998 to 2008.[103] Since there was screening in the whole country in 1998, one would not have expected such a dramatic increase. The screening programme was extended to the age group 65–70 years in 2001, but as most of these women had already been offered screening when they were younger, this extension cannot explain much of the increase.

Carcinoma *in situ* is also often treated by radiotherapy, although a carefully performed meta-analysis from 2000 predicted that radiotherapy increases overall mortality for women at particularly low risk, such as those who have their cancers found by screening.[4,96] Since the prognosis of carcinoma *in situ* is exceptionally good, one would expect radiotherapy of these cell changes to be particularly harmful.

The doubtful rationale for radiotherapy became apparent in a US study from 2004.[104] The authors considered it undertreatment that about half the women undergoing lumpectomy for ductal carcinoma *in situ* didn't get radiotherapy, arguing that radiotherapy reduces the risk of local recurrence and of subsequent development of invasive cancer. I noted that the 50–50 split likely reflected the considerable uncertainty and suggested a wait-and-see approach, as it is more important to survive than to reduce the risk of getting invasive cancer.[105] Other commentators mentioned that they had monitored patients who had not received radiation therapy for up to 20 years without witnessing recurrence in a substantial majority.[106] In reply, the author acknowledged that the relatively low rate of radiation after lumpectomy might reflect community equipoise with respect to its value and recommended randomised trials to resolve the issue.[107]

What this illustrates so clearly is that clinicians have great difficulty accepting that cancer is a very different disease today, when we have screening. Much of what we call breast cancer is not even a disease, but cell changes that women do not benefit from having detected and treated. A surgeon exemplified this difficulty when he described the meta-analysis of radiotherapy[96] in the *Läkartidningen* with the telling title: 'Best utility of radiotherapy in early breast cancer in young women'.[108] We explained to the surgeon that the meta-analysis suggested that radiotherapy of low-risk cancers *increased* mortality,[109] but our paedagogical initiative failed, as the title of his reply was: 'The meta-analysis was not about screening'.[110]

The technique has improved and the irradiation is more focused on the cancer today.[111] However, it is not possible to use radiotherapy without harms, and there are no large long-term studies that can tell us what the extent of the harms are with modern radiotherapy. As noted earlier, the paper usually quoted in support of the improvement only reports on 13 deaths from ischaemic heart disease in one group and 12 in the other,[112] which is far too little for making any judgement about the harms of modern radiotherapy. It has been suggested that radiotherapy may double not only the mortality from heart disease but also from lung cancer,[113] which may take many years to develop. Most recently, in 2010, a randomised trial of a single dose of intraoperative radiotherapy for invasive breast cancer resulted in the same low level of recurrence of the cancer as the standard of several weeks of repeated radiotherapy.[114] This is promising, as the dose is much lower for the intraoperative therapy.

Given the massive harms related to diagnosing and treating carcinoma *in situ* in screening programmes, it is unacceptable that the women have not been informed about carcinoma *in situ* when they are invited to screening (*see* Chapter 19). It is also unacceptable that they are informed that screening saves breasts. In 2011, we confirmed, using data from the Norwegian screening programme, that screening increases mastectomies.[115]

References

1 Schwartz LM, Woloshin S, Sox HC, *et al*. US women's attitudes to false positive mammography results and detection of ductal carcinoma in situ: cross sectional survey. *BMJ*. 2000; **320**(7250): 1635–40.

2 Jørgensen KJ, Gøtzsche PC. Overdiagnosis in publicly organised mammography screening programmes: systematic review of incidence trends. *BMJ*. 2009; **339**: b2587.

3 Vainio H, Bianchini F. *Breast Cancer Screening. IARC Handbooks of Cancer Prevention, Vol* 7. Lyon, France: IARC Press; 2002.

4 Gøtzsche PC, Nielsen M. Screening for breast cancer with mammography. *Cochrane Database Syst Rev*. 2009; (4): CD001877.

5 Welch HG. *Should I Be Tested for Cancer? Maybe not and here's why*. Berkeley: University of California Press; 2004.

6 Nielsen M, Thomsen JL, Primdahl S, *et al*. Breast cancer atypia among young and middle-aged women: a study of 110 medicolegal autopsies. *Br J Cancer*. 1987; **56**(6): 814–19.

7 Serrano M. Cancer regression by senescence. *N Engl J Med*. 2007; **356**(19): 1996–7.

8 Fox MS. On the diagnosis and treatment of breast cancer. *JAMA*. 1979; **241**(5): 489–94.

9 Janzon L, Andersson I. The Malmö mammographic screening trial. In: Miller AB, Chamberlain J, Day NE, *et al*., editors. *Cancer Screening*. Cambridge: Cambridge University Press; 1991. pp. 37–44.

10 Tindall G. Behind the screens. *Time*. 1994 Oct 8.

11 Zahl P-H, Andersen JM, Mæhlen J. Spontaneous regression of cancerous tumors detected by mammography screening. *JAMA*. 2004; **292**(21): 2579–80.

12 Fryback DG, Stout NK, Rosenberg MA, *et al*. The Wisconsin Breast Cancer Epidemiology Simulation Model. *J Natl Cancer Inst Monogr*. 2006; (36): 37–47.

13 Zahl P-H, Mæhlen J. Do model results suggest spontaneous regression of breast cancer? *Int J Cancer*. 2006; **118**(10): 2647.

14 Jonsson H, Johansson R, Lenner P. Increased incidence of invasive breast cancer after the introduction of service screening with mammography in Sweden. *Int J Cancer*. 2005; **117**(5): 842–7.

15 Jonsson H, Johansson R, Lenner P. Comments to the letters by Per-Henrik Zahl and Jan Mæhlen and by Peter C. Gotzsche concerning our article: Increased incidence of invasive breast cancer after the introduction of service screening with mammography in Sweden. *Int J Cancer*. 2006; **118**: 2649.

16 Zahl P-H, Mæhlen J, Welch HG. The natural history of invasive breast cancers detected by screening mammography. *Arch Intern Med*. 2008; **168**(21): 2311–16.

17 Zahl P-H, Gøtzsche PC, Mæhlen J. Natural history of breast cancers detected in the

Swedish mammography screening program: a cohort study. *Lancet Oncol*. Epub 2011 Oct 11.

18 Forrest P, editor. *Breast Cancer Screening: report to the health ministers of England, Wales, Scotland & Northern Ireland*. London: Department of Health and Social Science; 1986.

19 Day NE, Baines CJ, Chamberlain J, *et al*. UICC project on screening for cancer: report of the workshop on screening for breast cancer; meeting held in Helsinki, Finland, on April 7–9, 1986. *Int J Cancer*. 1986; **38**(3): 303–8.

20 Duffy SW, Tabár L, Fagerberg G, *et al*. Breast screening, prognostic factors and survival: results from the Swedish two county study. *Br J Cancer*. 1991; **64**(6): 1133–8.

21 Tabár L, Fagerberg CJ, Gad A, *et al*. Reduction in mortality from breast cancer after mass screening with mammography: randomised trial from the Breast Cancer Screening Working Group of the Swedish National Board of Health and Welfare. *Lancet*. 1985; **1**(8433): 829–32.

22 Skrabanek P. The debate over mass mammography in Britain: the case against. *BMJ*. 1988; **297**(6654): 971–2.

23 Woodman CBJ, Threlfall AG, Boggis CRM, *et al*. Is the three year breast screening interval too long? Occurrence of interval cancers in NHS breast screening programme's north western region. *BMJ*. 1995; **310**(6974): 224–6.

24 Skrabanek P. Mass mammography: the time for reappraisal. *Int J Technol Assess Health Care*. 1989; **5**(3): 423–30.

25 Schmidt JG. The epidemiology of mass breast cancer screening: a plea for a valid measure of benefit. *J Clin Epidemiol*. 1990; **43**(3): 215–25.

26 Schmidt JG. Response to Dr Shapiro's dissent. *J Clin Epidemiol*. 1990; **43**: 235–9.

27 Gøtzsche PC, Nielsen M. Screening for breast cancer with mammography. *Cochrane Database Syst Rev*. 2006; (4): CD001877.

28 Gøtzsche PC, Olsen O. Is screening for breast cancer with mammography justifiable? *Lancet*. 2000; **355**(9198): 129–34.

29 Olsen O, Gøtzsche PC. Cochrane review on screening for breast cancer with mammography. *Lancet*. 2001; **358**(9290): 1340–2.

30 Olsen O, Gøtzsche PC. Systematic review of screening for breast cancer with mammography. *Lancet*. 2001 Oct 20. Available at: http://image.thelancet.com/extras/fullreport.pdf (accessed 5 May 2010).

31 Nattinger AB, Hoffmann RG, Kneusel RT, *et al*. Relation between appropriateness of primary therapy for early-stage breast carcinoma and increased use of breast-conserving surgery. *Lancet*. 2000; **356**(9236): 1148–53.

32 Barratt A, Howard K, Irwig L, *et al*. Model of outcomes of screening mammography: information to support informed choices. *BMJ*. 2005; **330**(7497): 936–8.

33 Douek M, Baum M. Mass breast screening: is there a hidden cost? *Br J Surg*. 2003; **90** (Suppl. 1): (Abstract Breast 14).

34 Ries LAG, Eisner MP, Kosary CL, *et al*. *SEER Cancer Statistics Review, 1973–1999*. Available at: http://seer.cancer.gov/csr/1973_1999 (accessed 26 June 2003).

35 Fletcher SW, Elmore JG. Clinical practice: mammographic screening for breast cancer. *N Engl J Med*. 2003; **348**(17): 1672–80.

36 Gøtzsche PC. On the benefits and harms of screening for breast cancer. *Int J Epidemiol*. 2004; **33**(1): 56–64.

37 Zahl P-H, Strand BH, Mæhlen J. Incidence of breast cancer in Norway and Sweden during introduction of nationwide screening: prospective cohort study. *BMJ*. 2004; **328**(7445): 921–4.

38 Kricker A, Smoothy V, Armstrong B. *Ductal Carcinoma In Situ in New South Wales Women in 1995 to 1997*. Available at: www.nbcc.org.au (accessed 26 April 2000).
39 Miller AB, To T, Baines CJ, *et al*. The Canadian National Breast Screening Study-1: breast cancer mortality after 11 to 16 years of follow-up; a randomized screening trial of mammography in women age 40 to 49 years. *Ann Intern Med*. 2002; **137**(5 Pt. 1): 305–12.
40 Moss S. Overdiagnosis and overtreatment of breast cancer: overdiagnosis in randomised controlled trials of breast cancer screening. *Breast Cancer Res*. 2005; **7**(5): 230–4.
41 Zackrisson S, Andersson I, Janzon L, *et al*. Rate of over-diagnosis of breast cancer 15 years after end of Malmö mammographic screening trial: follow-up study. *BMJ*. 2006; **332**(7543): 689–92.
42 Welch HG. How much overdiagnosis? *BMJ*. 2006 Mar 10. Available at: www.bmj.com/content/332/7543/689/reply (accessed 4 May 2006).
43 Gøtzsche PC, Jørgensen KJ. Estimate of harm/benefit ratio of mammography screening was five times too optimistic. *BMJ*. 2006 Mar 27. Available at: http://bmj.bmjjournals.com/cgi/eletters/332/7543/691 (accessed 5 May 2010).
44 Jørgensen JJ, Johansen HK, Gøtzsche PC. Flaws in design, analysis and interpretation of Pfizer's antifungal trials of voriconazole and uncritical subsequent quotations. *Trials*. 2006; **7**: 3.
45 Paci E. Quantification of overdiagnosis: simple solutions are not necessarily true. *BMJ*. 2006 Apr 15. Available at: www.bmj.com/content/332/7543/689/reply (accessed 5 May 2010).
46 Biesheuvel C, Barratt A, Howard K, *et al*. Effects of study methods and biases on estimates of invasive breast cancer overdetection with mammography screening: a systematic review. *Lancet Oncol*. 2007; **8**(12): 1129–38.
47 Zahl P-H, Jørgensen KJ, Mæhlen J, *et al*. Biases in estimates of overdetection due to mammography screening. *Lancet Oncol*. 2008; **9**(3): 199–201.
48 Jørgensen KJ, Gøtzsche PC. Overdiagnosis in publicly organised mammography screening programmes: systematic review of incidence trends. *BMJ*. 2009; **339**: b2587.
49 Morrell S, Barratt A, Irwig L, *et al*. Estimates of overdiagnosis of invasive breast cancer associated with screening mammography. *Cancer Causes Control*. 2010; **21**(2): 275–82.
50 Baum M. Attitudes to screening locked in a time warp. *BMJ*. 2009 Jul 12. Available at: www.bmj.com/cgi/eletters/339/jul09_1/b2587 (accessed 5 May 2010).
51 Havercroft D. Let women decide for themselves. *BMJ*. 2009 Jul 19. Available at: www.bmj.com/cgi/eletters/339/jul09_1/b2587 (accessed 5 May 2010).
52 Vaidya JS. Women undergoing screening mammography experience a higher incidence of invasive breast cancer, without a corresponding reduction in symptomatic breast cancer. *BMJ*. 2009 Jul 20. Available at: www.bmj.com/cgi/eletters/339/jul09_1/b2587 (accessed 5 May 2010).
53 Jørgensen KJ, Gøtzsche PC. It is time for a new paradigm for overdiagnosis with screening mammography. *BMJ*. 2009 Aug 20. Available at: www.bmj.com/cgi/eletters/339/jul09_1/b2587 (accessed 5 May 2010).
54 Shapiro S. Discussion II. *J Natl Cancer Inst Monogr*. 1985; **67**: 75.
55 Atterstam I. [Mammography will be scrutinised after new study] [Swedish]. *Svenska Dagbladet*. 2009 Jul 11.
56 Johnson K. Softer mammography screening and breast exam guidelines draw mixed reactions. *Elsevier Global Medical News*. 2009 Nov 20.
57 Aschwanden C. Rational argument: convincing the public to accept new medical

guidelines. *Miller McCune*. 2010 Apr 20. Available at: www.miller-mccune.com/health/convincing-the-public-to-accept-new-medical-guidelines-11422 (accessed 5 May 2010).
58 National Breast and Ovarian Cancer Centre. *In the News: over-diagnosis from mammography screening*. 2009 Jul 11. Available at: www.nbocc.org.au/resources/in-the-news/over-diagnosis-mammography-screening.html (accessed 5 August 2009).
59 Bratt A. [Self-examination of the breasts rejected by researchers] [Swedish]. *Dagens Nyheter*. 2009 Oct 1.
60 Kösters JP, Gøtzsche PC. Regular self-examination or clinical examination for early detection of breast cancer. *Cochrane Database Syst Rev*. 2003; (2): CD003373.
61 Jørgensen KJ, Zahl P-H, Gøtzsche PC. Overdiagnosis in organised mammography screening in Denmark: a comparative study. *BMC Womens Health*. 2009; **9**: 36.
62 Salleh A. 1 in 4 breast cancers 'not threatening'. 2009 Nov 11. Available at: www.abc.net.au/science/articles/2009/11/11/2739398.htm (accessed 14 November 2009).
63 Oreskes N, Conway EM. *Merchants of Doubt*. New York: Bloomsbury Press; 2010.
64 Michaels D. *Doubt Is Their Product*. Oxford: Oxford University Press; 2008.
65 Topol EJ. Failing the public health: rofecoxib, Merck, and the FDA. *N Engl J Med*. 2004; **351**(17): 1707–9.
66 Nesi T. *Poison Pills: the untold story of the Vioxx drug scandal*. New York: St. Martin's Press; 2008.
67 Gøtzsche PC, Jørgensen KJ, Mæhlen J, *et al*. Estimation of lead time and overdiagnosis in breast cancer screening. *Br J Cancer*. 2009; **100**(1): 219.
68 Day NE, Walter SD. Simplified models of screening for chronic disease: estimation procedures from mass screening programmes. *Biometrics*. 1984; **40**(1): 1–14.
69 Boer R, Warmerdam P, de Koning H, *et al*. Extra incidence caused by mammographic screening. *Lancet*. 1994; **343**(8903): 979.
70 Sundhedsstyrelsen (National Board of Health). [*Early detection and treatment of breast cancer. Status report*] [*Danish*]. Copenhagen: Sundhedsstyrelsen; 1997.
71 [*General advice. Mammography screening – for early detection of cancer*] [*Swedish*]. Stockholm: Socialstyrelsen, SoS rapport; 1986: 3.
72 [*Mammography screening*] [*Swedish*]. Stockholm: Socialstyrelsen, SoS rapport; 1998: 17.
73 Yen M-F, Tabár L, Vitak B, *et al*. Quantifying the potential problem of overdiagnosis of ductal carcinoma in situ in breast cancer screening. *Eur J Cancer*. 2003; **39**(12): 1746–54.
74 Smith RA, Duffy SW, Gabe R, *et al*. The randomized trials of breast cancer screening: what have we learned? *Radiol Clin North Am*. 2004; **42**(5): 793–806.
75 Paci E, Warwick J, Falini P, *et al*. Overdiagnosis in screening: is the increase in breast cancer incidence rates a cause for concern? *J Med Screen*. 2004; **11**(1): 23–7.
76 Duffy SW, Agbaje O, Tabár L, *et al*. Overdiagnosis and overtreatment of breast cancer: estimates of overdiagnosis from two trials of mammographic screening for breast cancer. *Breast Cancer Res*. 2005; **7**(6): 258–65.
77 Olsen AH, Agbaje OF, Myles JP, *et al*. Overdiagnosis, sojourn time, and sensitivity in the Copenhagen mammography screening program. *Breast J*. 2006; **12**(4): 338–42.
78 Welch HG, Black WC. Using autopsy series to estimate the disease 'reservoir' for ductal carcinoma in situ of the breast. *Ann Intern Med*. 1997; **127**(11): 1023–8.
79 Gøtzsche PC, Jørgensen KJ. Stephen Duffy's claims on the benefits and harms of breast screening are seriously wrong. *BMJ*. 2009 May 1. Available at: www.bmj.com/cgi/eletters/338/jan27_2/b86#212985 (accessed 22 May 2011).

80 Gøtzsche PC. Increased incidence of invasive breast cancer after the introduction of service screening with mammography in Sweden. *Int J Cancer*. 2006; **118**(10): 2648.
81 Duffy SW, Tabár L, Olsen AH, *et al*. Absolute numbers of lives saved and overdiagnosis in breast cancer screening, from a randomised trial and from the breast screening programme in England. *J Med Screen*. 2010; **17**(1): 25–30.
82 Duffy SW, Lynge E, Jonsson H, *et al*. Complexities in the estimation of overdiagnosis in breast cancer screening. *Br J Cancer*. 2008; **99**(7): 1176–8.
83 Olsen AH, Jensen A, Njor S, *et al*. Breast cancer incidence after the start of mammography screening in Denmark. *Br J Cancer*. 2003; **88**(3): 362–5.
84 Törnberg S, Kemetli L, Lynge E, *et al*. Breast cancer incidence and mortality in the Nordic capitals, 1970–1998: trends related to mammography screening programmes. *Acta Oncol*. 2006; **45**(5): 528–35.
85 Svendsen AL, Olsen AH, von Euler-Chelpin M, *et al*. Breast cancer incidence after the introduction of mammography screening: what should be expected? *Cancer*. 2006; **106**(9): 1883–90.
86 Tabár L, Fagerberg G, Duffy SW, *et al*. The Swedish two county trial of mammographic screening for breast cancer: recent results and calculation of benefit. *J Epidemiol Community Health*. 1989; **43**(2): 107–14.
87 Swedish Cancer Society and the Swedish National Board of Health and Welfare. Breast-cancer screening with mammography in women aged 40–49 years. *Int J Cancer*. 1996; **68**(6): 693–9.
88 Westerholm B. [Shocking view on the worth of middle-aged women] [Swedish]. *Läkartidningen*. 1988; **85**(47): 4056–7.
89 Jørgensen KJ, Gøtzsche PC. Presentation on websites of possible benefits and harms from screening for breast cancer: cross sectional study. *BMJ*. 2004; **328**(7432): 148–51.
90 Jørgensen KJ, Gøtzsche PC. Content of invitations to publicly funded screening mammography. *BMJ*. 2006; **332**(7540): 538–41.
91 Dent J. Researchers question benefits of breast cancer screening. *Guardian*. 2006 Oct 18.
92 Tabár L, Smith RA, Vitak B, *et al*. Mammographic screening: a key factor in the control of breast cancer. *Cancer J*. 2003; **9**(1): 15–27.
93 Paci E, Duffy SW, Giorgi D, *et al*. Are breast cancer screening programmes increasing rates of mastectomy? Observational study. *BMJ*. 2002; **325**(7361): 418.
94 Gøtzsche PC. Misleading paper on mastectomy rates in a screening programme. *BMJ*. 2002 Aug 27. Available at: http://bmj.com/cgi/eletters/325/7361/418#24972 (accessed 22 May 2011).
95 Gøtzsche PC. Trends in breast-conserving surgery in the southeast Netherlands: comments on article by Ernst and colleagues. Eur J Cancer 2001, 37, 2435–2440. *Eur J Cancer*. 2002; **38**(9): 1288.
96 Early Breast Cancer Trialists' Collaborative Group. Favourable and unfavourable effects on long-term survival of radiotherapy for early breast cancer: an overview of the randomised trials. *Lancet*. 2000; **355**(9217): 1757–70.
97 Thornton H. Inappropriate use of evidence? *BMJ*. 2002 Aug 24. Available at: http://bmj.com/cgi/eletters/325/7361/418#24972 (accessed 22 May 2011).
98 Spence D. Confounding factor. *BMJ*. 2002 Aug 27. Available at: http://bmj.com/cgi/eletters/325/7361/418#24972 (accessed 22 May 2011).
99 Paci E, Duffy SW. Re: Botticelli's 'Birth of Venus'. *BMJ*. 2002 Oct 24. Available at: http://bmj.com/cgi/eletters/325/7361/418#24972 (accessed 22 May 2011).

100 Olsen AH, Schwartz W, Vejborg I. [Mammography screening: advantages and disadvantages] [Danish]. *Ugeskr Læger*. 2007; **169**(36): 2977–9.
101 May DS, Lee NC, Richardson LC, *et al*. Mammography and breast cancer detection by race and Hispanic ethnicity: results from a national program (United States). *Cancer Causes Control*. 2000; **11**(8): 697–705.
102 NHS Cancer Screening Programmes. *BASO Breast Audit 1999/2000*. Available at: www.cancerscreening.nhs.uk/breastscreen/publications.html (accessed 12 December 2001).
103 Dixon JM. Breast screening has increased the number of mastectomies. *Breast Cancer Res*. 2009; **11**(Suppl. 3): S19.
104 Baxter NN, Virnig BA, Durham SB, *et al*. Trends in the treatment of ductal carcinoma in situ of the breast. *J Natl Cancer Inst*. 2004; **96**(6): 443–8.
105 Gøtzsche PC. Re: Trends in the treatment of ductal carcinoma in situ of the breast. *J Natl Cancer Inst*. 2004; **96**(16): 1257.
106 Schwartz GF, Lagios MD, Silverstein MJ. Re: Trends in the treatment of ductal carcinoma in situ of the breast. *J Natl Cancer Inst*. 2004; **96**(16): 1258–9.
107 Baxter NN. Reponse Re: Trends in the treatment of ductal carcinoma in situ of the breast. *J Natl Cancer Inst*. 2004; **96**(16): 1259–60.
108 Liljegren G. [Best utility of radiotherapy in early breast cancer in young women] [Swedish]. *Läkartidningen*. 2000; **97**: 4423.
109 Gøtzsche PC, Olsen O. [Postoperative radiotherapy increases mortality in women who are diagnosed with breast cancer by screening] [Swedish]. *Läkartidningen*. 2001; **98**: 347.
110 Liljegren G. [The meta-analysis was not about screening] [Swedish]. *Läkartidningen*. 2001; **98**: 347–8.
111 Korreman SS, Pedersen AN, Aarup LR, *et al*. Reduction of cardiac and pulmonary complication probabilities after breathing adapted radiotherapy for breast cancer. *Int J Radiat Oncol Biol Phys*. 2006; **65**(5): 1375–80.
112 Hojris I, Overgaard M, Christensen JJ, *et al*. Morbidity and mortality of ischaemic heart disease in high-risk breast-cancer patients after adjuvant postmastectomy systemic treatment with or without radiotherapy: analysis of DBCG 82b and 82c randomised trials. *Lancet*. 1999; **354**(9188): 1425–30.
113 Darby S, McGale P, Taylor C, *et al*. Long-term mortality from heart disease and lung cancer after radiotherapy for early breast cancer: prospective cohort study of about 300 000 women in US SEER cancer registries. *Lancet Oncol*. 2005; **6**(8): 557–65.
114 Vaidya JS, Joseph DJ, Tobias JS, *et al*. Targeted intraoperative radiotherapy versus whole breast radiotherapy for breast cancer (TARGIT-A trial): an international, prospective, randomised, non-inferiority phase 3 trial. *Lancet*. 2010; **376**(9735): 91–102.
115 Suhrke P, Mæhlen J, Schlichting E, *et al*. Effect of mammography screening on surgical treatment for breast cancer in Norway: comparative analysis of cancer registry data. *BMJ* 2011; **343**: d4692.

17

Ad hominem attacks: a measure of desperation?

Years ago, I was hauled over the coals by mammography advocates for writing about research raising the potential for screening to do harm. It wasn't an issue they wanted even mentioned in public.

Melissa Sweet[1]

Anyone who dares challenge the sacred cow of screening has a terrible time.

Michael Baum[2]

PEOPLE PUBLISHING UNWELCOME RESULTS ARE OFTEN MOST haunted in their home country, likely because they are most influential there. Our Danish opponents have remarked that it is our 'fault' that the introduction of screening in Denmark has been so much delayed. This is undoubtedly correct, as political statements over the years have referred to our research as the reason the politicians doubted the value of screening and hesitated to introduce it.

The most vicious personal attacks we have been exposed to – apart from those of Peter Dean who is in a category of his own – have come from Danish colleagues. The debate started at a reasonable academic level, and with good manners, but already after the first article, the level of the debate was as low as in Sweden, and from there, it only became worse.

Two surgeons, Jens Peter Garne and Ib Hessov, started by praising the Two-County trial highly while criticising the Canadian trials in the *Ugeskrift for Læger* in July 2000,[3] and we responded with our usual arguments.[4]

Six months later,[5] just as predicted by Schopenhauer, Garne and Hessov no longer commented on the scientific substance but used erroneous *ad hominem* arguments. They considered it bad manners to go to the press before colleagues had seen our research and blamed us for a news story raising doubt about screening. We had not contacted the press.[6] A journalist who knew about the report we had submitted to the Danish National Board of Health in May 1999 had acquired it through the Freedom of Information Act and wrote about it. Garne and Hessov also claimed that my statement in an interview that more women lose a breast when they attend screening originated from unpublished reports. This was not true. We had published our data in the *Lancet* in January 2000,[7] and the Malmö trial had reported more mastectomies with screening 12 years earlier, in 1988.[8]

After our 2001 *Lancet* and Cochrane reviews came out, a journalist reported on the reactions.[9] Mogens Blichert-Toft from the Danish Breast Cancer Group characterised much of what we had written as 'pure misinformation', based on 'wrong assumptions' that 'cannot be used for anything'. Walter Schwartz, head of the Funen breast screening unit, dismissed our findings of overdiagnosis entirely, saying it didn't happen where he worked. He also noted that in his experience, fewer of the small tumours had metastasised than the large ones. True, but this cannot tell us anything about screening.

Garne and Hessov reappeared with unwarranted accusations.[10] The *Ugeskrift for Læger* wrote about our review 2 days after it appeared in the *Lancet*, which was perfectly legitimate of course. But Garne and Hessov found it unacceptable that the readers of the *Ugeskrift for Læger*, and subsequently the whole population of Denmark, should get informed about such a sensitive issue from a journalist, before it had been possible for decision-makers and experts to read and discuss the research reports. Most of all, it reflected badly on the *Ugeskrift for Læger*. This line of reasoning is also used by Peter Dean, Daniel Kopans, Nick Day and other screening advocates. Journals and newspapers that publish something they don't like are always irresponsible it seems, and these publications include the *Lancet*, the *BMJ* and the *New York Times*. Rather good company to be in, I would say. According to Duffy, Tabár and Smith, my findings, which they call 'claims', are not only irresponsible but even reckless.[11]

I explained that such were the conditions for medical publishing.[12] Garne and Hessov's foolish remarks are nevertheless interesting. Scientific debates should not be postponed by requiring that decision-makers and experts should be given time to read and discuss research reports before researchers are 'allowed' to say anything about their research. And who exactly should 'authorise' the researchers, and when? A journalist captured the situation aptly when she called an earlier article that came out just after our first *Lancet* review in 2000, 'Sensitive research'.[13] Indeed.

Ironically, although we had done nothing wrong, Garne and Hessov didn't make a similar comment when, in fact, the embargo rules *had* been violated by one of their allies. This speaks volumes of the double standards screening advocates have. Three weeks before Nyström and colleagues[14] published their meta-analysis of the Swedish trials in the *Lancet* in 2002, one of the authors discussed the effect on total mortality and on breast cancer mortality in a Danish national newspaper, and Elsebeth Lynge explained what it meant.[15] This was a serious violation of *Lancet*'s embargo rules, and the misconduct effectively impeded any scientific debate on the research. The newspaper journalist asked me to comment, but I couldn't, as I didn't have access to the report! Journalists always send me the reports when they ask for a comment, as they can access them 2 days before they are published, but this wasn't possible in this case.

UK statistician publishes in Danish

In January 2002, Nick Day, who did the statistical analysis of the Two-County trial, criticised our work in the *Ugeskrift for Læger*.[16] In response, a female general practitioner published a letter with the title 'May one write anything when the purpose is to promote screening?'[17] Day's article appeared in a theme issue about screening, but she was surprised with the unusual tone of his paper, e.g. Day described our criticism of the trials as utterly incompetent and worthless. Both the British and the Danes are usually more polite; we are certainly not used to such incivility in our medical journal.

She also noted that Day's paper was translated by Iben Holten of the Danish Cancer Society, who was not impartial, and she wanted to know who ordered the paper. She didn't see a need to participate in screening because we had shown it didn't affect total mortality or total cancer mortality, and she considered it immaterial which diagnosis would be written on her own death certificate when the time of death was not changed. Finally, she thanked us for our courage despite the humiliating and contemptuous way with which we were being treated from some quarters. The editors explained that they had approached another person who suggested they contact Nick Day.

Day's paper is full of errors. I wrote 'No' nine times in the margin and replied that most of his criticism was unwarranted and that we had already responded to the remainder in our reviews.[18] Day didn't quote our Cochrane review or its equivalent on the *Lancet* website, although they could have answered most of his points. I noted it was rather generous that the authors of the 1993 meta-analysis of the Swedish trials claimed that the cluster randomisation in the Two-County trial wasn't biased, with reference to an unpublished lecture.[19] Furthermore, I noted that a reference to the randomisation method in Nyström's thesis from 2000 led to an empty reference,[20] and that when we asked Nyström about it, he sent an unpublished letter that didn't describe the method either.

We had plenty of such experiences related to the Two-County trial, which had not increased our confidence in it. After Day's paper in the *Ugeskrift for Læger*, I didn't have much confidence in his analysis of the trial either. Most curiously, Day criticised us for not having paid attention to the clustering when we included it in our meta-analysis. Day hadn't paid attention to the clustering himself when he analysed the trial,[18] and the results weren't affected by it. Day also criticised the Canadian trials for having allowed breast examinations but did not mention that the trial protocol for the Two-County trial also described breast examinations, which was not revealed in the publications on the trial.

Finally, Day said the *Lancet*'s decision to publish our paper was regrettable and irresponsible and that we hadn't paid attention to any of the many critical comments that had been raised. We surely had – a lot of attention.

Inappropriate name-dropping

Garne and Hessov returned a fourth time. In June 2002, they published an article in the *Ugeskrift for Læger* defying a rational discourse on screening. The title was: 'WHO and *The Lancet*: yes to mammography screening'.[21] What a puzzling title. How could a medical journal say yes or no to anything that is a political decision? It didn't make sense.

There were only two references to the *Lancet* in their paper and one was Nyström's 2002 meta-analysis[14] that didn't (and couldn't) express the *Lancet*'s views. The other reference was to an anonymous *Lancet* editorial. The *Lancet*'s editor sometimes writes anonymous editorials, and I therefore thought it was one of Richard Horton's. That didn't make sense. Horton had spent a lot of time examining our research before he published it in 2001 and he was convinced we were right. He could therefore hardly have written an editorial 6 months later saying there was no longer any doubt about the value of screening. Furthermore, a competent editor wouldn't take an authoritative stance in a situation where there is no clear right or wrong.

When I looked up the so-called anonymous *Lancet* editorial, I found that in fact it was *not* anonymous. Although there were no authors in Garne and Hessov's citation, there were two authors, both of whom worked at the British Columbia Cancer Agency.[22] This was very slick. In their paper, Garne and Hessov spoke of a 'solid editorial comment', but it wasn't an editorial comment in the sense that it expressed the *Lancet*'s views. And it didn't even say unequivocally yes to screening. It noted, 'The latest analysis does not tell us whether the massive effort to develop screening programmes in at least 22 countries and to encourage participation is worthwhile. That issue must be honestly confronted by those organisations and individuals with an interest in maintaining programmes for mammography screening.'[3]

Garne and Hessov's claim that the World Health Organization (WHO) had said yes to screening seemed also to be uncompelling. They referred to a press release,[23] but the press release wasn't about WHO's recommendations, or, in fact, anyone's recommendations. It described a meeting convened by the International Agency for Research on Cancer (IARC) with 24 experts who had agreed that mammography screening of women between 50 and 69 years of age reduced breast cancer mortality. The press release noted, 'The consensus on the value of mammography screening has recently been challenged by Danish investigators associated with the Cochrane Collaboration.' So the whole idea seemed to have been to get experts to agree that screening worked. That must have been an easy task, as the majority of the invited experts were well-known screening advocates. Furthermore, it was not a WHO statement but a statement from the IARC. The homepage of the IARC states, 'As a WHO Agency, IARC follows the general governing rules of the UN family. It is governed by its own Governing bodies, however.' I was later informed by one of the 24 participants in the meeting that the process had not been satisfactory and that when he had argued that our research had been incredibly important for raising pertinent issues about the trials, some participants had been intemperate in disagreeing. So much for WHO saying yes to screening.[24]

The IARC meeting was published in a 229-page book that I reviewed for the *International Journal of Epidemiology*.[25] I noted that the book was comprehensive, very well written and highly relevant for everyone with an interest in cancer screening. But I also mentioned that the authors had left out essential issues. They noted that overdiagnosis and overtreatment is an inevitable consequence of screening, but omitted to mention the data in our *Lancet* review that documented a considerably increased use of radiotherapy, tumourectomy and mastectomy. I also noticed that there was no reference to a recent systematic review by the Early Breast Cancer Trialists' Collaborative Group.[26] It showed that radiotherapy in women who have their cancers identified by screening is likely to increase overall mortality, but since these women die from heart problems, they are not counted as breast cancer deaths. The authors acknowledged – in contrast to most of the screening advocates that had attacked us – that misclassification of cause of death could bias the results in the screening trials in favour of screening. But they didn't mention that overall cancer mortality – including breast cancer mortality – is the same in the screened groups as in the control groups, contrary to what one would expect, given the large mortality reductions in breast cancer the IARC working group claimed in the book.

There were other important omissions in the book. Curiously, for example, the book concluded that the flawed New York trial was valid and argued that prior breast cancers (existing before the randomisation date) were adequately excluded from both the study group and the control group. As mentioned in the previous chapter, this is not correct.

A Danish epidemiologist later wrote about the book that he wondered why the experts who had written it had not commented on the original and important observations we had made in our Cochrane review. He concluded amusingly that Heisenberg's uncertainty principle was not only valid in nuclear physics but also for meta-analyses.[27] The act of observation seems to change what is being observed, namely the magnitude of the effect of screening.

I noted in my book review that what I had missed most was a discussion of ethical issues. This is particularly relevant for Garne and Hessov's misleading headline. There is a difference between what we can do (science) and what we should do (ethics), which they ignored completely.

Garne and Hessov continued to deny that screening increases mastectomies and quoted Nyström's recent meta-analysis for saying that our criticism of the Swedish trials was 'misleading and unfounded'. However, as we showed a month later in the *Lancet*,[28] our criticism was appropriate and relevant, and it is therefore also published in our updated Cochrane review.

The IARC's press release stated that screening could reduce breast cancer mortality by 35%, and the director of the Danish Cancer Society repeated this percentage.[29] Ole Hartling and I explained that it was misleading, as it referred to women who attend for screening, which constitute a subgroup with a good prognosis. We also discussed ethics, namely the lack of fully informed consent, and noted again that screening leads to more mastectomies.[30]

Garne shot back at us for the fifth time, insinuating that we were unethical, as he wasn't aware of studies that documented that screening leads to more mastectomies.[31] In our reply to his second letter, we told him it was documented in the randomised trials.[6] We referred to this fact again; to the fact that carcinoma *in situ* is often treated with mastectomy; and to the Dutch study that showed that screening had increased mastectomies more than tumourectomies.[32,33]

Repetition doesn't help when people won't listen. Garne and Hessov wrote a sixth letter,[34] arguing that *studies specifically designed to detect the 'possible existence' of overdiagnosis didn't exist*. This nonsense means that if I performed a large asthma trial and noted that 30 times as many patients died when they received the drug as when they received placebo, I shouldn't really care because the study was designed to look at symptoms, not deaths. Furthermore, the IARC book Garne and Hessov referred to in an earlier letter[21] states that overdiagnosis is an obvious source of harm and the book refers to both randomised trials and observational studies documenting substantial overdiagnosis. Nonetheless, Garne and Hessov called it a scandal that 'without evidence' we had said that two women lose a breast unnecessarily for every 1000 women who are screened.

This debate provided convincing support to the recommendation by the Danish Council of Ethics that the screening programme should be evaluated by laypeople and professionals who are not directly involved with the programme.[35] We should not be led by people with vested interests.

Further *ad hominem* arguments

After the Garne-Hessov attacks, the debate in Denmark took a vicious turn. Two doctors from my own hospital, Ilse Vejborg, head of the mammography screening unit, and Niels Kroman, chief physician at the department of breast surgery, started a series of petty personal attacks in 2004.

First, they wrote a letter in a newspaper[36] claiming that our review was very controversial (although the only other comprehensive review of the trials, performed by the US Preventive Services Task Force, came to similar findings),[37] and they compared it with Bjørn Lomborg's book *The Skeptical Environmentalist*. This is a dubious honour for any scientist, because his book is filled with selective quotations of data that speak against global warming and it omits supportive data from the same sources.[38]

Next, in the *Ugeskrift for Læger*,[39] they cited a famous Danish comedy by Ludvig Holberg from 1723.[40] In the comedy, a learned person, Erasmus, argues that a stone cannot fly, and as his mother cannot fly, it follows that she is a stone. They argued that we had done similarly, using circuitous reasoning to prove a postulate from the postulate itself in our 'continued crusade against mammography screening'. Well, first, Erasmus's reasoning has nothing to do with circular reasoning; it was an example of the logical fallacy that one cannot prove something based on two negatives. Second, Vejborg and Kroman succeeded in just three lines to mix the characters from two different comedies by Holberg and a novel by another author. Third, our unforgivable sin was that we had published a paper where one-quarter of the references were to our own publications. There is nothing wrong with that and nothing circular either. We had translated our *BMJ* paper on the presentation of possible benefits and harms from screening on websites (*see* Chapter 19) and had republished it in the *Ugeskrift for Læger*,[41] and none of the two sets of editors had objected that we quoted relevant work by ourselves.

Vejborg and Kroman accused me of having published deliberately misleading and even erroneous citations and noted that they had previously drawn attention to this 'dishonest behaviour'. They referred to two previous letters I had written but failed to explain what the alleged problems were, and in actual fact, there are no misleading or erroneous citations in these letters. They gave just one concrete example, which was wrong. They claimed that my statement that the US Preventive Services Task Force was sceptical towards mammography screening was 'directly untrue'. We replied that the Task Force had written: 'What emerges as a more important concern, across all age groups, is whether the magnitude of benefit is sufficient to outweigh the harms.'[37] This was what we had translated into Danish and I believe it expresses scepticism towards screening.[42]

Lynge's unholy mixture of politics and science

In 2005, we published a review in the *Ugeskrift for Læger* suggesting that breast screening is a double-edged sword.[43] We mentioned the flawed observational study that claimed that screening had reduced breast cancer mortality in Copenhagen by 25% (*see* Chapter 15).[44] The senior author, Elsebeth Lynge, had used this result for a political purpose, declaring to the media that the importance of extending screening to the whole country could no longer be doubted. Such a statement is inappropriate for a researcher to make, as it transgresses the fine line not only between science and politics, but also between science and ethics.

In ethics, one cannot deduce an 'ought' from an 'is'. David Hume (1711–76) raised the 'is-ought' problem in his *Treatise of Human Nature*. He noted that many writers make claims about what ought to be, on the basis of statements about what is, often in ways that are imperceptible and get unnoticed. Hume cautions against such inferences in the absence of any explanation of how the ought-statements follow from the is-statements. For example, although we might be able to keep a seriously brain-damaged person alive for decades in a respirator, it doesn't follow that this is what we ought to do. Decisions about general screening are made by politicians, not by scientists, and it is a value judgement whether the benefits exceed the harms.

In our review, we noted that Lynge and colleagues,[44] both in their paper and to the media, had given a misleading picture of the harms. For example, they said that cancer precursors only constituted 11% of the cases, thus ignoring all the slow-growing and harmless cases of overdiagnosed invasive cancer.

Lynge had also said to the media that it is possible to screen without overdiagnosis, citing another paper she had published with Anne Helene Olsen (*see* Chapter 16).[45] We explained in our review that this claim was so heavily criticised by two of the examiners at Olsen's subsequent PhD defence that it should be regarded as academically non-approved. We added that it was therefore misleading when the authors in their more recent paper concluded that the mortality from breast cancer was reduced without serious adverse effects.[44]

At the PhD defence, the American examiner, Noel Weiss, pointed out that Olsen couldn't exclude that there was overdiagnosis in Denmark; he also noted that there were actually more cancer cases in the screened group. Another examiner, Niels Keiding, professor of biostatistics at our university, noted that considering that Olsen was a statistician it was curious that there were no numbers and no statistical analyses in her paper, but only some graphs. He also commented that the data were too weak to support her strong conclusion about the lack of overdiagnosis. Both examiners asked Olsen for her opinion on this, but even more curiously, she avoided replying both times. It is biologically impossible to screen without overdiagnosis and also impossible to prove that something does *not* exist. It would have been more honest for her to reply that her conclusion was unjustified.

I believe these events illustrate the undue influence of politics on research on mammography screening and, conversely, the undue influence of poor research on politics. Olsen's tutor was Elsebeth Lynge, who was responsible for the voluminous 1997 report from the Danish National Board of Health that recommended introduction of screening in Denmark.[46]

Finally, we noted in our review that the attendance at screening in Copenhagen was so low (63%) that it may be an argument for stopping screening, since the minimum uptake recommended is 70%.

The dean of the university and the chairman for the examiners reacted to our review and replied that Olsen had been granted a PhD and that this wouldn't have happened if the examiners had rejected one of her articles.[47] But that was a technical remark. We hadn't said that the whole article had been rejected, only that one of its claims hadn't been accepted by the examiners, which was true.

Lynge's political manoeuvres worked. The minister of health asked the Danish National Board of Health to look at her Danish study claiming a 25% mortality reduction to judge whether screening should be extended to the whole country within the next few years. The Board of Health had published the 1997 report that recommended screening, and Lynge was behind both reports and was an advisor to the Board of Health on screening. Therefore, the question from the ministry was pretty much like asking Lynge whether she believed in a study published by Lynge.

Other events showed that Lynge, although being a professor at our university, did not separate science from politics. The university selected Lynge as chair for the evaluation committee when Karsten Juhl Jørgensen submitted his doctoral thesis in 2010. As all three members had clear conflicts of interest in relation to mammography screening, and as the university guidelines stated that, 'no one can participate in the evaluation of a thesis in the presence of circumstances that may be suitable to raise doubt regarding the impartiality of that individual', we complained to the university about the composition of the committee, noting that Lynge had already denigrated Karsten's work in the media and that his work represented a serious criticism of her own papers. This made no impression on Lynge, who replied that she was not conflicted, as did the other examiners, which the university accepted. We therefore complained again, also referring to the law of public administration. This time, we cut in stone what we meant:

> Mammography screening is a controversial intervention and a major international political topic of dissent involving huge economical interests and career investments . . . Any researcher will naturally wish to defend their own work against criticism, and in this case, we are concerned that the examiners could be tempted to 'find an excuse' for rejecting the submitted thesis, as such a move could be used as a very effective political tool in the ongoing dispute.

The university accepted our appeal this time and appointed a new committee without conflicted members.

Mette Kalager in Norway was also sceptical but accepted Lynge as one of the examiners on her PhD thesis, which cost her dearly. One of her three papers had demonstrated considerable overdiagnosis in the Norwegian screening programme, but the examiners – of which only Lynge had expertise in mammography screening – rejected this paper for no good reason. I have seen the paper as a peer reviewer and it is outrageous that it was rejected. Mette's main tutor, Professor Hans-Olov Adami from Harvard and Karolinska, advised her to accept withdrawing the paper in order not to cause additional delays, but he wrote a most damning letter to the dean of the University of Oslo in March 2011. In it, he noted that the quality of the evaluation committee's comments was astoundingly low with limited scientific substance and indeed an element of vested interests and biased views. He also found that excluding Kalager's paper on overdiagnosis was a lost opportunity to have a rich scholarly discussion about an issue of enormous relevance and methodologic complexity. Referring to Lynge's own paper on overdiagnosis, he noted that there was a need for methodologic improvements of the type Kalager and colleagues had attempted.

Mette Kalager told me that because one of her papers was published in the *New England Journal of Medicine*, it should not be a problem to get her thesis approved with only two papers. She therefore omitted her study on overdiagnosis, revised her thesis and resubmitted it. To her great surprise, it was rejected in September 2011 by the same committee that had recommended her to withdraw the paper on overdiagnosis and resubmit the thesis, and yet again, for no good reason, and in a reject letter with little scientific substance.

What is perhaps most amazing in all this is Lynge's double standards. Her own PhD student, Anne Helene Olsen, obtained her PhD despite the fact that her article that claimed there was no overdiagnosis in Denmark did not support this strong claim.

Ad hominem attacks *ad infinitum*

Vejborg and Kroman returned to the *Ugeskrift for Læger*, with enhanced authority in the persons of Chairman Peer Christiansen and Secretary General Henning Mouridsen, both from the Danish Breast Cancer Group, and Chairman Henrik Flyger of the Danish Breast Surgery Society.[48] This addition of authors didn't lift the level of the debate. They claimed again that we had published 'a number of untruthful statements'. This accusation contrasted unequivocally with the evidence.[42,43]

What they wrote about the science was unbelievable. They said that updated results from the trials from Malmö and Canada had shown an effect in line with other trials. This was wrong, as the Canadian trials showed relative risks of 0.97 and 1.02 after 13 years of follow-up,[49] i.e. no effect of screening. Continuing from this error, they proceeded to claim that there was no basis for our conclusion in the Cochrane review. And their errors continued. They argued that the US Preventive Services Task Force had found scientific evidence for introducing mammography screening, and that it was therefore 'directly misleading' when I left an impression of the opposite. I hadn't. The Task Force had noted that, 'in absolute terms, the mortality benefit of mammography screening is small enough that biases in the trials could erase or create it.'

Could it become worse? Yes, and it did. Vejborg, Kroman and their allies remarked for the second time that we should not have quoted ourselves (our results in the *Lancet* on overdiagnosis) because, 'to prove a postulate by itself is not scientifically correct'.[48] Such claims are foolish and even absurd because they didn't apply this 'rule' to themselves, as they quoted their own research in their letter! They also had the audacity to underline how unacceptable it was that we had disregarded the rules for academic debate in our propaganda against screening. Words fail me.

We were told that the extent of overdiagnosis we had reported was 'totally undocumented'; that the rapid responses on the webpages of the *BMJ*, to which we had referred, were just an 'uncensored chatroom'; and that we had misunderstood the numbers on breast cancer mortality. Finally, they couldn't resist the temptation of ending their letter with the 'time to move on' mantra, referring to the editorial in the *Lancet* that Garne and Hessov had described as anonymous, although it wasn't.[22]

We responded to all this nonsense and noted that, according to Statistics Denmark, using the same 10-year periods as those used by our critics, the mortality from breast cancer in Copenhagen had fallen by 12% in the age group 50–69 years (that is invited to screening), and by 17% in the group aged 40–49 years (that is not invited). But despite the falsehoods and the defamatory personal attacks, we were not allowed to publish our reply, not even after we had appealed to the editor. He published a note that there had been so much debate about mammography screening that it should continue elsewhere, unless there were new decisive data.

What is most devastating and depressing about these debates is that it doesn't matter that you prove your opponents wrong; they simply ignore it and repeat their mistakes.

The deception of the public continued. In 2005, Peer Christiansen from the Danish Breast Cancer Group said in an interview that the national screening programmes in England, the Netherlands and Sweden had all shown a reduction of 20%–25% in breast cancer mortality due to screening.[50] None of this is true.

At the time, the *Ugeskrift for Læger* had a tradition for republishing interesting papers that had appeared in prestigious international journals. In 2006, we republished our *BMJ* paper on the contents of invitations for publicly funded screening mammography (*see* Chapter 19). Our paper was widely commended internationally, but all hell broke loose in Denmark when we translated it.[51] The same five people attacked us again. The fact that their criticims were groundless didn't deter them. We were castigated in the title of their letter: 'Mammography screening – ideology contra science',[52] and we were told that it was not appropriate to conduct an ideologic discussion under the guise of science. We had a good laugh. They were the ideologues.

We were also told that when healthy people were invited to screening, it was important that they were informed soberly about both advantages and drawbacks, and that what we had just published in the *BMJ* was anything but sober. This remark was hypocritical and surreal. What we showed in our paper was that the women are *not* being informed about the most important harms of screening. We also showed, with verbatim quotations, that the Danish invitations to screening were very far from being balanced and from providing an adequate basis for informed consent.[51]

Short of arguments, our opponents again resorted to personal attacks and untrue statements. They claimed that our paper in the *BMJ* hadn't been peer-reviewed (which it had); complained that it hadn't been peer-reviewed in the *Ugeskrift for Læger* (which wasn't needed, as it was a translation); claimed that the paper contained factual errors and exemplified this with a statement that it was wrong that carcinoma *in situ* was often treated by mastectomy and radiotherapy (which is what actually happens); and they were dissatisfied that we had referenced two studies in an insufficient way (which we simply had to, as the journal allowed only 10 references, in contrast to our 24 references in the *BMJ*). I was also reprimanded for misusing my position as a member of the scientific panel of our journal to propagate untruthful statements that were so gross that the dean had had to intervene. Wrong again. My statement that Olsen's conclusion about the lack of overdiagnosis was rejected by the examiners at her PhD defence was absolutely correct.

Fortunately, the editor allowed us to respond this time. We rejected their arguments and noted that they paid no attention to the fact that two of the three Danish standard invitations contained nothing about harms, although this is a legal requirement, and that none of them mentioned overdiagnosis.[53] We also noted that they gave no indication as to what they intended to do about this. This reaffirmed our recommendation that the responsibility for the programmes should be separated from the responsibility for the information material.[51]

One might wonder why people would engage in kamikaze-like attacks that are very likely to taint their reputation. I think the answer is that propaganda is highly effective. Lies work when they are repeated often enough, particularly if propagated by people in authority and if they defame people. Propaganda can make us believe in just about anything. This phenomenon was clearly evident when Niels Kroman at an international breast conference in Copenhagen showed a portrait of me during his presentation with the text: 'Who doesn't fear this man'.

The collective stupidity continued. Even in June 2008, Garne, Lynge, Kroman and the two heads of the Danish screening units, Ilse Vejborg and Walter Schwartz, still questioned whether screening leads to overdiagnosis and repeated that the source of this was ourselves – namely, our Cochrane review. Furthermore, they considered it 'grotesque' that we said screening leads to more mastectomies.[54] We explained that others had shown that in Norway, Sweden and the United Kingdom the increase in diagnoses was only compensated to a minor degree when the women were no longer screened due to advanced age, and that data from the Danish Cancer Registry showed the same.[55] Furthermore, other registry data from Denmark showed a marked increase in mastectomies when screening was introduced, which wasn't compensated for later. Finally, we noted that we found it remarkable that Garne and colleagues, who are experts in this area, didn't seem to know these data.

Two months later, also in 2008, a weird letter was published in the *Ugeskrift for Læger* by Mette Kalager, the head of the Norwegian breast screening programme.[56] To begin with, the title was wrong: 'Unclear whether there is overdiagnosis of breast cancer'. That has never been unclear, only its extent can be debated. Kalager quoted Garne and colleagues but not our reply. She also made a serious calculation error. We found that 10 women of 2000 were overdiagnosed, and she compared this rate with a rate of 12.8 women per 2000 diagnosed with cancer or carcinoma *in situ* in the Norwegian programme. Kalager overlooked that our number referred to 10 years of screening and her own number to only one screening session. Based on this error, she calculated that about 80% (10/12.8) of all diagnoses were overdiagnoses and said we had claimed that 'nearly all cases of breast cancer in a screening programme are overdiagnosed'. We have never said such a foolish thing. She also claimed that the author of a Norwegian report should have modified his estimate of 25% overdiagnosis after being criticised, but she didn't document this, and he hadn't done it, which he confirmed when we asked him.[57] Later, Kalager changed her mind about screening. The punishment from the screening community was harsh. People at the Norwegian Cancer Registry, where she worked, accused her of scientific misconduct, a completely groundless accusation, which was rejected by the Norwegian Ombudsman. She quit her job at the registry and went to Harvard in Boston, where she finished her PhD. In 2010, she published a study that failed to find an effect of screening in Norway (*see* Chapter 15) and called for a reassessment of the rationale for screening.[58]

Of course our troubles didn't end there. A week later, Garne and colleagues[59] complained that we had not taken lead time into account. We explained that there is something fundamentally wrong with the lead-time models some researchers have used to conclude that there is very little overdiagnosis,[60] and that we had instead looked at the incidence of cancers when the women were no longer screened,[61] which is a much more reliable method.

All the people who attacked us so viciously had conflicts of interest. In

2007, I saw to my surprise an advertisement for a complete guide to breast self-examination on DVD, to which Ilse Vejborg and Mogens Blichert-Toft had contributed.[62] It had been known for quite some time that regular self-examination was harmful[63] and there were other problems. The advertisement declared that self-examination can prevent breast cancer, which of course it cannot, it can only detect cancer that is already there. Furthermore, it noted that 'it is important that all women make it a habit to regularly examine whether they have lumps in the breast'. No, it is important that they *don't* do this. Not even the American Cancer Society recommends it any longer; it changed its guidelines in 2003.[64]

References

1 Sweet M. Scare factor in health messages. *Australian Doctor*. 2003 Jan 24: 25.
2 Lister S. NHS accused over women's breast cancer screening risks. *The Times*. 2009 Feb 19.
3 Garne JP, Hessov I. [Good reasons for mammography screening: about misunderstood criticism of underlying investigations!] [Danish]. *Ugeskr Læger*. 2000; **162**(31): 4165–6.
4 Gøtzsche PC, Olsen O. [Good reasons for mammography screening: about misunderstood criticism of underlying investigations!] [reply]. *Ugeskr Læger*. 2000; **162**(31): 4166–7.
5 Hessov I, Garne JP. [Do more women lose their breast after screening?] [Danish]. *Ugeskr Læger*. 2001; **163**(4): 446–7.
6 Olsen O, Gøtzsche PC. [Do more women lose their breast following screening: and when are we supposed to discuss it?] [Danish]. *Ugeskr Læger*. 2001; **163**(11): 1576.
7 Gøtzsche PC, Olsen O. Is screening for breast cancer with mammography justifiable? *Lancet*. 2000; **355**(9198): 129–34.
8 Andersson I, Aspegren K, Janzon L, *et al*. Mammographic screening and mortality from breast cancer: the Malmö mammographic screening trial. *BMJ*. 1988; **297**(6654): 943–8.
9 Jungersen D. [Mammography – the best we can offer] [Danish]. *Ugeskr Læger*. 2001; **163**: 6162–3.
10 Hessov I, Garne JP. [Cochrane report on mammographic screening] [Danish]. *Ugeskr Læger*. 2001; **163**(48): 6767–8.
11 Smith RA, Duffy S, Tabár L. The authors reply. *J Surg Oncol*. 2002; **81**: 164–6.
12 Gøtzsche PC. [Cochrane report on mammographic screening] [Danish]. *Ugeskr Læger*. 2001; **163**: 6768.
13 Jungersen D. [Sensitive research] [Danish]. *Ugeskr Læger*. 2000; **162**: 381–3.
14 Nyström L, Andersson I, Bjurstam N, *et al*. Long-term effects of mammography screening: updated overview of the Swedish randomised trials. *Lancet*. 2002; **359**(9310): 909–19.
15 Skovmand K. [Screening saves more from dying in breast cancer] [Danish]. *Politiken*. 2002 Feb 22: 6.
16 Day NE. [Breast cancer screening] [Danish]. *Ugeskr Læger*. 2002; **164**(2): 207–9.

17 Hvas AC. [Is it allowed to write anything to promote screening?] [Danish]. *Ugeskr Læger*. 2002; **164**(7): 919–20.
18 Gøtzsche PC. [Criticism of the Cochrane review on mammographic screening is not justified] [Danish]. *Ugeskr Læger*. 2002; **164**(5): 653–4.
19 Nyström L, Rutqvist LE, Wall S, *et al*. Breast cancer screening with mammography: overview of Swedish randomised trials. *Lancet*. 1993; **341**(8851): 973–8.
20 Nyström L. *Assessment of Population Screening: the case of mammography* [dissertation]. Umeå, Sweden: Umeå University Medical Dissertations; 2000.
21 Garne JP, Hessov I. [WHO and *The Lancet*: yes to mammographic screening] [Danish]. *Ugeskr Læger*. 2002; **164**(23): 3081–2.
22 Gelmon KA, Olivotto I. The mammography screening debate: time to move on. *Lancet*. 2002; **359**(9310): 904–5.
23 International Agency for Research on Cancer. *Mammography Screening Can Reduce Deaths from Breast Cancer*. Press release no. 139. Lyon, France: International Agency for Research on Cancer; 19 March 2002. Available at: www.iarc.fr/en/media-centre/pr/2002/pr139.html (accessed 19 December 2009).
24 Gøtzsche PC. [WHO and *The Lancet*: yes to mammographic screening] [Danish] [reply]. *Ugeskr Læger*. 2002; **164**(23): 3082–3.
25 Gøtzsche PC. Breast cancer screening: International Agency for Research on Cancer (IARC) Handbooks of Cancer Prevention (book review). *Int J Epidemiol*. 2003; **32**: 472.
26 Early Breast Cancer Trialists' Collaborative Group. Favourable and unfavourable effects on long-term survival of radiotherapy for early breast cancer: an overview of the randomised trials. *Lancet*. 2000; **355**(9217): 1757–70.
27 Olsen J. [Breast cancer screening: re-evaluation] [Danish]. *Ugeskr Læger*. 2003; **165**(6): 588.
28 Gøtzsche PC. Update on effects of screening mammography. *Lancet*. 2002; **360**(9329): 338–9.
29 Rolighed A. [The Danish Cancer Society, screening and trustworthiness] [Danish]. *Ugeskr Læger*. 2003; **165**: 612.
30 Gøtzsche PC, Hartling O. [Is information on breast cancer screening reliable?] [Danish]. *Ugeskr Læger*. 2003; **165**: 1068–70.
31 Garne JP. [Do women unnecessarily lose the breast following breast cancer screening?] [Danish]. *Ugeskr Læger*. 2003; **165**(22): 2314–15.
32 Gøtzsche PC, Hartling O. [Reply to the debate on 'Do women unnecessarily lose the breast following breast cancer screening?'] [Danish]. *Ugeskr Læger*. 2003; **165**(25): 2586–7.
33 Gøtzsche PC. Trends in breast-conserving surgery in the Southeast Netherlands: comments on article by Ernst and colleagues. Eur J Cancer 2001, 37, 2435–2440. *Eur J Cancer*. 2002; **38**(9): 1288.
34 Garne JP, Hessov I. [No evidence that mammographic screenings result in overtreatment] [Danish]. *Ugeskr Læger*. 2003; **165**(31): 3025–6.
35 [*Screening – an account*] [*Danish*]. Copenhagen: Det Etiske Råd; 1999.
36 Vejborg I, Kroman NT. [Screening saves lives and breasts] [Danish]. *Weekendavisen*. 2004 Sep 3–9: 10.
37 Humphrey LL, Helfand M, Chan BK, *et al*. Breast cancer screening: a summary of the evidence for the U.S. Preventive Services Task Force. *Ann Intern Med*. 2002; **137**(5 Pt. 1): 347–60.
38 Oreskes N, Conway EM. *Merchants of Doubt*. New York: Bloomsbury Press; 2010.

39 Vejborg I, Kroman N. [Mammography screening: again] [Danish]. *Ugeskr Læger*. 2005; **167**(7): 783.
40 Andersen D. [Mammografi and Holberg] [Danish]. *Ugeskr Læger*. 2005; **167**: 1057–8.
41 Jørgensen KJ, Gøtzsche PC. [Information about breast cancer screening presented on websites is biased and insufficient: a secondary publication] [Danish]. *Ugeskr Læger*. 2005; **167**(2): 174–8.
42 Gøtzsche PC, Jørgensen KJ, Hartling O. [Mammography screening: again] [Danish] [reply]. *Ugeskr Læger*. 2005; **167**(7): 783–4.
43 Gøtzsche PC, Jørgensen KJ. [Screening for breast cancer – a double-edged sword] [Danish]. *Ugeskr Læger*. 2005; **167**: 1312–14.
44 Olsen AH, Njor SH, Vejborg I, *et al*. Breast cancer mortality in Copenhagen after introduction of mammography screening: cohort study. *BMJ*. 2005; **330**(7485): 220–4.
45 Olsen AH, Jensen A, Njor S, *et al*. Breast cancer incidence after the start of mammography screening in Denmark. *Br J Cancer*. 2003; **88**(3): 362–5.
46 Sundhedsstyrelsen (National Board of Health). [*Early detection and treatment of breast cancer. Status report*] [*Danish*]. Copenhagen: Sundhedsstyrelsen; 1997.
47 Hemmmingsen R, Keiding N. [Effect of mammography screening for breast cancer] [Danish]. *Ugeskr Læger*. 2005; **167**(16): 1772–3.
48 Vejborg I, Kroman NT, Christiansen P, *et al*. [Mammography screening: one more time] [Danish]. *Ugeskr Læger*. 2005; **167**(16): 1767–8.
49 Gøtzsche PC, Nielsen M. Screening for breast cancer with mammography. *Cochrane Database Syst Rev*. 2009; (4): CD001877.
50 Jensen UJ. [Debate about mammography screening] [Danish]. NYHS: 2005 Mar 13–15.
51 Jørgensen KJ, Gøtzsche PC. [Are invitations to mammography screening a reasonable basis for informed consent? Secondary publication] [Danish]. *Ugeskr Læger*. 2006; **168**(17): 1658–60.
52 Vejborg I, Kroman NT, Christiansen P, *et al*. [Mammography screening: ideology contra science] [Danish]. *Ugeskr Læger*. 2006; **168**(23): 2263.
53 Gøtzsche PC, Jørgensen KJ. [Mammography screening: ideology contra science] [Danish] [reply]. *Ugeskr Læger*. 2006; **168**(23): 2263–5.
54 Garne JP, Lynge E, Vejborg I, *et al*. [Overdiagnosis and overtreatment of breast cancer] [Danish]. *Ugeskr Læger*. 2008; **170**(23): 2044–5.
55 Gøtzsche PC, Hartling OJ, Nielsen M, *et al*. [Overdiagnosis and overtreatment of breast cancer] [Danish] [reply]. *Ugeskr Læger*. 2008; **170**(23): 2045–6.
56 Kalager M. [Unclear about overdiagnosis of breast cancer] [Danish]. *Ugeskr Læger*. 2008; **170**(33): 2473.
57 Gøtzsche PC, Hartling OJ, Nielsen M, *et al*. [Unclear about overdiagnosis of breast cancer] [Danish] [reply]. *Ugeskr Læger*. 2008; **170**(33): 2473–4.
58 Kalager M, Zelen M, Langmark F, *et al*. Effect of screening mammography on breast-cancer mortality in Norway. *N Engl J Med*. 2010; **363**(13): 1203–10.
59 Garne JP, Lynge E, Vejborg I, *et al*. [Overdiagnosis and overtreatment of breast cancer 2] [Danish]. *Ugeskr Læger*. 2008; **170**(34): 2596.
60 Zahl P-H, Jørgensen KJ, Mæhlen J, *et al*. Biases in estimates of overdetection due to mammography screening. *Lancet Oncol*. 2008; **9**(3): 199–201.
61 Gøtzsche PC, Hartling OJ, Nielsen M, *et al*. [Overdiagnosis and overtreatment of breast cancer 2] [Danish] [reply]. *Ugeskr Læger*. 2008; **170**(34): 2596.
62 [The breast – your complete guide to self-examination] [Danish] [advertisement]. *Dagens Medicin*. 2007 Oct 11: 23.

63 Kösters JP, Gøtzsche PC. Regular self-examination or clinical examination for early detection of breast cancer. *Cochrane Database Syst Rev*. 2003; (2): CD003373.
64 Role of breast self-examination: changes in guidelines; focus on awareness rather than detection. *American Cancer Society*. 2003 May 15.

18

US recommendations for women aged 40–49 years

IN PREPARATION FOR CHAPTER 19, 'WHAT HAVE WOMEN BEEN TOLD?,' I shall decribe first what women aged 40–49 years have been advised to do in the United States, as this is an interesting story of politics trumping both science and ethics.

The US recommendations for these women have followed a zigzag course over the decades, as described by Gina Kolata and Michael Moss of the *New York Times*.[1] The National Cancer Institute originally promoted screening to this age group, but then stopped recommending it in 1977, then recommended it again in the late 1980s, and then abandoned the recommendation in 1993. In Europe, it was much easier, as there was agreement that women under 50 years of age should not be screened; however, Tabár dissented and declared in 1993 that, 'biologically, there is no sense that breast cancer would be smart enough to respect a woman's 50th birthday.'[2] He also said that unless studies can unequivocally show that mammographic screening is not useful, it should be done. Tabár's arguments are empty. Instead of the 50th birthday, he could equally well have said the 40th, 30th or 20th birthday. And it is impossible to demonstrate that an effect of an intervention *does not* exist. There could be a miniscule effect that would require 10 billion women to detect in those aged 10–20 years, for example. And how should I demonstrate that the Loch Ness monster doesn't exist? By emptying the lake? If I did, someone may still claim it existed, somewhere in the universe.

In 1997, the National Institutes of Health convened a panel of neutral people who had not published in the area.[3] After having read more than 100 scientific papers, the panel concluded that screening should not be a blanket recommendation, but should be left to informed decision-making.

When the panel presented this reasonable conclusion to an audience packed with radiologists and other screening advocates, it was met with boos and hisses that punctuated the proceedings. Richard Klausner, director of the National Cancer Institute, created his own stir, as he said he disagreed with the panel. It seemed to be a matter of those who shouted the loudest and were most brutal winning: the radiologists, who also had the biggests conflicts of interest. The panel was accused of condemning American women to death and its report was described as fraudulent.[4]

Klausner criticised the report and said he was shocked by it, and a national television programme began its news with an apology to the American women for the panel's report.[4] There was a public outcry and the case was brought to Congress, where the US Senate unanimously overturned the panel's recommendations.[3]

The women paid attention to this debate of course, but it seemed to have been sufficiently blurred to confuse them, as many believed it was about money rather than the question of benefit.[5] Screening advocates also argued that money was the only reason for discouraging screening young women, but consider the counterargument, which is that people who advocate screening, specifically radiologists, do so for self-interest if not greed.[6]

For a European, and for my American friends, this was surreal. I have never experienced such uncivilised and rude behaviour at scientific meetings in Europe, although it does occur. People who get up at a conference and ask for greater honesty about the harms of cancer screening have been shouted down as heretics.[7]

President Clinton stated after this farce, 'Now, women in their 40's will have clear guidance based on science and action to match it.'[1] Clear guidance, after all this, and based on science? A journalist wrote that the government's 'get-a-mammogram-no-matter-what-you-hear' recommendation sounded more like a faith-based health policy than evidence-based medicine.[8]

After we had published our reviews in 2001, Suzanne Fletcher from Harvard, who chaired a 1993 federal panel that also reviewed mammography, said she would like to see 'an independent committee have access to and review the original data from all the trials, including patient records, so that answers might be obtained to the questions the Danish research raised.'[1]

Donald Berry put some perspective and fun into this saga when he noted that annual mammograms for women in their forties appeared to add 36 hours to their lifespan and that they would get more benefit from walking to the doctor's office.[9]

Fran Visco, president of the US National Breast Cancer Coalition, said: 'You can't make that determination by fiat' and added that although the government might want it to be a clear issue, it is not.[8] In 2002, the coalition wrote on its website:[10]

> There is insufficient evidence to support blanket recommendations for or against screening mammography in any age group of women. The decision to undergo screening must be made on an individual level based on a woman's personal preferences, family history, and risk factors.
>
> At best, mammography screening may offer only very small benefits to certain age groups of women. NBCC believes that there are public health interventions that could save more lives and use fewer health care resources than mammography screening programs.

It is thought-provoking that such announcements come from those who suffer from the disease.

One year earlier, the coalition had invited me to its annual meeting in Washington, where I gave a talk about The Nordic Cochrane Centre's findings. It was one of the most moving moments in my career. I had checked where the exit doors were, so that I could escape if hundreds of women started to throw tomatoes and eggs at me, but there was no need: I received a standing ovation. I could have cried. These brave women who fought so hard against their breast cancer welcomed being informed about the benefits and harms of screening from a researcher who had no conflicts of interest.

An analysis of six top-circulation US newspapers revealed how public opinion is shaped. Although the recommendation changed in 1993 into not recommending screening, this left little imprint on the articles, which were generally supportive of screening in the whole period 1990–97.[11] Quotes and recommendations were about twice as likely to support as to express reservation about screening, and 95% of the articles described the mortality reduction in relative terms and only 11% in absolute terms. Next after governmental institutions, the most quoted source was radiologists, one of which was particularly prominent (not named, but my guess is Daniel Kopans, who has always been 'particularly prominent' in debates on screening). The American Cancer Society came third, and this society and some radiologists were very successful in maintaining a high media profile.

In November 2009, the breast screening brawl started again. The US Preventive Services Task Force published new analyses in the *Annals of Internal Medicine* and changed its recommendations, making screening optional rather than routine in women aged 40–49 years.[12] It also noted that – for all women

– biennial intervals are more efficient and provide a much better balance of benefits and harms than annual intervals. These changes were minor and very rational. They reflected the evidence and would bring the United States in line with Europe, where we have never screened annually, and where most countries don't screen women in their forties.

But, although most of them come from Europe, Americans think they are different from Europeans. An avalanche of protests ensued. The *Wall Street Journal* hit the bottom of journalism when it declared in its headline that 'The mammogram decision is a sign of cost control to come.'[13] This newspaper isn't exactly a watchdog for conflicts of interest, and it noted that the panel at the Task Force didn't include any oncologists and radiologists 'who best know the medical literature'. I would say there is overwhelming evidence that the exclusion of such people is an advantage. Further, the *Wall Street Journal* called it myopic to recommend cutting off all screening in women over 75 years of age. Not much respect for evidence at Wall Street, which the global financial crisis has so eloquently demonstrated.

According to Elsevier Global Medical News, a panel of mammography experts at the annual meeting of the Radiological Society of North America said that the new recommendations would cost women's lives and Daniel Kopans argued that women in their forties could now go back to the 1950s, when they waited until a cancer was too large to ignore any more.[14] That is an interesting remark, as *breast cancer mortality has consistently fallen more in this age group in Europe, without screening, than in the screened age group* (*see* Chapters 5 and 15). To speak about going back to the 1950s is therefore unreasonable. Kopans should have spoken about going back to Europe, as this would have benefited American women.

Kopans also claimed that the Task Force had used selective science, which wasn't true. In the *Washington Post*, Kopans was quoted as saying, 'Tens of thousands of lives are being saved by mammography screening, and these idiots want to do away with it . . . It's crazy – unethical, really.'[15]

Radiologist Stephen Feig also earns his living from mammography, and in an interview[14] he referred to one of Tabár's 'beyond reason' studies.[16] The interview referred to an editorial by Feig in *Cancer* where he quotes Tabár's 63% reduction in breast cancer mortality and says: 'It is likely that screening, rather than advances in treatment, was responsible for nearly all the benefit.'[17] If we adopt the *Wall Street Journal*'s allegories about eye diseases, it must be tunnel vision when a radiologist suggests that the tremendous advances in treatment have had virtually no effect on breast cancer mortality.

It is noteworthy that Feig said this in 2009. As we have already seen, very little, if any, of the decline in breast cancer mortality can be due to screening. This makes Feig's assertion the strongest exaggeration I have ever seen. It is difficult to imagine a larger exaggeration than one that goes from close to zero to close to 100%.

Feig's shameless editorial must have been popular with the editors of *Cancer*, as they allowed him seven pages of text, which I haven't seen before; editorials usually take up one to two pages. Furthermore, as the editorial was accepted 1 day after it was received by the editors, I doubt it was peer-reviewed. In it, Feig noted that although the incidence of breast cancer increased by 31% between 1980 and 1990 in the United States, the mortality rate increased by only 4% over the same period. Thus, like so many other screening advocates, Feig doesn't seem to understand – or perhaps deliberately ignores – that overdiagnosed cancers have an excellent prognosis, and that such statements are therefore misleading. The last sentence in the editorial was: 'However, further gains may be anticipated as more women comply with American Cancer Society screening guidelines.' As *Cancer* is owned by the American Cancer Society, the whole thing looks a bit incestuous.

The end of Elsevier's news report was interesting:[14]

> The panelists also expressed concern about the effect of the recommendation on payment for screening mammograms. In particular, they cited concern that language in health care reform bills currently before Congress would give final authority to the USPSTF [US Preventive Services Task Force] on medical guidelines. In turn, this could prompt insurers to stop paying for screening mammography not recommended by the task force. Dr. Feig and Dr. Kopans reported that they have no relevant conflicts of interest.

So, people whose livelihood depends on mammography declare they have no relevant conflicts of interest in relation to recommendations that would reduce the number of screenings by more than half and that might lead insurers to refuse to continue to pay for the mammograms. Come on! In 1999, Maryan Napoli from the US Center of Medical Consumers informed the readers of the *Journal of the National Cancer Institute* that Kopans owned several patents on mammography-related methods and breast biopsy techniques and had not declared these conflicts, in clear violation of the journal's explicit policy.[18] Kopans replied that he received no 'direct benefit' from the patents, but that doesn't matter; the conflicts should be declared. Napoli explained she raised the issue because Kopans had publicly raised charges of fraud against colleagues who disagreed with his interpretation of the data about screening women in their forties.

The arrogance of the screening advocates towards the academic conventions is incredible. I don't recall having seen Kopans declare his conflicts even after this episode, and haven't seen Tabár do it either. For example, Kopans co-authored American Cancer Society guidelines for breast screening with magnetic resonance imaging in *Cancer* in 2008 without listing any conflicts,[19] and Duffy, Smith and Tabár did the same in a letter in the *Journal of the National Cancer Institute* in 2005.[20]

References

1 Kolata G, Moss M. X-ray vision in hindsight: science, politics and the mammogram. *New York Times*. 2002 Feb 11.
2 Vanchieri C. Europeans say screen only women age 50 and older. *J Natl Cancer Inst*. 1993; **85**(5): 350.
3 Ernster VL. Mammography screening for women aged 40 through 49: a guidelines saga and a clarion call for informed decision making. *Am J Public Health*. 1997; **87**(7): 1103–6.
4 Fletcher SW. Whither scientific deliberation in health policy recommendations? Alice in the Wonderland of breast-cancer screening. *N Engl J Med*. 1997; **336**(16): 1180–3.
5 Woloshin S, Schwartz LM, Byram SJ, *et al*. Women's understanding of the mammography screening debate. *Arch Intern Med*. 2000; **160**(10): 1434–40.
6 Baines C. Screening mammography in women 40–49 years of age: no. In: DeVita V, Hellman S, Rosenberg S, editors. *Important Advances in Oncology*. Philadelphia: Lippincott; 1995. pp. 243–51.
7 Burne J. More than you need to know? *Guardian*. 2003 Nov 15.
8 Trafford A. Second opinion: 'final word' on mammograms? Not yet. *Washington Post*. 2002 Mar 5: HE01.
9 Connolly C. Mammography review shatters the status quo. *Washington Post*. 2002 Feb 17: A01.
10 National Breast Cancer Coalition. The *Mammography Screening Controversy: questions and answers*. 2002 Feb 25. Available at: www.stopbreastcancer.org/bin/index.htm (accessed 18 March 2002).
11 Wells J, Marshall P, Crawley B, *et al*. Newspaper reporting of screening mammography. *Ann Intern Med*. 2001; **135**(12): 1029–37.
12 US Preventive Services Task Force. Screening for breast cancer: U.S. Preventive Services Task Force recommendation statement. *Ann Intern Med*. 2009; **151**(10): 716–26, W–236.
13 A breast cancer preview. *Wall Street Journal*. 2009 Nov 19.
14 Wachter K. New mammography screening guidelines will cost lives, RSNA experts say. *Elsevier Global Medical News*. 2009 Dec 3. Available at: www.oncologystat.com/news-and-viewpoints/news/New_Mammography_Screening_Guidelines_Will_Cost_Lives__RSNA_Experts_Say_US.html;jsessionid=B31F3F96EE6477D027567511DF091D39 (accessed 12 December 2009).
15 Stein R. Breast exam guidelines now call for less testing. *Washington Post*. 2009 Nov 17.
16 Duffy SW, Tabár L, Chen HH, *et al*. The impact of organized mammography service

screening on breast carcinoma mortality in seven Swedish counties: a collaborative evaluation. *Cancer*. 2002; **95**(3): 458–69.

17 Feig SA. Effect of service screening mammography on population mortality from breast carcinoma. *Cancer*. 2002; **95**(3): 451–7.

18 Napoli M. Re: Benefits and risks of screening mammography for women in their forties: a statistical appraisal. *J Natl Cancer Inst*. 1999; **91**(14): 1251–2.

19 Murphy CD, Lee JM, Drohan B, *et al*. The American Cancer Society guidelines for breast screening with magnetic resonance imaging: an argument for genetic testing. *Cancer*. 2008; **113**(11): 3116–20.

20 Duffy SW, Smith RA, Tabár L. Re: Efficacy of breast cancer screening in the community according to risk level. *J Natl Cancer Inst*. 2005; **97**(22): 1703.

19

What have women been told?

The public is left totally confused, and usually at the mercy of screening providers.

Lancet editorial[1]

Website information on screening

'Presentation on websites of possible benefits and harms from screening for breast cancer' was the first paper Karsten Juhl Jørgensen wrote with me, and his first scientific paper ever. He worked on it while a medical student, and we published it in the *BMJ* in 2004.[2] The background for it was a one-page review of 58 Australian leaflets from 1998 showing that the information presented to women invited for breast cancer screening was biased and insufficient and didn't allow fully informed consent.[3] Another Australian study showed that only 18% of 54 publications used to inform about screening mammography included anything on false positive and false negative results, and only 48% gave any information on the harms of screening.[4]

The success of a screening programme depends on the participation rate; therefore, it is obvious that information from governmental institutions and professional advocacy groups could be biased in order to enhance uptake. Industry funding of advocacy groups is another potential conflict of interest, which, although being very common, isn't always revealed.

The importance of balanced information is underlined by a study from New South Wales that found that 61% of women decided for themselves whether to have a screening mammogram, and a further 26% made the decision together with their doctor.[5] Another study showed that websites are important, as a quarter of the European population use the Internet to find information about health issues.[6]

We studied 27 websites from Australia, Canada, Denmark, New Zealand, Norway, Sweden, the United Kingdom and the United States and found that the information was generally not balanced.[2] Only three websites, all from consumer organisations, questioned the value of screening, whereas 13 sites from advocacy groups and 11 from governmental institutions all recommended screening.

All advocacy groups but one[2] accepted industry funding, apparently without restrictions. Some sites were outright shameless, e.g. 'Partnership with the Canadian Cancer Society can assist your company in reaching your commercial objectives'. In contrast, the three consumer organisations acknowledged the risk of bias related to industry funding and two of them didn't accept any industry donations.

Advocacy groups and governmental organisations favoured information items that shed positive light on screening, and only four of these groups mentioned the major harms of screening, overdiagnosis and overtreatment, in contrast to all three sites from consumer organisations. Furthermore, the chosen information was often misleading or erroneous and didn't reflect recent findings, apart from the consumer sites, which were much more balanced and comprehensive.

Even the information that *was* correct was usually framed in a fashion expected to increase uptake of screening. The benefit was given as a relative risk reduction three times as often as an absolute risk reduction, and scaring women with impressive numbers was common. For example, 12 sites mentioned the lifetime risk of developing breast cancer, which is irrelevant, as screening only takes place in certain age groups, and this was usually followed by the annual number of diagnoses, which can be very large in large countries. Only three sites mentioned the relatively reassuring message that women have more than a 50% chance of surviving breast cancer once it's diagnosed, and only four stated that the lifetime risk of dying from breast cancer is only about 3%–4%.

Usually, the beneficial effect on breast cancer mortality was related to a time span of many years, whereas the harms were related to only one screening round. Statements that about 5% of screened women would be recalled at each screening round for additional testing are far less disturbing than saying that the cumulated risk for suspecting cancer in the United States is 49% after 10 mammograms (in Europe, it is only half as much).[7] Furthermore, saying that false positive findings can sometimes create 'anxiety' is much more soothing than saying that more than 10% of screened women at some point will experience important psychological distress for many months.[8]

Most websites stated that the women's decision about participation should be based on informed consent, but the information they offered didn't allow this, which was a peculiar discrepancy. We also noted that if the concern was, as screening advocates have suggested, that too few women would participate if they were presented with the relevant issues, screening might not be justifiable. A woman who attends screening doesn't know what she is buying into, and the personnel at the screening centre don't know either, or don't tell.

Invitations to screening

In 2001, a long-awaited revision of the UK leaflet on breast screening was launched.[9] The prevailing paternalistic attitude to women, with little respect for their autonomy and for informed consent, was still the same, however. For example, the leaflet asked, 'Why do I need breast screening?' rather than, 'Do I need breast screening?'[9]

The leaflet was roundly criticised in the *Lancet*,[10] and the governmental website wasn't any better. It announced that the leaflet purported to ensure that women are told what screening can and cannot achieve so that they can 'make a genuinely informed choice about why they are attending for screening'. About *why* they are attending for screening? There wasn't room for an informed choice about *not* going to screening.

Hazel Thornton wondered why figures of 40%–50% reduction in breast cancer mortality from the Two-County trial were used instead of the findings from the Cochrane review.[11] Furthermore, she said that for those launching the information campaign to claim that the revised leaflet 'heralded a new relationship of trust and honesty between patients and the NHS [National Health Service]' was over-optimistic in the extreme. The leaflet didn't provide women with even the most basic details about the benefits, risks, limitations and consequences, or alternatives, when presenting for mammographic screening.

It was with this background that Karsten and I decided to study invitations to mammography screening. They are essential for informed choice, as they are the only source of information distributed to all women. We included the same countries as in our survey of websites, apart from the United States, which doesn't have a publicly organised screening programme.[12]

The 31 invitations we obtained weren't really invitations. They looked more like an offer you cannot refuse, as they were generally even more persuasive and unbalanced than the websites. Appeals for participation could be pronounced, e.g. 'We strongly recommend that you use this free service', or, 'I am writing to personally invite you'. This tone of familiarity was inappropriate and gave an association of being invited for dinner at grandma's house, which you cannot decline. Saying that 'the benefits of screening far outweigh the risks of any harm from the breastscreen' is a value judgement that an authority cannot make on behalf of others; only the invited women can make it.

Avoiding screening could become very inconvenient. 'If you would like to avoid participation, we ask you to fill out a form. You obtain this form by calling the breast-diagnostic centre.' This is entirely inappropriate for a voluntary examination, as it gives the impression that it is your duty to accept screening. Another invitation said, 'If the time is very inconvenient, we ask you to contact the mammography screening centre as soon as possible', which makes the women feel they are troublesome if the pre-allotted time is inconvenient.

Reminder letters often contained even stronger appeals, e.g. 'I am concerned that you have not yet responded to our recent invitation for a screening mammogram.' This is not only improper familiarity; it also induces guilt.

Most of the invitations gave an appointment date and time. In Denmark, this approach is illegal if it concerns merchandise. Tradesmen cannot assume that people have accepted to buy some merchandise that was sent to them without being asked, only because the 'customers' haven't actively said 'No'. The reason for this principle is pretty obvious, and it should also apply to something as precious as people's health.

In Sweden, the home country for screening, women weren't informed about anything that could be relevant for their decision to participate in screening.

All invitations but one mentioned the benefit of screening, seven gave the size of the benefit and all seven described it as a relative risk reduction in breast cancer mortality, which looks much more impressive than the absolute risk reduction.

Not a single invitation mentioned the major harms of screening, and one of the pamphlets was outright 'funny', as it noted, 'There has been a 26% increase in breast cancer cases in the last ten years.' This message may scare women into attending, but it is nothing else than a description of the harm created by those responsible for screening, as it reflects the level of overdiagnosis with screening over a 10-year period! The information could also be terribly wrong, e.g. 'Some of these studies have been going on for 30 years and none have found any serious side effects from the mammography', and 10 invitations claimed that screening leads to less invasive surgery or simpler treatment. *None of the invitations mentioned the uncertainties related to treatment of carcinoma* in situ.

The most commonly mentioned harm was pain associated with the procedure, and even though this is probably the least serious harm, as it is transient, it was often downplayed, e.g. 'Any discomfort should only last a few seconds.'

As for websites, the lifetime risk of developing breast cancer was often noted. Half the invitations recommended regular self-examination, clinical breast examinations, or both, although regular self-examination is harmful and we don't know anything about clinical breast examinations, as they haven't been tested in randomised trials.[13]

One screening unit wasn't even shy about its conflict of interest: 'You can take a positive step to decrease your own risk, and help us achieve our goal, by deciding to take part.'

When our paper came out in the *BMJ* in 2006, Julietta Patnick, director of the UK Cancer Screening Programmes, said to the BBC: 'I would strongly encourage all women to make an informed choice to attend for screening when invited',[14] and she repeated it when our updated Cochrane review came out 6 months later.[15] Fairly interesting. How can strong encouragement from an authority have anything to do with free, informed choice? Three years later, after we had published our criticism of the UK leaflet in use in 2009 (*see* the section 'Breast screening: the facts, or maybe not' below), Patnick stated: 'Questioned whether women were truly given a choice over breast screening, she said breast screening was a choice – but that she wanted women to choose to have it.'[16] That remark is almost Shakespearean. To choose or not to choose. Patnick cannot have it both ways. One cannot respect autonomy and be paternalistic at the same time.

In the same issue of the *BMJ* where we published our paper on the content of invitations to screening, there was an editorial by consultant breast surgeon J Michael Dixon. Curiously, he didn't comment on our paper, but the title encapsulated his opinion: 'Screening for breast cancer: time to accept that, despite limitations, it does save lives'.[17] His argumentation followed an odd zigzag course, however. He first wondered how it had been possible to detect sufficient numbers of small cancers to reduce the mortality from breast cancer with the mammographic equipment available when the trials were performed, to which he gave a thumbs down. But then he argued that there had been important improvements; namely, better mammography machines, higher-resolution film, an increase in the number of views at each screening round and double reading (thumbs up). He referred to a recent report that summarised the results from the English breast screening programme (thumbs up),[18] but cautioned that although the authors were respected members of the 'breast scientific community', they cannot be considered to be independent because they are involved in the delivery and organisation of the programme (thumbs down).

He then quoted that report – with no caveats – as saying that screening saves 1400 lives per year, which means that for every 400 women screened over a 10-year period, one less woman dies from breast cancer than would have died had they not been screened (thumbs up).[18] We have been unable to find any evidence for this exaggerated estimate in reports from the NHS Breast Screening Programme or elsewhere. Dixon also quoted the report as saying that screening leads to fewer mastectomies (thumbs up). He admitted that he couldn't find the evidence for this in the report (thumbs down), but then added that 'other studies have reported similar findings', quoting only one, which is the small flawed study by Duffy and Paci from Florence described in Chapter 16.[19] He concluded that 'this counters another concern aired by the sceptics of breast screening' (thumbs up).

Dixon noted that the official report gives no reliable data on interval cancers and mentioned that although it stated that the expected rate in the first year is 0.45 per 1000 women screened, a large study in the United Kingdom reported a higher rate, 0.82 per 1000 women, which suggests that the programme doesn't do what it is supposed to do (all thumbs down). Dixon quickly swung the pendulum back again as he said that 'the current national leaflet presents not only the benefits but also the limitations of screening' (thumbs up). Thus, although the leaflet says absolutely nothing about overdiagnosis, Dixon did not accept the criticism that the UK screening programme has persuaded women to attend rather than allowing them to choose on the basis of the potential benefits and risks.

Without presenting any data on overdiagnosis, Dixon concluded that 'it is finally time to accept that although breast screening by mammography is far from perfect it is worth while. Criticisms about the early trials are no longer relevant. Breast screening has moved on and is looking to the future, and so should the sceptics' (thumbs up, final verdict). Dixon's conclusion wasn't supported by the evidence he provided; it merely offered his opinion.

Dixon's editorial must have left many readers confused. Michael Baum responded to it and wrote that, back in 1987, while he was professor of surgery at King's College in London, he was given the task of establishing the first mammographic screening unit in southeast England.[20] This followed the findings of the Forrest committee, announced by Prime Minister Margaret Thatcher, rather conveniently 2 weeks before a general election. Baum took great pride in setting up the unit, and was appointed to the national steering committee of the NHS Breast Screening Programme. However, he soon learned first-hand the 'toxic side effects' of the process and became increasingly disturbed by the failure of true informed consent among the innocent women who accepted the summons to the screening centre. He added that he quickly worked out that the 25% relative risk reduction in breast cancer mortality headlined in the invitations could be framed in another way that described the absolute benefit.

Baum realised that he had become a thorn in the side of the programme's committee, and things came to a head in 1997 when he found himself 'in a minority of one' in demanding that the information leaflets express benefits in absolute numbers and describe harms in an open and fair way. The concern of the committee was that such information would deter women from attending and the target of more than 70% acceptance, on which the programme was predicated, would be missed. He noted that this perfectly illustrated the conflict of interest that we had just described in the *BMJ*. Baum 'did the honourable thing' and resigned from the committee. He concluded: 'As a surgeon I have a legal and ethical commitment to describe to my patients the harms and the benefits of my interventions, but a double standard clearly exists among the screening community, who seem to be in denial.' Baum's testimony says it all:

> *Those who are responsible for mammography screening don't care the least that the way they sell it is blatantly and indisputably unethical.*

Hazel Thornton argued that rather than end the debate about screening and look to the future, as Dixon had suggested, it would be preferable to raise the level of the debate:[21]

> If breast screening is to move on, then it is time the proponents of breast screening moved on, not just to the future, but to the present. Women today do not want to be patronised, or fobbed off with unbalanced, insufficient information, but to be treated with respect, so that they can make up their own minds.

In Germany, the government didn't pay attention to sensible advice about respecting women. Instead, it passed a bill penalising cancer patients financially if they have failed to undergo regular cancer screening.[22] This law is so disrespectful of citizens who have made a rational decision *not* to be screened that jaws dropped in disbelief all over the world. The law also penalises the weakest of the weak in our societies – namely, those who don't attend because they fail more or less everything in life that is expected of them.

A scandalous revision of the Danish screening leaflet

The problems with the invitations to screening were also major in Denmark. In 2001, the Danish Medical Association stated that women should be informed about both benefits and harms.[23] The association argued that women needed to know that 20%–25% of women who are screened will be recalled for further testing because of a suspicion of cancer. It also noted – clearly addressing those responsible for screening – that some had claimed that full information would only create anxiety and confusion. The association found that this can only apply to people in a state of crisis or psychologically out of control. People who are healthy and can take care of themselves have a right to full information.

The association's concerns had no immediate effect, but 5 years later – only 10 days after our review of invitations to screening had been published – the director of the Danish National Board of Health declared that the leaflet should be revised so that it would be correct and balanced.[24] The board held a meeting in November 2006 asking for suggestions for revisions. The invitees were mainly people with a conflict of interest, but there were four of us without such conflicts: Margrethe Nielsen, co-author of the 2006 and 2009 Cochrane review; Ole Hartling, chairman of the Danish Council of Ethics; general practitioner John Brodersen, who had studied the psychosocial effects of false positive findings; and me. We were all worried about the dominance of those with vested interests, including people from the board whom we predicted would defend the status quo. We therefore asked for guidance before the meeting and suggested that the contents of the leaflet should be based on the best available evidence and that data for benefits and harms should be given as absolute numbers with the same denominator, for example per 1000 women. We received no reply.

After the meeting, the board informed us that as it had not been possible to achieve consensus, it would finalise the leaflet itself together with a 'Committee for Health Information' I had never heard about. The four of us replied that we hoped we would get the opportunity to comment on the next draft – particularly as the current draft was far from balanced. Furthermore, we questioned why there was such a large discrepancy between what we had agreed at the meeting – even with the screening advocates – and the content and wording of the draft. Finally, we noted that we assumed that the board would use the best available evidence and would therefore take the comments we had offered in writing into consideration.

Again we received no reply from the board, but we did receive the final version 6 months later. It was a disaster. The leaflet was not evidence-based, our suggestions had been completely ignored and the leaflet reflected the views of the screening advocates.

We consulted an expert in health law, who supported our view that the revised leaflet didn't comply with Danish law, which it is the task of the Board of Health to enforce. Very interesting. The Board of Health is supposed to be the watchdog of the Board of Health, just like Elsebeth Lynge was supposed to evaluate the research by Elsebeth Lynge. That is really something of a conflict of interest. Furthermore, the leaflet didn't live up to what was written in the board's own report from 1997 that paved the way for screening: 'The offer of participation in the programme should include very careful information to women mentioning advantages and disadvantages.'[25] There were no fewer than 13 main problems with the leaflet:

1. There is very little information about harms.
2. Women are given an appointment without having asked for it and receive dunning letters if they fail to attend, which puts pressure on them.
3. The board recommends screening after weighing its advantages and disadvantages, which gives the impression that it is better to attend screening than not to attend.
4. Harms are called inconveniences. It can be inconvenient to arrive late at a meeting but it is a catastrophe to be treated for a cancer disease one doesn't have and wouldn't have acquired in the rest of one's lifetime were it not for screening.
5. Screening leads to more gentle treatment and a greater chance of a breast-conserving operation. This is wrong.
6. It is uncertain how often overtreatment occurs. This was the official reason for not saying anything about its size, although the beneficial effect was not determined with any greater certainty.
7. Mammography is unpleasant. This understates that half of the women perceive it as painful.
8. One feels more secure when the mammogram is normal. This is misleading as (i) many cancers occur between screening rounds, (ii) the chance of not having breast cancer is more than 99% both before and after the investigation, and (iii) screening can also cause insecurity.
9. Every year, about 4000 women will get the disease and about 1300 will die. Such numbers are unnecessarily frightening and also misleading, as they refer to all women and not just those who are invited to screening.
10. Screening reduces breast cancer mortality by 25%. This claim comes from the small observational study from Copenhagen discussed in Chapter 15.
11. The leaflet mentions the beneficial effect among those who attend. This is

misleading because they are healthier than other women; furthermore, the harms would increase similarly if we only look at attenders.
12. All six papers in the reference list are to Danish publications, and the four most important ones have been written by people with a conflict of interest in relation to screening.
13. There were no references to the best avaible evidence, e.g. the Cochrane review or the review by the US Preventive Services Task Force.[26,27]

The leaflet looked like a sales brochure. It is difficult to imagine more flagrant disregard for conflicts of interest, sound science, informed consent and women's needs. *Nowhere* were absolute numbers presented, such as one woman benefiting out of 2000 screened.

The scandal led to several questions in parliament to the minister in 2008, but to no effect. The minister replied that it was his perception that the board had acted in an exemplary way, including describing openly the advantages and disadvantages of screening. This is what Harry Frankfurt would have called pure bullshit.[28] Guess who informed the minister about what he should say? The Board of Health of course. A system immune to criticism is not a healthy one.

All the leaflets we'd examined had been inadequate. But we were so intensely disappointed with the Danish National Board of Health that we realised we needed to write a leaflet ourselves to provide the information women needed to make a rational decision.

Our screening leaflet

At The Nordic Cochrane Centre, we wrote our leaflet in Danish at first. It describes benefits and harms in numbers that are readily understood using the same denominator,[29] as advised by Australian researchers.[30] Our leaflet is evidence-based and explains the basis for our numbers and why more optimistic numbers provided by others are less reliable.

We tested draft versions among general practitioners in three Nordic countries and among laypeople, which led to considerable improvements. The leaflet starts with a summary (the full leaflet is reproduced in English in Appendix 2):

> It may be reasonable to attend for breast cancer screening with mammography, but it may also be reasonable not to attend, as screening has both benefits and harms.
>
> If 2000 women are screened regularly for 10 years, one will benefit from

> the screening, as she will avoid dying from breast cancer. At the same time, 10 healthy women will, as a consequence, become cancer patients and will be treated unnecessarily. These women will have either a part of their breast or the whole breast removed, and they will often receive radiotherapy, and sometimes chemotherapy.
>
> Furthermore, about 200 healthy women will experience a false alarm. The psychological strain until one knows whether or not it was cancer, and even afterwards, can be severe.

As noted in Chapter 16, it is remarkable that epidemiologist Johannes Schmidt in 1990 reported exactly the same balance between harm and benefit as we did. Schmidt's observation was ignored for 16 years, until we published the same ratio.[26]

We acquired funding from a small Danish cancer foundation (KræftFonden) that allowed us to print and distribute the leaflet to general practitioners and gynaecologists in Denmark in March 2008. As it became very popular, we translated it into English and published it in the *BMJ* (*see* next section). Maryann Napoli, from the US Center for Medical Consumers, called it 'the first honest mammography information for women written by health professionals',[31] and I think this is the reason that volunteers have translated it into other languages so that it now exists in 13 languages (available at: www.cochrane.dk).

We presented the leaflet on prime-time television that devoted more than 20 minutes to the subject.[32] The journalists went to great lengths when preparing the programme and ultimately were persuaded by our scientific arguments, rather than the message from the Board of Health. But we didn't get there easily. I had to explain repeatedly the background for our numbers and what the differences are between randomised trials and observational studies, and I felt at times I was being interrogated. Clearly, the journalists wanted to be absolutely certain they bet on the right horse when they went against the all-powerful Board of Health.

Breast screening: the facts, or maybe not

Our *BMJ* papers on websites and invitations didn't have much impact, if any, on the way women were being informed about screening throughout the world. The UK leaflet was particularly misleading, and as those updating it had been completely resistant to good arguments, we decided to write a paper solely about the shortcomings of the UK leaflet.[33]

This was not news, or at least so we thought. You usually have a fairly good idea whether your scientific work will be of minor or major interest, but it can be unpredictable. Your most important work may receive little recognition initially, only to be 'rediscovered' years later, whereas at other times, when you don't expect much to happen, all of a sudden it does.

The UK leaflet has the authoritative title *Breast Screening: the facts*,[34] which suggests that here's something you can trust. However, it is full of persuasion, short on fact and is often erroneous. We called our paper 'Breast screening: the facts – or maybe not'.[33]

As advised by the editors, our 2006 article on the content of invitations had included a box with recommended information (*see* Figure 19.1):[12]

Main benefits and harms, assuming a 15% reduction in breast cancer mortality and overdiagnosis of 30%

If 2000 women are screened regularly for 10 years:

- 1 woman will avoid dying from breast cancer
- 10 healthy women, who would not have been diagnosed without screening, will have breast cancer diagnosed and be treated unnecessarily; 4 of these will have a breast removed, 6 will receive breast conserving surgery, and most will receive radiotherapy
- 1800 will be alive after 10 years; without screening 1799 will be alive.

Other main points

Of 2000 women (in Europe) who participate in 10 rounds of screening

- 500 will be recalled for additional investigations because cancer is suspected; about 125 will have a biopsy
- 200 will experience psychological distress for several months related to a false positive finding.

Screening can provide false reassurance. Up to 50% of cancers among women in screening programmes are detected between two screening rounds, and these interval cancers are the most dangerous.

Mammography is painful for about a third of women.

FIGURE 19.1 Key elements in information leaflets as recommended by us in 2006 in *BMJ*

The UK leaflet had been updated after we published this box, but its contents remained essentially the same, although the National Screening Committee agreed already in 2000 that the purpose of information was not to recruit women but to allow them to choose whether to participate.[35] It is too late to start asking questions on arrival at the screening unit, as the leaflet suggests, as it would be difficult to decline screening in that situation.

The leaflet followed the usual pattern. Scare through big numbers, e.g. screening saves 'an estimated 1400 lives each year in this country' and failure to mention the major harm of screening. The guidelines from the UK General Medical Council state, 'You must tell patients if an investigation or treatment might result in a serious adverse outcome, even if the likelihood is very small.'[36] The likelihood of being overdiagnosed after mammography is not very small; it is 10 times larger than the likelihood of benefit.[26,33]

The leaflet implied that screening leads to fewer mastectomies: 'Around half the cancers that are found at screening are still small . . . This means that the whole breast does not have to be removed.'

It noted that about one in every 20 women screened will be recalled for more tests, but didn't explain that this 5% rate applies to only one round of screening. The summary downplayed the recalls further, as it said they could 'cause worry', although we know that the psychosocial strain of a false alarm can be severe and may continue after women are declared free from cancer. Many women experience anxiety, worry, despondency, sleeping problems, a negative impact on sexuality and behaviour, and changes in their relationships and existential values.[8,37] This can go on for months; some women will feel more vulnerable about disease and will see a doctor more often.[38]

It is also misleading to say that a mammogram 'involves a tiny dose of radiation, so the risk to your health is very small' when the women are not told that the much bigger dose used in radiotherapy is very harmful when given to healthy people.

Carcinoma *in situ* wasn't mentioned, although it constitutes about 20% of the diagnoses made at screening sessions. A patient representative described her experience of gaining this information as trying to 'uncover a closely guarded state secret'.[35]

A correspondent noted that, 'If the recipient does not wish to attend and ignores the invitation they will be labelled a 'DNA' ('Did Not Attend'), so they must either write or telephone to express their wishes and give their reasons, which can feel intimidating and stressful.'[39]

We published our leaflet (reproduced at the end of this book) on the *BMJ* website.[33]

When our paper on the UK leaflet came out in February 2009, 23 people from the United Kingdom, the United States, Canada, Australia and France published a letter in *The Times* calling for action.[40] The signatories included epidemiologists, practising physicians, patient representatives, journalists and a breast surgeon, and the message was strong. I reproduce it in its entirety, as it had political implications:

> Sir, Most people could be forgiven for believing that one of the vital weapons in the war against breast cancer is early detection – even before there are any symptoms of breast cancer present. This belief has generated a Europe-wide consensus that screening healthy women for breast cancer will save lives. In the vanguard of this campaign, the NHS screening programme for breast cancer (NHS BSP) by mammography has been lauded as a triumph and has laid claim to the responsibility for the dramatic decline in breast cancer mortality since its initiation 20 years ago. An alternative view is that such success might equally well be attributed to improvements in treatment that anteceded the launch of the NHS BSP.
>
> However, there are harms associated with early detection of breast cancer by screening that are not widely acknowledged. For example, there is evidence to show that up to half of all cancers and their precursor lesions that are found by screening, if left to their own devices, might not do any harm to the woman during her natural lifespan. Yet, if found at screening, they potentially label the woman as a cancer patient: she may then be subjected to the unnecessary traumas of surgery, radiotherapy and perhaps chemotherapy, as well as suffer the potential for serious social and psychological problems. The stigma may continue to the next generation as her daughters can face higher health-insurance premiums when their mother's overdiagnosis is misinterpreted as high risk. We believe that women should be clearly informed of these harms in order to make their own choice about whether to attend for screening.
>
> The subject has now come to a head with the publication in the next issue of the British Medical Journal of Breast screening: the facts – or maybe not by Peter C. Gøtzsche and his colleagues from the independent Nordic Cochrane Centre. They describe a synthesis of published papers that quantify the benefits and harms of screening using absolute rather than relative numbers that make it easier to comprehend. They conclude as follows: if 2,000 women are screened regularly for ten years, one will benefit from the screening, as she will avoid dying from breast cancer. At the same time, ten healthy women will, as a consequence, become 'cancer patients' and will be treated unnecessarily. While there is debate about exactly what these numbers are (some data shows more women benefit and fewer healthy women treated unnecessarily) the overall picture is clear.
>
> The most disturbing statistic is that none of the invitations for screening comes close to telling the truth. As a result, women are being manipulated,

> albeit unintentionally, into attending. It is therefore imperative that the NHS BSP rewrites the information leaflets, for example by using the template provided by the Nordic Cochrane Centre, and leave it to the properly informed woman to accept the invitation or not.

However, patronising attitudes don't disappear easily. Peter Johnson, chief clinician at Cancer Research UK, said that it was dangerous to scare people away from a programme that had brought substantial benefits.[41] I explained on the BBC that women couldn't make an informed choice because of the one-sided propaganda they received.[42] Stephen Duffy said in the same programme that my numbers were 'completely inaccurate' and talked about an 'atmosphere of hysteria'. I wondered who was being hysterical.

This time, however, the usual mantras from the screening advocates had little effect. The monster wouldn't go away. Only 2 days later, an article in *The Times* announced that the NHS was tearing up its leaflet and writing a new one from scratch.[43] Mike Richards, the National Cancer Director, said a formal review was in progress and would be tested against the best available evidence.

This was completely new. Nowhere in the world had screening organisations been the least troubled by the fact that the information they provided contradicted the best available evidence. Julietta Patnick, director of the NHS cancer screening programmes, didn't seem prepared to abandon her paternalism. She said that, according to research, 'putting too much numerical information meant women just put the leaflet down.'[43] In actual fact, an abundance of research has shown that the great majority of cancer patients want as much information as possible, and it is highly likely that healthy women who run a risk of being made cancer patients unnecessarily would also want information. If the research Patnick refers to was conducted on women who have been brainwashed into believing that screening can only be beneficial (which seems to be the case in the United Kingdom), it is not surprising that such women may not want more information.

A group of Norwegian researchers was equally careless with science. They interviewed 69 women in focus groups about their decision to participate in mammography screening and found that they were content with the programme and with the invitations, which directly encouraged participation and included a pre-specified time of appointment.[44] However, the premises of their enquiry were flawed.[45] The invitations were seriously biased in favour of participation, there was no information about the major harms of screening and the decision to attend had already been made for the women by a public authority.

There were many other flaws. The researchers had explored 'the decision to attend', leaving out the option not to attend, and they didn't interview those who chose not to participate. Moreover, the headline of the leaflet given to the women was: 'Why should you participate in the mammography programme? Mammography can save lives'. The women 'expected mammography results to be clear and unambiguous', and they expressed 'sincere trust in a normal mammogram as proof of healthy breasts'. The researchers therefore found that the women's views 'seemed to be in accordance with the information in the leaflets'. *Thus, they simply confirmed that women could replicate flawed information.* Screening mammograms are far from being 'unambiguous'.

The authors mentioned that 'the decision to opt out would have taken more effort'. This is to say the least. To avoid participation and further invitations, Norwegian women have to call the screening unit to obtain a form, complete it and send it back. I doubt medical ethicists would find this an acceptable procedure.

Although their paper was published in the *Journal of Medical Ethics*, the Norwegian authors presented an astonishingly primitive view on ethics.[44] They argued that informed consent assumes that individuals are rational actors. They also said that feminists have emphasised that what it means to be rational describes women's decision processes wrongly, and that risk statistics are 'limiting rationality in ways that fit with traditional male values'. The authors used such arguments for defending the paternalistic status quo that information is really not what the women need. In our comment on their paper,[45] we acknowledged that emotions are often far more important for human decisions than facts, but this applies also to males, and it cannot be used as an argument for secrecy about harms of interventions.

Thornton has noted that the women cannot make a decision if they are not given the necessary facts.[46] Many won't want the information; others will want every last statistic. But assumptions shouldn't be made about what 'all women' want; it doesn't treat women with dignity and women are different. Women's groups do the same thing when they purport to speak for women, which can be disrespectful and terribly patronising.

What Thornton said has been said many times before, and it shouldn't be necessary to repeat the obvious. But the Norwegian study reminds us that it *is* necessary.

In 'Behind the headlines', produced by the NHS Knowledge Service, Julietta Patnick said that the ratio – instead of being one life saved to 10 receiving unnecessary treatment, as had been stated in *The Times* – was much nearer to a one to one ratio.[47] In the *New York Times*, Patnick 'dismissed the Cochrane figures as inaccurate'.[48] We were perplexed by this. Our numbers are accurate and it seems impossible to get the ratio wrong by a factor of 10.

Sir Mike Richards repeated the one to one ratio and said, 'There are no doubts in my mind about the benefits.' Richards, being the British 'Cancer Tsar', said what was expected of him, but it is the women who need to decide whether the benefit outweighs the harms, not Richards. But of course, those who sing from the same hymnbook might get a knighthood, like Commander of the Order of the British Empire Dame Valerie Beral from the NHS Breast Screening Programme recently did. Julietta Patnick is Commander of the British Empire. As there is no longer any Empire, we should perhaps interpret this as the Empire of Cancer Screening. Being knighted seems to be important for the British, although knights became extinct centuries ago. As they say in the BBC's *Yes Minister* series: 'The Prime Minister doesn't want the truth, he wants something he can tell Parliament.'

In November 2009, a survey of eight leaflets in Germany, Italy, France and Spain showed similar results to ours.[49] None of them mentioned overdiagnosis; four recommended breast self-examination, and they attempted to directly influence women with suggestive phrases to pressure them into participating.

People in charge are unwilling to admit their mistakes. Per-Henrik Zahl mentioned in 2009 that even though it is very rare that women get a thrombosis when they take oral contraceptives, they are nevertheless informed about this risk.[50] In contrast, the risk of overdiagnosis is very large, but Norwegian women are not informed about it. In her reply, Rita Steen from the Norwegian Cancer Registry offered this remarkable statement:

> The reason that we now include this information is not that we think overdiagnosis is a large problem in the programme, but because the problem has received so much attention in the debate about mammography.

What arrogance! Were it not for our research, Norwegian women would have been kept in the dark.

In June 2009, we published a paper in the *Ugeskrift for Læger* listing the major problems with the new leaflet from the Danish National Board of Health.[51] We sent this paper, our own leaflet and our criticism of the UK leaflet to the new director of the Board of Health, suggesting that a revision of the Danish leaflet was necessary. He replied that he was aware that there were disagreements among the experts, but that the board's leaflet reflected the views discussed at the meeting. This was yet another case of bullshit, short of lying, as Frankfurt defined it.[28] I assume the director had been misinformed by his staff. He promised the available literature would be assessed in 2010, including the papers we had quoted in our letter, and that the leaflet would then be reviewed.

I haven't heard anything more from the Danish National Board of Health.

And after the events in 2009, I was so disappointed that I didn't expect anything to happen in any country in the foreseeable future. I think I am right. In December 2010, shortly before Christmas when people had other things on their mind, the revised UK leaflet was published. It was devastating. Spokespeople for the NHS's programme had stuck to the beliefs about benefit that prevailed 25 years ago and still questioned the issue of overdiagnosis.[52] The programme's 2010 Annual Review was equally misleading and remained largely unaffected by repeated criticism and pivotal research questioning the benefits of screening and documenting substantial harms.[53] The only hint at overdiagnosis in the leaflet was this ambiguous sentence: 'Screening can find cancers which are treated but which may not otherwise have been found during your lifetime.' Some women could interpret this as, 'Great! Screening finds cancers that are hard to find – that's why I go for screening.' I therefore subjected the ambiguous sentence to a test among fourth-year medical students. They were unprepared – just as women invited to screening are – as they had not been lectured about screening. Most of them couldn't tell what it meant and most felt that laypeople would perceive the message as positive, e.g. a chance of cure.

We published our observations in the *Journal of the Royal Society of Medicine* in August, 2011,[54] and although we had carefully documented with Danish data that screening increases mastectomies, the usual untruthful and misleading statements were offered to the media by Julietta Patnick: 'We know that 97 per cent of women with screen-detected cancers are alive five years later compared to just over 80 per cent of women diagnosed without screening, and screening lowers a woman's risk of having a mastectomy.'[55]

American Cancer Society

> *When anybody says 'It's not the money, it's the principle' they mean it's the money.*
>
> *Yes Minister* (BBC series)

> *You don't ask a barber whether you need a haircut.*

Cancer societies are fundraising institutions, which creates an obvious conflict of interest. Their messages are often carefully tailored to maximise donations from the public,[56] and it is important to realise that information from cancer societies may not always be truthful, or in the citizens' best interest.

The American Cancer Society (ACS) is a prime example of this.[56] It is the primary promoter of cancer screening in the United States and it benefits from a hard sell of breast screening.[56] In 1999, the ACS announced in a leading newspaper that early detection of breast cancer results in a cure 'nearly one hundred percent of the time'.[57] Upon being questioned about this figure by a reporter, a communications director from the ACS replied, 'When you make an advertisement, you just say what you can to get women in the door . . . You exaggerate a point.' As the reporter noted, on the other side of that door is a mammogram machine that draws US$125 per patient (the reporter did in fact say 'patient', although healthy women are *not* patients, a distinction that is often forgotten).

The aggressiveness with which the ACS has marketed breast screening in the United States is illustrated by a disrespectful advertisement that appeared, for example, in a cancer journal in 2000 (*see* Figure 19.2).[58]

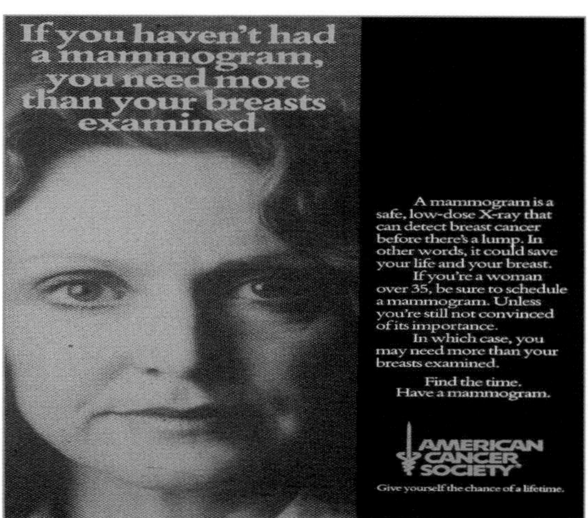

FIGURE 19.2 Advertisement from the American Cancer Society in *HemOnc Today*, 2000

There have also been offers of a mammogram as a Mother's Day present,[59] and at one time, the ACS claimed that 80% of women aged 35–50 years were at high risk and were recommended to get a baseline mammogram, which made epidemiologist John Bailar say that it's mathematically absurd to claim that more than half can be at high risk.[56]

If the ACS starts telling people they should *not* get screened, there will likely be a huge drop in donations. This could be an important reason why the ACS for a long time didn't follow through with its idea of stopping telling men to have regular PSA tests for detection of prostate cancer.

In 2002, the ACS recommended monthly breast self-examination from age 20.[60] These girls had barely left high school before being asked to worry about dying from cancer and to examine their breasts regularly for the rest of their lives, with all it entails in terms of anxiety and disfiguring biopsies. Young girls and their partners have more pleasant things on their mind than worries about cancer. Good sex, for example. And why worry when only 12 women died from breast cancer before age 30 in the United Kingdom in 2008?[61]

Brian Cox and others reported in 1993 that breast cancer mortality – unexpectedly – was a little *higher* in the first 7 years of screening among young women than among similar women in the control groups in the randomised trials.[62] Michael Retsky, from Boston, and colleagues[63] observed bimodal relapse patterns in two breast cancer databases that were unexplainable with the accepted continuous tumour growth paradigm. They suggested that metastatic breast cancer growth commonly includes periods of temporary dormancy at both the single cell phase and at the avascular micrometastasis phase, and that surgery to remove the primary tumour may terminate dormancy by initiating formation of new blood vessels (angiogenesis), resulting in accelerated relapses.[64,65] On the basis of their findings, they suggested a new paradigm for early-stage breast cancer that might involve new types of treatments meant to stabilise and preserve dormancy rather than attempting to kill all cancer cells, as is currently done.

Retsky noted in an interview in 2005[66] that surgery might unleash breast cancer growth. He emphasised that his hypothesis was based on indirect evidence and he didn't suggest any changes in clinical practice based on this, but hoped it would entice researchers to test the hypothesis, which he thought was a key to understanding the biology of breast cancer. However, in the same news article, Robert Smith of the ACS said that the findings were based on a misreading of the data.[66]

It's difficult to see how that could be the case, and Smith's other arguments were equally misleading. He noted, 'When you first invite women to screening, you get some with tumours that are already advanced.' Of course you do, but the same occurs in a control group of women who are not screened. He continued, 'And not all of the women will respond to the invitation to screening. They may die next year or the year after, and because they were invited, they will be counted as a death in the screening group.' Of course they will, but the same occurs in the control group. 'So you really can't look at this pattern and make any sense out of it.' Interesting, as we perform randomised trials to make sense of the results we obtain. Furthermore, Smith said that young women tend to get more aggressive breast cancers. Are we supposed to think that the same doesn't happen in the control group? 'So the idea these women became worse after surgery may stem from the fact that their prognosis may have been poorer to begin with', Smith said. Such women exist to the same extent in the control group. This is why we randomise, to make sure that women in the two groups are comparable.

A UK colleague wrote to me and said: 'I fail to understand; is Dr. Smith plain dumb or playing games using people's lack of knowledge?' Very few Americans know enough about randomised trials to see through Smith's fallacious arguments. But it doesn't matter, it seems, whether what was said is right or wrong, as long as it looks good and is repeated frequently.

In October 2009, the ACS's chief medical officer, Otis Brawley, admitted in an interview in the *New York Times* that the advantages to screening had been exaggerated and said the Society worked on putting a message on its website in early 2010 to emphasise that screening for breast and prostate cancer and certain other cancers can come with a real risk of overtreating many small cancers while missing cancers that are deadly.[67]

This mutiny didn't last long. Only a month later, when the US Preventive Services Task Force had come up with its new recommendations about decreasing the amount of screening, Brawley issued a long press release that left no doubts: 'The American Cancer Society feels that . . . the lifesaving benefits of screening outweigh any potential harms. Surveys of women show that they are aware of these limitations, and also place high value on detecting breast cancer early.'[68] This wasn't correct. Very few women are aware that screening can harm them,[69] and their opinion about screening should be considered in light of the one-sided propaganda they have systematically been exposed to. One of Brawley's colleagues said to a journalist that 'he's trying to save his job' and that 'he was broiled at home for the interview'.[70]

In the middle of the political turmoil in November 2009, a politician said she was very concerned that the recommendations from the Task Force conflicted 'with those of other authorities, like the American Cancer Society'.[71] When did the ACS become an 'authority'? It is an 'interest' organisation, with its own goals and with obvious financial conflicts of interests. The society's board of trustees includes corporate executives from the pharmaceutical industry, and the ACS receives huge donations from the mammography industry and many other industries, including chemical ones. This may explain why it is consistently hostile to cancer prevention.[72] Gigantic corporations, which profit handsomely from polluting the air, water and food with a wide range of carcinogens, appreciate the passivity of the ACS. It has repeatedly rejected or ignored requests from Congressional committees, regulatory agencies, unions and environmental organizations to provide scientific testimony critical to efforts to legislate and regulate a wide range of occupational and environmental carcinogens. The ACS has actively campaigned against laws that ban deliberate addition to food of additives known to cause cancer in animals or humans. In 1992, the ACS issued a joint statement with the Chlorine Institute in support of the continued global use of organochlorine pesticides – despite clear evidence that some were known to cause breast cancer. Zeneca Pharmaceuticals, which sells tamoxifen (a drug used against breast cancer), is a spin-off of Imperial Chemical Industries, one of the world's largest manufacturers of chlorinated and other industrial chemicals, including those incriminated as causes of breast cancer. Zeneca has been the sole multimillion-dollar funder of the US National Breast Cancer Awareness Month since its inception in 1984.

By 1989, the cash reserves of the ACS were worth more than US$700 million. At that time, 26% of its budget was spent on medical research and programmes; the rest covered 'operating expenses', including about 60% for generous salaries, pensions, executive benefits and overhead. Most contributors believe their donations are being used to fight cancer, not to accumulate financial reserves. Yet fundraising appeals routinely state that the ACS needs more funds to support its cancer programmes, pleading poverty and lamenting lack of funds for cancer research. The ACS also makes donations to political parties, although tax experts have warned that these donations may be illegal, because the ACS is a non-profit organisation.

On its website, the ACS states, rather shamelessly:[73]

> A new era of corporate outreach for the American Cancer Society has been launched through its Employer Initiative. Its goal is to build lasting relationships with major U.S. companies by offering and implementing products and services that help employers meet their business goals while increasing mission and income returns to the Society.

The new 2009 guidelines from the US Preventive Services Task Force didn't leave any footprints at the ACS's headquarters. Robert Smith said that his organisation stuck with the current guidelines, 'because we not only looked at the evidence that the task force looked at, but we also looked at newer, modern data'.[74] Smith then cited one of Tabár's 'beyond reason' studies that Smith himself had co-authored, showing that breast cancer deaths declined by 19% among women who didn't get regular mammograms and by 48% among those who did. He also said, 'We want women to understand the shortcomings of screening but we don't want to be dissuading them from doing it.' The ACS cannot have it both ways, and it should not make decisions on behalf of women.

Information from other cancer societies

On its website, the Danish Cancer Society offers information about mammography screening, and a few lines down, there is a figure (*see* Figure 19.3).[75]

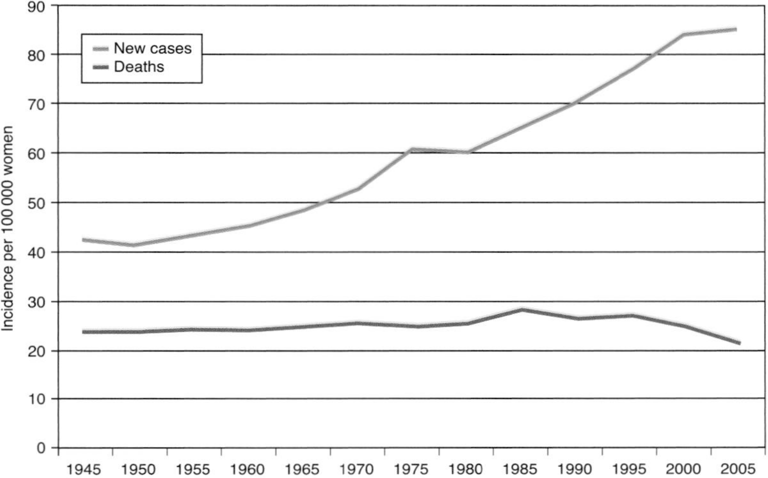

FIGURE 19.3 Misleading graph in information piece about mammography screening on the Danish Cancer Society's website (redrawn)

The text at the bottom of the graph says that the distance between the two curves grows because an increasing number of women with breast cancer live longer or are cured. This is the only explanation there is. Visual displays exert a strong influence on how we perceive things, and the figure represents strongly misleading propaganda for screening. What cannot be seen in the figure is that the incidence has increased substantially because of overdiagnosis and that the decline in breast cancer mortality was largest in young age groups that were not invited to screening (*see* Chapter 15).

In 2000, a major Danish newspaper reported that 5-year survival was now somewhat better than previously for some cancers, and Hans Storm from the Danish Cancer Society was quoted as saying, 'This can only be due to improved treatment.'[76] However, it can also be due to advancement of the time of diagnosis, which can lead to better 5-year survival even when there is no reduction in mortality (*see* Chapter 2).

In 2002, the front page of another major Danish newspaper touted that 'Mammography saves women.'[77] The 5-year survival was 83% in a Danish county with screening and 77% in two counties without. This information came from a PhD dissertation supported by the Danish Cancer Society, and the author said that the numbers speak for themselves. The results were also believed by the top politician on health in the Danish counties, who advised that screening be introduced in the whole country, supported by the director for the Danish Cancer Society. However, one of the official examiners for the dissertation noted 6 days later that such comparisons are 'problematic', and I explained that they are not only problematic but completely misleading.[78] Even if screening has no effect, 5-year survival from time of diagnosis will *always* be better in a region with screening than in a region without. I also remarked that the Danish Cancer Society, being a research-intensive organisation, should be more concerned about its credibility so that there would be no need of fire extinguishers afterwards.

In 2008, a third major Danish newspaper announced that 'five-year survival has increased from 60% to 80% in 30 years.'[79] According to spokespeople from the Danish Breast Cancer Group and the Danish Cancer Society – Henning Mouridsen and Hans Storm, respectively – this was due to better treatments and screening. There was no explanation that 5-year survival rates over a time span of 30 years are extremely misleading. It is easy to explain this to laypeople, but I have never seen such explanations in newspapers, likely because oncologists and their organisations prefer to keep quiet about it and pretend the changes are all due to their own expertise.

Also in 2008, an article from the Danish Cancer Society showed that after the politicians had donated a substantial amount of money for improved diagnosis and treatment of cancer, the survival had improved.[80] Although two of the authors were statisticians and the third an epidemiologist, they interpreted this as evidence that the plan had worked. I therefore noted that the survival data were useless for saying anything about the effect of the donation and that they should have looked at annual number of cancer deaths instead.[81] The authors replied that my attack on cancer researchers only showed that behind my cool manner and my critical-scientific palisades, 'other feelings were hidden, which evidently drove my commitment'.[82]

In December 2009, a national newspaper reported that Denmark had the highest death rate in breast cancer among the OECD countries.[83] The Danish Cancer Society didn't miss the golden opportunity. Chief physician Iben Holten said that the most important reason was that we find cancer later, and chief statistician Susanne Møller added that the one thing that comes to mind is that Denmark hasn't had nationwide screening. She added that in Sweden, which has screened for many years, the women are diagnosed earlier and therefore also have better survival. Two of the five regions in Denmark had still not been able to get screening off the ground, and Holten noted that she was very sorry about this, as those women who are not found by screening have a far worse prognosis.

I find this totally dishonest. Key people in the Cancer Society must be aware that no one knows why some countries have much higher breast cancer mortality rates than others. As noted in Chapter 15, other people from the Cancer Society were more truthful. They wrote in 2004 that the difference in relative survival comparing breast cancer patients in Denmark and Sweden had existed even before mammographic screening began in either country.[84]

In 2010, when we had reported that there was no visible effect of screening in Denmark,[85] and had also reminded people about the considerable overdiagnosis, Iben Holten remarked on the society's website that 'there are no women who are treated for breast cancer unless the doctors are 100% ['certain', I assume; a word was missing] of the diagnosis.'[86] I am confident that Holten, being a pathologist, knows that doctors are far from being 100% accurate in their diagnoses (*see* Chapter 2). Furthermore, it is dishonest to dismiss overdiagnosis as a problem.

In the United Kingdom, there were similar problems. In May 2009, Susan Mayor announced in the News section of the *BMJ* that 'UK deaths from breast cancer fall to lowest figure for 40 years.'[87] Cancer Research UK had collated the data from government statistics, and they showed that deaths from breast cancer increased steadily, reached a peak in 1989 and then fell by 36%. Peter Johnson, Cancer Research UK's chief clinician, said, 'It's incredibly encouraging to see fewer women dying from breast cancer now than at any time in the last 40 years, despite breast cancer being diagnosed more often.'

Thus, the spokesperson from the charity used all the overdiagnosed healthy women to the charity's advantage, as few readers would realise that his comparison was seriously misleading. The good news was accompanied by a graph from the charity's website (*see* Figure 19.4).

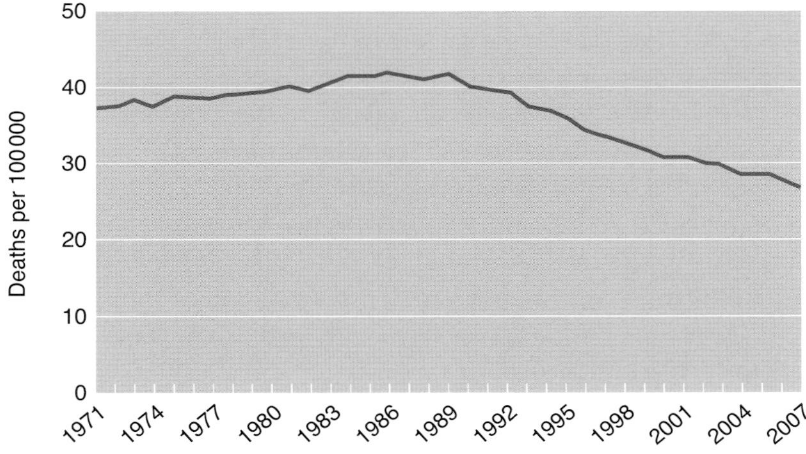

FIGURE 19.4 Breast cancer deaths per 100 000 women in the UK (all ages)

But there was a problem. Mayor had noted that the decline had occurred in all age groups and that it was 41% in women aged 40–49 years (who had not been invited to screening), and also 41% in women aged 50–64 years. Johnson acknowledged the effect of improved treatments and better management, but he also said screening had contributed, which one couldn't see. We checked the website of the charity.[88] Just below the graph that was published in the *BMJ*, there was a much more relevant graph, divided into age groups (*see* Figure 19.5).

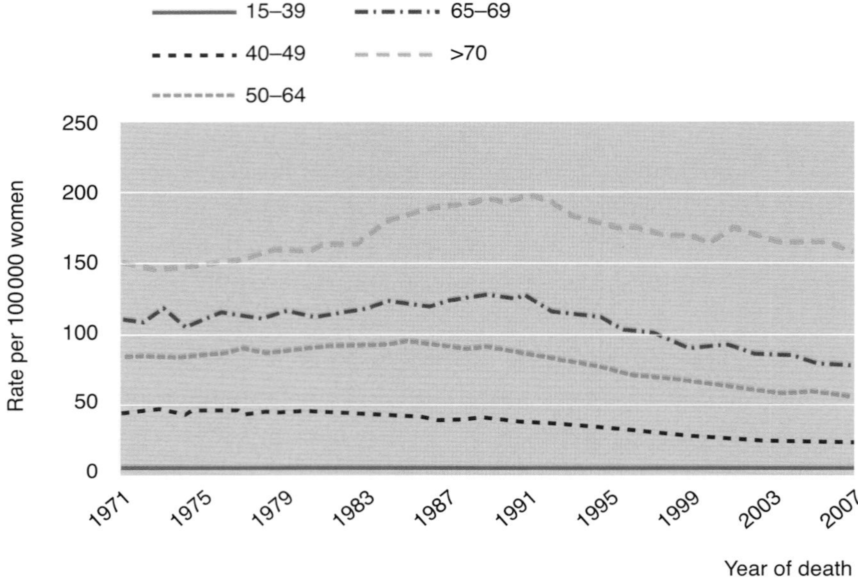

FIGURE 19.5 Breast cancer deaths per 100 000 women in the UK, by age group

This was revealing. The mortality rate in women who were at least 70 years old continued to rise and didn't peak until 1991, and this trend had therefore concealed the fact that the decline in mortality in the most relevant age group, 50–64 years, had started 3 years before screening started, and in the youngest age group already in the 1970s. The percentage decline in the age group 40–49 years was the largest of any of the age groups if the whole observation period is considered. Furthermore, the calculations quoted in the news article of the percentage declines in the various age groups didn't use any data before 1989, which is misleading. It seems that the cancer society cherry-picked the graph and the years that were politically expedient.

In Australia, the deception was just the same. Liz Wylie, medical director of BreastScreen WA, argued similarly to Peter Johnson when she said, 'In Australia our mortality rates are falling even though the incidence of breast cancer is rising and that's because of early detection.'[89] In 2009, after publication of the study that showed that screening had led to substantial overdiagnosis in New South Wales,[90] Sally Crossing, founding member of the NSW Breast Cancer Action Group, noted that while she agreed that women needed to be informed, she was worried that evidence on overdiagnosis would be used to restrict publicly funded screening and undermine early detection of breast cancer.[91]

Norwegian screening advocates also had a loose regard for truth. When Mæhlen and Zahl noted in a leading newspaper that many women are overdiagnosed, Steinar Thoresen from the Cancer Registry strongly rejected their findings.[92] He claimed that the proportion of women with metastases had been halved since the programme was introduced (which can only be true if there is massive overdiagnosis of harmless cancers). *A physician working with diagnosing breast cancer declared that it wasn't necessary to give information about the negative aspects of screening because there aren't any.*[93] It is appalling that the doctors we entrust to take care of the women can be so unprofessional.

A final word of caution against misleading scare campaigns. Notices in London's Underground once warned that women have a 1 in 12 risk of developing breast cancer, and women in the United States have been warned that their risk is 1 in 8.[94] Consequently, fear of breast cancer is so pervasive among US women that it is causing them to ignore far more serious health threats. Such risks are uninterpretable unless they are related to age, and when they are, they become much less frightening. I give here some numbers:[95] A UK woman who is 30 has a lifetime risk of 1 in 12 of developing breast cancer and 1 in 24 of dying from it. For a woman who is 70, these risks are only 1 in 29 and 1 in 37, respectively. The risk of dying from cardiovascular disease is much more tangible. It is 1 in 3 for all ages.

One might also ask: What is the risk of getting cardiovascular disease? Surely higher than dying from it, i.e. higher than 1 in 3. And the risk of getting diabetes or osteoarthritis? Very high, indeed. The meaninglessness of frightening the healthy population in this way can be seen if we imagine the ultimate scare campaign, with big posters in the underground saying: 'People have a risk of 1 in 1 of dying!' Or, as a wit once put it: birth is a uniformly fatal disease.

Getting funding or not getting funding

I once asked a famous tumour biologist during a coffee break at an international breast screening meeting whether he agreed with me that it was impossible to lower breast cancer mortality by 30% with screening, based on our knowledge of tumour biology. He agreed. I then asked why people like him didn't participate in the scientific debate. He didn't reply and it is not difficult to imagine why. It is not wise to point out that your colleagues are wrong when you are on the receiving end of major funds from a cancer charity. It has long been suspected, although difficult to prove, that donations from such charities tend to favour those in the funding committee or their friends, and those who share existing beliefs.

Samuel Epstein reported that most members of the board of the American Cancer Society (ACS) are closely tied in with the US National Cancer Institute. Many board members and their colleagues obtain funding from both organisations, and substantial National Cancer Institute funds go to ACS directors who sit on key National Cancer Institute committees. Although the Cancer Society asks board members to leave the room when the rest of the board discusses their funding proposals, this is a token formality. Easy access to funding is one of the 'perks' and a significant amount of Cancer Society research funding goes to this extended membership.[72]

It is not easy to get funding if one has views or results that are not mainstream. It is much easier if one produces results people like to see. For example, Elsebeth Lynge opened a centre for epidemiology and cancer screening a couple of years ago at the University of Copenhagen and has received millions of Danish kroner from the Danish Cancer Society. Her most important results – that screening is possible without overdiagnosis and that the effect of screening is 25% in Copenhagen – are both wrong,[85,96] but this doesn't seem to matter, as long as the prevailing belief system is fed reinforcing results. Most of those who publish on screening earn a living from it or have conflicts of interest in other ways. This is not the best starting point for production of reliable results.

What do women believe?

The propaganda about breast screening has been highly effective and has resulted in grave misconceptions about its effects. A study of American and European women[97] found that 68% believed screening reduced their risk of getting breast cancer (which it doesn't, it just detects cancer), 62% believed that screening at least halved mortality (screening has no documented effect on total mortality)[26] and 75% believed that 10 years of screening saved 10 of 1000 participants (which is 10 times the most optimistic estimate and 20 times the Cochrane estimate).

Other studies have shown that only 8% of women were aware that participation has the potential to harm healthy women[69] that 94% doubted the possibility of non-progressive breast cancers[69] and that one-third thought screening detects more than 95% of breast cancers[98] (screening only detects between half and two-thirds of the cancers, and the most dangerous ones are usually detected between two screening rounds).

An earlier study from 1995 of American women aged 40 to 50 years found even bigger misconceptions.[99] The women overestimated their probability of dying from breast cancer within 10 years 20-fold and the absolute risk reduction obtained with screening 100-fold.

Women die from many causes other than breast cancer. Assuming an effect of screening of 15%, this means that 90.30% of the women will be alive after 10 years of screening, and 90.25% will be alive if there is no screening.[26] Such sobering numbers wouldn't sell many tickets to the 'screening lottery', so it's not an oversight that we never see them. An absolute effect of screening of only 0.05% may seem strangely low, but screening cannot have an effect on the survival of women who were already diagnosed with breast cancer before they were randomised. These women are therefore not included in the results of the trials. In a 10-year period, relatively few women will both get the diagnosis and die from it.

I'm sure cancer screening wouldn't have been so popular if people had known the facts about its benefits and harms.[69,97–101]

References

1 The trouble with screening. *Lancet*. 2009; **373**(9671): 1223.
2 Jørgensen KJ, Gøtzsche PC. Presentation on websites of possible benefits and harms from screening for breast cancer: cross sectional study. *BMJ*. 2004; **328**(7432): 148–51.
3 Slaytor EK, Ward JE. How risks of breast cancer and the benefits of screening are communicated to women: analysis of 58 pamphlets. *BMJ*. 1998; **317**(7153): 263–4.
4 Croft E, Barratt A, Butow P. Information about tests for breast cancer: what are we telling people? *J Fam Pract*. 2002; **51**(10): 858–60.
5 Davey HM, Barratt AL, Davey E, *et al*. Medical tests: women's reported and preferred decision-making roles and preferences for information on benefits, side-effects and false results. *Health Expect*. 2002; **5**(4): 330–40.
6 European Opinion Research Group. *European Union Citizens and Sources of Information about Health*. 2003. Available at: http://europa.eu.int/comm/health/ph_information/documents/eb_58_en.pdf (accessed 3 October 2003).
7 Elmore JG, Barton MB, Moceri VM, *et al*. Ten-year risk of false positive screening mammograms and clinical breast examinations. *N Engl J Med*. 1998; **338**(16): 1089–96.
8 Brodersen J. *Measuring Psychosocial Consequences of False-Positive Screening Results: breast cancer as an example*. Copenhagen: University of Copenhagen, Department of General Practice; 2006. Available at: http://publichealth.ku.dk/staff/?id=ecd7a9b0-6c37-11dc-bee9-02004c4f4f50&vis=publikation (accessed 11 November 2011).
9 NHS. *Breast Screening, the Facts*. London: Health Promotion England; 2001. Available at:

www.cancerscreening.nhs.uk/breastscreen/publications/ia-02.html (accessed 2 February 2003).

10 Dixon-Woods M, Baum M, Kurinczuk JJ. Screening for breast cancer with mammography. *Lancet*. 2001; **358**(9299): 2166–7.

11 Thornton H. Breast screening seems driven by belief rather than evidence. *BMJ*. 2002; **324**(7338): 677.

12 Jørgensen KJ, Gøtzsche PC. Content of invitations to publicly funded screening mammography. *BMJ*. 2006; **332**(7540): 538–41.

13 Kösters JP, Gøtzsche PC. Regular self-examination or clinical examination for early detection of breast cancer. *Cochrane Database Syst Rev*. 2003; (2): CD003373.

14 Breast screen treatment concerns. *BBC News*. 2006 Mar 3.

15 Breast screen 'wrong care' fears. *BBC News*. 2006 Oct 18.

16 McCartney M. Are women being misled about pros and cons of breast screening? *Pulse*. 2009 Apr 1.

17 Dixon JM. Screening for breast cancer: time to accept that, despite limitations, it does save lives. *BMJ*. 2006; **332**(7540): 499–500.

18 Advisory Committee on Breast Cancer Screening. *Screening for Breast Cancer in England: past and future*. NHSBSP publication No 61. Sheffield: NHS Cancer Screening Programmes; 2006. Available at: www.cancerscreening.nhs.uk/breastscreen/publications/nhsbsp61.pdf (accessed 27 February 2006).

19 Paci E, Duffy SW, Giorgi D, *et al*. Are breast cancer screening programmes increasing rates of mastectomy? Observational study. *BMJ*. 2002; **325**(7361): 418.

20 Baum M. Ramifications of screening for breast cancer: consent for screening. *BMJ*. 2006; **332**(7543): 728.

21 Thornton H. Ramifications of screening for breast cancer: more debate and better information still needed. *BMJ*. 2006; **332**(7543): 728.

22 Tuffs A. Germany will penalise cancer patients who do not undergo regular screening. *BMJ*. 2006; **333**(7574): 877.

23 [Screening and information duties] [Danish]. *Ugeskr Læger*. 2001; **163**: 2678.

24 Skovmand K. [Invitations to be reviewed] [Danish]. *Politiken*. 2006 Mar 14: 5.

25 Sundhedsstyrelsen (National Board of Health). *[Early detection and treatment of breast cancer. Status report] [Danish]*. Copenhagen: Sundhedsstyrelsen; 1997.

26 Gøtzsche PC, Nielsen M. Screening for breast cancer with mammography. *Cochrane Database Syst Rev*. 2006; (4): CD001877.

27 Humphrey LL, Helfand M, Chan BK, *et al*. Breast cancer screening: a summary of the evidence for the U.S. Preventive Services Task Force. *Ann Intern Med*. 2002; **137**(5 Pt. 1): 347–60.

28 Frankfurt H. *On Bullshit*. Princeton, NJ: Princeton University Press; 2005.

29 Gøtzsche PC, Hartling OJ, Nielsen M, *et al*. *Screening for Breast Cancer with Mammography*. 2008 Jan. Available at: www.cochrane.dk (accessed 22 December 2009).

30 Barratt A, Howard K, Irwig L, *et al*. Model of outcomes of screening mammography: information to support informed choices. *BMJ*. 2005; **330**(7497): 936–8.

31 Center for Medical Consumers. *Make an Informed Decision about Mammography*. Available at: http://medicalconsumers.org/2009/03/01/make-an-informed-decision-about-mammography (accessed 27 September 2009).

32 Praxis. *TV2*. 2008 Mar 11.

33 Gøtzsche P, Hartling OJ, Nielsen M, *et al*. Breast screening: the facts – or maybe not. *BMJ*. 2009; **338**: 446–8.

34 Department of Health, NHS Cancer Screening Programmes. *Breast Screening: the facts*. 2006. Available at: www.cancerscreening.nhs.uk/breastscreen/publications/ia-02.html (accessed 20 March 2008).
35 Raffle A, Gray M. *Screening: evidence and practice*. Oxford: Oxford University Press; 2007.
36 General Medical Council. *Consent Guidance: patients and doctors making decisions together*. London: GMC, 2008. Available at: www.gmc-uk.org/guidance/ethical_guidance/consent_guidance/index.asp (accessed 2008).
37 Brodersen J, Thorsen H, Kreiner S. Validation of a condition-specific measure for women having an abnormal screening mammography. *Value Health*. 2007; **10**(4): 294–304.
38 Barton MB, Moore S, Polk S, *et al*. Increased patient concern after false-positive mammograms: clinician documentation and subsequent ambulatory visits. *J Gen Intern Med*. 2001; **16**(3): 150–6.
39 Blennerhassett MAJ. Unhealthy paternalism. *BMJ*. 2009 Feb 20. Available at: www.bmj.com/cgi/eletters/338/jan27_2/b86#212985 (accessed 22 May 2011).
40 Baum M, Vaidya JS, Thornton H, *et al*. Breast cancer screening peril: negative consequences of the breast screening programme. *The Times*. 2009 Feb 19.
41 Lister S. NHS accused over women's breast cancer screening risks. *The Times*. 2009 Feb 19.
42 Are we being provided with the full facts? Interview with Peter Gøtzsche, Paul Pharoah and Stephen Duffy. *BBC Radio*. 2009 Feb 20. Available at: www.bbc.co.uk/radio4/womanshour/01/2009_07_fri.shtml (accessed 22 February 2009).
43 Smyth C. NHS rips up breast cancer leaflet and starts all over again. *The Times*. 2009 Feb 21.
44 Østerlie W, Solbjør M, Skolbekken JA, *et al*. Challenges of informed choice in organised screening. *J Med Ethics*. 2008; **34**(9): e5.
45 Jørgensen KJ, Brodersen J, Hartling OJ, *et al*. Informed choice requires information about both benefits and harms. *J Med Ethics*. 2009; **35**(4): 268–9.
46 Saul H. 'The tide is turning' in the breast screening debate. *Eur J Cancer*. 2010; **46**: 261–5.
47 National Health Service. *Breast Cancer Screening*. 2009. Available at: www.nhs.uk/news/2009/02February/Pages/Breastcancerscreening.aspx (accessed 23 February 2009).
48 Rabin RC. Benefits of mammogram under debate in Britain. *New York Times*. 2009 Mar 30.
49 Gummersbach E, Piccoliori G, Zerbe CO, *et al*. Are women getting relevant information about mammography screening for an informed consent: a critical appraisal of information brochures used for screening invitation in Germany, Italy, Spain and France. *Eur J Public Health*. 2010; **20**(4): 409–14.
50 Brækhus LA. [No information on risk of mammography] [Danish]. *ABC Nyheter*. 2009 Apr 20. Available at: www.abcnyheter.no/node/87263 (accessed 27 April 2009).
51 Gøtzsche PC, Hartling O, Nielsen M, *et al*. [Invitation to breast cancer: propaganda or information?] [Danish]. *Ugeskr Læger*. 2009; **171**: 1963.
52 NHS Breast Screening Programme. *NHS Breast Screening* [leaflet]. Sheffield: Department of Health; 2010. Available at: www.cancerscreening.nhs.uk/breastscreen/publications/ia-02.html (accessed 27 December 2010).
53 NHS Breast Screening Programme. *NHS Breast Screening Programme Annual Review 2010: Overcoming barriers*. Available at: www.cancerscreening.nhs.uk/breastscreen/publications (accessed 22 May 2011).

54 Gøtzsche PC, Jørgensen KJ. The Breast Screening Programme and misinforming the public. *J R Soc Med.* 2011; **104**(9): 361–9.
55 Lakhan N. Claims of breast cancer screening success are dishonest, say critics. *Independent*. 2011 Sep 1.
56 Lerner BH. *The Breast Cancer Wars*. Oxford: Oxford University Press; 2001.
57 Sturgeon B. Breast cancer detection: trick or treatment? *Senior News*. 1999; **18**: 7 Oct.
58 Dotts T. Debate persists over mammography's benefits. *HemOnc Today*. 2000: 11, 14.
59 Skrabanek P. Mass mammography: the time for reappraisal. *Int J Technol Assess Health Care*. 1989; **5**(3): 423–30.
60 Smith RA, Cokkinides V, von Eschenbach AC, *et al*. American Cancer Society guidelines for the early detection of cancer. *CA Cancer J Clin*. 2002; **52**(1): 8–22.
61 Cancer Research UK. *Breast Cancer: UK mortality statistics*. Available at: http://info.cancerresearchuk.org/cancerstats/types/breast/mortality (accessed 7 April 2010).
62 Elwood JM, Cox B, Richardson AK. The effectiveness of breast cancer screening by mammography in younger women. *Online J Curr Clin Trials*. 1993; Doc no. 32.
63 Retsky M, Demicheli R, Hrushesky W, *et al*. Surgery triggers outgrowth of latent distant disease in breast cancer: an inconvenient truth? *Cancers*. 2010; **2**(2): 305–37.
64 Demicheli R, Retsky MW, Hrushesky WJ, *et al*. The effects of surgery on tumor growth: a century of investigations. *Ann Oncol*. 2008; **19**(11): 1821–8.
65 Retsky MW, Demicheli R, Hrushesky WJ, *et al*. Dormancy and surgery-driven escape from dormancy help explain some clinical features of breast cancer. *APMIS*. 2008; **116**(7–8): 730–41.
66 DeNoon DJ. Surgery may unleash breast cancer growth. 2005 Sep 13. Available at: www.mombu.com/medicine/cancer/t-webmd-surgery-may-unleash-breast-cancer-growth-1902287.html (accessed 22 May 2011).
67 Kolata G. In shift, cancer society has concerns on screenings. *New York Times*. 2009 Oct 20.
68 American Cancer Society. *American Cancer Society Responds to Changes to USPSTF Mammography Guidelines*. Press Release. Atlanta, GA: American Cancer Society; 16 Nov 2009. Available at: http://pressroom.cancer.org/index.php?s=43&item=201 (accessed 22 May 2011).
69 Schwartz LM, Woloshin S, Sox HC, *et al*. US women's attitudes to false positive mammography results and detection of ductal carcinoma in situ: cross sectional survey. *BMJ*. 2000; **320**(7250): 1635–40.
70 Crewdson J. Rethinking the mammogram guidelines. *Atlantic*. 2009 Nov 19.
71 Sack K, Kolata G. Screening policy won't change, U.S. officials say. *New York Times*. 2009 Nov 18.
72 Epstein SS. American Cancer Society: the world's wealthiest 'nonprofit' institution. *Int J Health Serv*. 1999; **29**(3): 565–78.
73 American Cancer Society. Available at: www.cancer.org/docroot/AA/AA_4_Corporate_Recognition.asp (accessed 25 May 2010).
74 Debating benefits, risks of routine mammograms. *National Public Radio USA*. 2009 Nov 20.
75 Kræftens Bekæmpelse. [Screening for breast cancer – mammography] [Danish]. Available at: www.cancer.dk/Hjaelp+viden/kraeftformer/kraeftsygdomme/brystkraeft/screening+for+brystkraeft/ (accessed 12 April 2011).
76 Grund J. [Cancer patients live longer] [Danish]. *Jyllandsposten*. 2000 May 25: 2.
77 Hagerup A. [Mammography saves women] [Danish]. *Berlingske Tidende*. 2002 Dec 23: 1.

78 Gøtzsche PC. [The Danish Cancer Society, screening and trustworthiness] [Danish]. *Ugeskr Læger*. 2003; **165**: 611–12.

79 Tougaard H. [More women survive breast cancer] [Danish]. *Politiken*. 2008 May 22: 5.

80 Storm HH, Gislum M, Engholm G. [Cancer survival before and after initiating the Danish Cancer Control plan] [Danish]. *Ugeskr Læger*. 2008; **170**(39): 3065–9.

81 Gøtzsche PC. [Non-useful cancer survival statistics following the Danish Cancer Control Plan] [Danish]. *Ugeskr Læger*. 2008; **170**(43): 3442.

82 Storm HH, Engholm G, Gislum M. [Non-useful cancer survival statistics following the Danish Cancer Control Plan] [Danish] [reply]. *Ugeskr Læger*. 2008; **170**(43): 3442–3.

83 Hansen JH. [Denmark has the highest death rate for breast cancer] [Danish]. *Information*. 2009 Dec 9.

84 Christensen LH, Engholm G, Ceberg J, *et al*. Can the survival difference between breast cancer patients in Denmark and Sweden 1989 and 1994 be explained by patho-anatomical variables? A population-based study. *Eur J Cancer*. 2004; **40**(8): 1233–43.

85 Jørgensen KJ, Zahl P-H, Gøtzsche PC. Breast cancer mortality in organised mammography screening in Denmark: comparative study. *BMJ*. 2010; **340**: c1241.

86 Danish Cancer Society. [*Danish researchers: screening for breast cancer has no effect*] [*Danish*]. Danish Cancer Society; 2010 Mar 27. Available at: www.cancer.dk/Cancer/Nyheder/2010kv1/screeningharingeneffekt.htm (accessed 27 March 2010).

87 Mayor S. UK deaths from breast cancer fall to lowest figure for 40 years. *BMJ*. 2009; **338**: b1710.

88 Jørgensen KJ, Brodersen J, Nielsen M, *et al*. Fall in breast cancer deaths: a cause for celebration, and caution. *BMJ*. 2009; **338**: b2126.

89 O'Leary C. Breast tests 'a risk' for women. *West Australian*. 2006 Oct 19.

90 Morrell S, Barratt A, Irwig L, *et al*. Estimates of overdiagnosis of invasive breast cancer associated with screening mammography. *Cancer Causes Control*. 2010; **21**(2): 275–82.

91 Salleh A. 1 in 4 breast cancers 'not threatening'. 2009 Nov 11. Available at: www.abc.net.au/science/articles/2009/11/11/2739398.htm (accessed 14 November 2009).

92 Gjerding ML, Solstad F. [Mammography doesn't reduce mortality] [Norwegian]. *Verdens Gang*. 2006 Nov 25.

93 Dregelid S. [Receive unnecessary cancer treatment] [Norwegian]. *Aftenposten*. 2006 Oct 18.

94 Bunker JP, Houghton J, Baum M. Putting the risk of breast cancer in perspective. *BMJ*. 1998; **317**(7168): 1307–9.

95 Haybittle J. Women's risk of dying of heart disease is always greater than their risk of dying of breast cancer. *BMJ*. 1999; **318**(7182): 539.

96 Jørgensen KJ, Gøtzsche PC. Overdiagnosis in publicly organised mammography screening programmes: systematic review of incidence trends. *BMJ*. 2009; **339**: b2587.

97 Domenighetti G, D'Avanzo B, Egger M, *et al*. Women's perception of the benefits of mammography screening: population-based survey in four countries. *Int J Epidemiol*. 2003; **32**(5): 816–21.

98 Barratt A, Cockburn J, Furnival C, *et al*. Perceived sensitivity of mammographic screening: women's views on test accuracy and financial compensation for missed cancers. *J Epidemiol Community Health*. 1999; **53**(11): 716–20.

99 Black WC, Nease RF Jr, Tosteson AN. Perceptions of breast cancer risk and screening effectiveness in women younger than 50 years of age. *J Natl Cancer Inst*. 1995; **87**(10): 720–31.

100 Schwartz LM, Woloshin S, Fowler FJ Jr, *et al*. Enthusiasm for cancer screening in the United States. *JAMA*. 2004; **291**(1): 71–8.
101 Gigerenzer G, Mata J, Frank R. Public knowledge of benefits of breast and prostate cancer screening in Europe. *J Natl Cancer Inst*. 2009; **101**(17): 1216–20.

20

Extraordinary exaggerations

There seems to be no study too fragmented, no hypothesis too trivial, no literature citation too biased or too egoistical, no design too warped, no methodology too bungled, no presentation of results too inaccurate, too obscure, and too contradictory, no analysis too self-serving, no argument too circular, no conclusions too trifling or too unjustified, and no grammar and syntax too offensive for a paper to end up in print.

Drummond Rennie[1]

Those who selectively present inadequate evidence to support a belief will ultimately lose the trust of the public at large.

Hazel Thorton[2]

CONFLICTS OF INTEREST ARE COMMON IN BIOMEDICAL RESEARCH. Best known are the financial conflicts of interest when doctors collaborate with the drug industry. Mammography screening is also a large industry and there are passionate beliefs involved. One would therefore expect the literature on breast screening to be influenced by conflicts of interest, and we confirmed this in a 2007 study.

Karsten Juhl Jørgensen searched for articles on mammography screening that mentioned a benefit or a harm, or both, and included 143 papers from 2004, most of which reported original research results.[3] Fifty-five articles mentioned only benefits, whereas seven mentioned only harms. Overdiagnosis was more often downplayed or rejected in articles whose authors worked directly with mammography screening programmes (40%), compared with authors who worked in screening-affiliated specialties or were funded by cancer charities (17%) and authors in specialties unrelated to mammography screening (7%). Benefit was provided as a relative risk reduction in breast cancer mortality 10 times as often as an absolute risk reduction.

What is the ratio between benefits and harms?

> *Every public criticism of screening has to be countered with ever more positive assertions in order that public confidence is not shaken.*
>
> Angela Raffle[4]

People supporting screening tend to exaggerate its benefits and downplay its harms. When they describe the benefits and harms in the form of a ratio, the numerator will be too large and the denominator too small. One would therefore expect such ratios to be particularly misleading. Influential UK researchers are second to none in this pseudo-scientific game, which manifests itself in getting as far from the truth as possible and yet still succeeding in having the ratio published.

The flawed ratios were much welcomed in the pro-screening community, particularly by Robert Smith of the American Cancer Society, who contributed to their production. I shall devote quite some space to discussing the issues around this.

In line with Angela Raffle's quotation at the beginning of this section, Arthur Schopenhauer mentions in his book *The Art of Always Being Right* that being contradicted provokes people into exaggerating their statements beyond their proper limits. He argued that by showing a man quite quietly that he is wrong, and that what he says and thinks is incorrect, you embitter him more than if you use some rude or insulting expression. We published our most important papers in the *Lancet* and the *BMJ*, and they contradicted prevailing beliefs and clearly irritated the screening advocates.

When people have maintained unsustainable beliefs for some time, it seems that the more evidence you present showing they are wrong, the more bizarre their responses become. An Australian colleague, Vivienne Miller, wrote to me that it is crucial for people to maintain their beliefs because they are related to their view of themselves as a person (self-esteem) and to their sense of how others perceive them. We noticed that the debate became more embittered after we published our review of the contents of invitations for screening in the *BMJ* on 4 March 2006.[5] Therefore, this paper must have hit the self-esteem of the screening advocates particularly hard.

Three weeks after we published the paper, Henrik Møller and Elizabeth Davies from the Thames Cancer Registry reported a benefit to harm ratio of 1 to 2.[6] This is five times more optimistic than the 1 to 10 ratio we had just reported:[5]

> If 2000 women are screened regularly for 10 years, one woman will avoid dying from breast cancer, and 10 healthy women, who would not have been diagnosed without screening, will have breast cancer diagnosed and be treated unnecessarily.

Even though Møller and Davies' paper wasn't original research but just an editorial, we felt compelled to tell the readers what was wrong with their approach.[7]

First, Møller and Davies had extrapolated the benefit in the screening trials to the remaining lifespan of the invited women and had used lifetime breast cancer mortality after age 50 in their calculation of benefit. This approach is invalid. The effect of screening cannot continue many years after screening has ceased; all the new cancers in this period will be detected clinically, which means that the 'effect' of screening on these cancers will be zero. Furthermore, they also ignored that breast cancer mortality increases with age. By their inappropriate extrapolations, they estimated the number needed to screen to save one life at only 250. The number was much higher, 1000 after 10 years, in the meta-analysis of the Swedish trials,[8] and it was 2000 if based on the Cochrane review[9] or the review from the US Preventive Services Task Force.[10]

Second, their estimate of overdiagnosis was much too low, as they used the 10% reported by the Malmö investigators without correction for the dilution and contamination biases (*see* Chapter 16).

Three years later, we irritated the screening advocates again, when we published our criticism of the UK leaflet in the *BMJ* in 2009. A wealth of rapid responses were published on the *BMJ* website, and the exaggerations were now monstrous.

Nicholas Wald and Malcolm Law, who are epidemiologists, started off by claiming that over 10 years of screening, six women per 2000 would avoid dying from breast cancer.[11] We noted that if based on the randomised trials, Wald and Law's estimate could only be correct if one assumed screening reduced breast cancer mortality by 90% (*see* next section).[12] However, they didn't use data from the randomised trials. They derived their estimate in a curious way that involved erroneous use of observational data. They used the official death rates for women who died aged 55–74 years and estimated a hypothetical, higher death rate in the absence of screening, assuming the effect of screening was 30%. They then calculated the benefit, again assuming an effect of 30%. Thus, by using a wrong estimate twice, they inflated their estimate twice.

They also overlooked that many women who die aged 55–74 years die from slow-growing cancers diagnosed before the women became eligible for screening, as they were too young. This error is somewhat like tallying the number of deaths from myocardial infarction in a country, and then using the effect of streptokinase to calculate the number of lives saved, which disregards that many die before they reach hospital and others are never treated because too many hours have elapsed since the start of symptoms.

Finally, Wald and Law multiplied their 10-year estimate by two and said that 12 will benefit after 20 years. This is also problematic. There are no trial data spanning 20 years of screening with an unscreened control group, and it is a bias-prone method to extend estimates far beyond the time period covered by the data. Worst of all perhaps they didn't consider the harms, which will also increase with time. The balance between benefits and harms would therefore not be expected to change much from 10 to 20 years.

Duffy's 'funny' numbers

After Wald and Law's astonishing approach to science, Stephen Duffy joined the debate and said that using a 10-year period may overestimate harms.[13] This isn't correct. The uncertainty related to deciding whether a suspicious mammogram or biopsy is cancer is substantial. This means that the more years women go to screening, the more borderline cases and therefore the more overdiagnosis there will be. Overdiagnosis will be greater after 20 years of screening than after 10 years also for another reason; namely, because many cancers detected by screening would have regressed if left alone without treatment.[14] Such cancers will of course also appear after the first 10 years.

A woman who described herself as a former patient had apparently had enough of the manipulation of numbers, as she wrote:[15]

> As a reasonably numerate member of the public, I find it curious that a number of 'experts' differ in their assessment of the benefit of breast cancer screening

> by a factor of nearly 10. This is such a huge difference that, clearly, someone must be wrong . . . I know whose figures I believe. Is this those of the Professor of Cancer Screening who, of course, has a vested interest in exaggerating screening benefits? Or his colleague, perhaps, who makes the fairly basic error of assuming that, because x women benefit over 10 years, 2x women must benefit over 20 years? Or, finally, the party raising uncomfortable truths about how flawed the UK screening programme really is? I'll leave you to guess.

The patient's letter was the 24th comment published in reply to our criticism of the UK leaflet. We were as disturbed as the patient. So we wrote a lengthy reply to Duffy, explaining all the errors he had made.[16] Since Duffy disagreed substantially with our estimates – both of the benefits and of the harms – we first described which data sources and methods he had used compared to ours (Table 20.1).

TABLE 20.1 Data sources and methods used to generate estimates of benefits and harms of screening

Disagreement	Duffy's approach	Our approach	Advantage of our approach
Research design	Unsystematic reviews of randomised trials and observational studies	Systematic reviews of randomised trials and observational studies	Reliable, and therefore the recommended method
Statistical methods	Involves models and assumptions	Does not involve models and assumptions	Transparent, easy to understand, and data massage is not possible
Statistical methods	Extrapolation far beyond what the data support	No undue extrapolations	Reliable, and therefore the recommended method
Statistical methods	Subgroup analysis of attenders (like 'per protocol analysis' in drug trials)	No subgroup analysis (like 'intention-to-treat analysis' in drug trials)	Reliable, and therefore the recommended method

As usual, it required detective work to find out what Duffy had done. He didn't offer any numbers in support of the calculations by Wald and Law, but he quoted a paper by himself, Tabár, Robert Smith and others. I looked it up and found that it was obfuscated. It referred to the number of breast cancer deaths in the Two-County trial but it didn't state which publication they came from. This is typical of Duffy and Tabár. Given the many papers on this trial and the varying numbers reported, it would be difficult and very labour-intensive for most people to find the missing reference, but we found it. We weren't the least surprised that the missing reference reported a 24% reduction in Östergötland (whereas researchers using the Swedish cause-of-death register only found a 10% reduction). Duffy claimed that our reply to Wald and Law contained 'inaccuracies', but the reference he cited in support of this was to an unsystematic review by himself, Tabár and Smith.[17] This paper stated that in the Two-County trial, 'Cause of death was determined on blind review', which, as I have explained, is false in relation to the purported 24% reduction in Östergötland.

Duffy claimed that our estimate of a 15% reduction in breast cancer mortality had 'no basis in empirical data'. In contrast to Duffy, I believe that data from randomised trials are empirical.

Duffy stated that the calculation by Wald and Law was 'reasonable and simple' and 'involves fewer assumptions' than ours. More nonsense. Our estimate required no assumptions, and it was based directly on the trials, in contrast to the curious and erroneous methods used by Wald and Law.

Duffy wrote that our assertion that Wald and Law's estimate entails a 90% reduction in breast cancer mortality with screening was clearly wildly inaccurate and was 'presumably based on flawed logic'. Therefore, I explained how I had derived the 90%, using the Swedish meta-analysis of the Swedish trials.[8] A little knowledge of elementary school algebra suffices to work it out:[16]

> After 9 years there were 2.6 and 3.3 deaths, respectively, per 1000 women, in the invited and control groups, and after 12 years, the numbers were 3.9 and 5.1. Thus 2 breast cancer deaths per 2000 women were avoided after 10 years of screening, and not 6 as Duffy claims. There were 425 breast cancer deaths in the control groups of 125,866 women after a mean of 9 years of follow-up. If the effect of screening were a 90% reduction in breast cancer mortality, there would be 43 breast cancer deaths in a screened group of the same size. The risk difference then becomes 425/125,866 – 43/125,866 = 0.00338 – 0.00034 = 0.00304, which gives a number needed to invite to screening of 1/0.00304 = 328 to avoid one breast cancer death. This is very close to the 333 that Wald and Law reported (6 deaths avoided per 2000 in 10 years). Thus, if we were to try to generate the numbers provided by Wald and Law, but now based on the randomised trials, we would have to postulate that the effect of screening were a 90% reduction in breast cancer mortality.

This calculation shows better than anything how terribly flawed the methods are that Duffy, Wald and Law advocate.

We were also accused of a 'highly selective interpretation of the published results on overdiagnosis', but it is not selective to perform a systematic review of the reliable studies, which leads to exclusion of Duffy's flawed studies on overdiagnosis that relied on complicated models with dubious assumptions and his propensity for multiple adjustments (*see* Chapter 16). Using the same simple algebra as for mortality, which we have done in our Cochrane review,[18] it is easy to see that 30% overdiagnosis means that 10 women are overdiagnosed per 2000.

Since randomised trials provide the most reliable evidence, I fail to understand why many epidemiologists and statisticians repeatedly use observational data and complicated statistical models, unless the very idea with these manoeuvres is to produce wrong results in favour of screening. Duffy doesn't even follow his own advice about models:[19]

> When there is disagreement between direct results from empirical data and modelled estimates derived by combining information from disparate sources, it would be wise to trust the former.

In June 2009, Fiona Godlee published an editor's choice in the *BMJ*,[20] noting that general practitioner Iona Heath had turned down mammography screening because she thought the evidence was pretty clear that the potential harms of overdiagnosis outweighed the potential benefits.[21] Heath worried, though, that her decision was based on information that her patients cannot easily find because the invitation leaflet doesn't mention harms.

Godlee also noted that Wald, Law and Duffy had criticised us for substantially underestimating the survival benefit of screening and that nearly 2 months on, after we had replied in extensive detail, we had not been challenged again. Furthermore, Godlee said that *in private emails to the BMJ, advocates of the NHS Breast Screening Programme had criticised the editors for not adequately presenting the facts in support of screening.* Godlee mentioned that the *BMJ* would welcome a balanced article on this subject, but also that, for the moment, what is being asked for is simply that women should be made aware of the potential for harm from overdiagnosis so they can make a more informed decision.

A month later, Wald, Law and Duffy had joined forces and published a letter in the *BMJ*, 'Breast screening saves lives',[22] where there was nothing about overdiagnosis, and therefore no contribution to an informed decision, as Godlee had called for. The exaggeration was now extreme. *Wald, Law and Duffy wrote that over 20 years of screening, one woman per 100 screened would avoid dying from breast cancer.*[22] This is 20 times more optimistic than the estimate for 10 years of screening based on the comprehensive systematic reviews of the randomised trials![9,10] Duffy generally supports an approach of calculating the effect among those who actually attend screening, based on the effect among those invited and the attendance rate. However, because of roundings, it doesn't matter whether we use invited women or women actually screened as the denominator for our estimate.

Clearly, if Wald, Law and Duffy had been right, it would have been very easy to see an effect of breast screening in UK mortality statistics in the relevant age groups, but there is none (*see* Figure 19.5).[23]

It seems to me that screening advocates rather consistently underestimate the intelligence of their audience. Or perhaps they are just knowingly spreading misleading numbers, as the politicians cannot judge who is right and who is wrong and therefore tend to rely on authority rather than on sound science. Doctors and scientists saw through Duffy's smoke and mirrors. One noted that 'intelligent, unbiased analysis of the numerous existing studies ought to lead one to conclude that breast screening is of little or no value in reducing breast cancer mortality',[24] and another asked: 'Would we accept such extremely rosy extrapolations and assumptions from the pharmaceutical industry?'[25]

The criticisms did not perturb Wald, Law and Duffy, and they continued with their exaggerations on the *BMJ* website.[26] We countered, with a simple calculation, that their estimate of one woman saved for every 100 women screened over 20 years means that 2850 women per year will be saved in the United Kingdom. This is twice as many as the 1400 lives the NHS Breast Screening Programme claims are saved each year, which is already much too optimistic.[27]

There were other problems,[27,28] and one of their statements was particularly startling: 'The decline in breast cancer mortality over time has occurred despite a concurrent increase in incidence; it would have been greater had incidence remained the same.' This remark shows that Wald, Law and Duffy still denied that screening leads to substantial overdiagnosis.

They used a 'generally accepted' 24% reduction in mortality from breast cancer and inflated this estimate, assuming it would have been 31% if all invited women had attended, which is like saying that if only everybody with meningitis had been treated earlier, more would have been saved, or if more people had stayed at home, fewer would have been killed in car crashes. Life is not like that, and the authors also ignored that attendees are healthier than non-attendees (self-selection bias).

More seriously, Wald, Law and Duffy used mortality rates from 1988 – when screening started in the United Kingdom – to calculate the effect of screening. This is misleading as it disregards that most of the decline in breast cancer mortality since 1988 has been due to improved treatment and not to screening. Using their false premise, we showed that their claim is much closer to a 73% reduction in breast cancer mortality than to a 47% reduction among women who attend screening, both being implausibly large.

Wald, Law and Duffy gave some numbers as the basis for their calculations. As is typical for Duffy's approach to science, there were no references as to where they came from, but we nevertheless discovered that the numbers were wrong. They claimed that in 1988, the risk of dying from breast cancer in the age group 55–74 years was 3%, but using national statistics,[29] we found only 2.1%. They also claimed that 60% of breast cancer deaths occurred in the age group 55–74 years in 1988, but we found only 44.3% in 1988. Their erroneous estimates had a huge inflating impact on their results; the first error alone, for example, amounts to 43% (3 divided by 2.1).

Duffy consistently calls my calculations inaccurate – and sometimes even completely inaccurate or wildly inaccurate – but it seems to be he who has a problem. I thought it was a prerequisite for being a statistician that one can handle numbers, but I have learned this is not necessarily so. Despite Duffy's routine derogatory remarks about my calculations, I haven't made any errors, and he hasn't demonstrated any, in spite of his incessant claims. The errors are in Duffy's numbers and in his methods.

We agreed with Wald, Law and Duffy that 'proof of efficacy comes from the trial evidence, not from changes in mortality over time', but they didn't follow their own advice.

Exaggerating 25-fold

> *Bad science is where data have been cherry-picked – when some data have been deliberately left out – or it's impossible for the reader to understand the steps that were taken to produce or analyze the data. It is a set of claims that can't be tested, claims that are based on samples that are too small, and claims that don't follow from the evidence provided.*
>
> Naomi Oreskes and Erik Conway[30]

The exaggerations escalated. In March 2010, Duffy, Tabár, Smith, Anne-Helene Olsen and others published a paper estimating that between 2 and 2.5 lives are saved for every overdiagnosed case.[31] Compared with the estimate from the randomised trials, the ratio of 2.5 to 1 is wrong by a factor of 25.[18]

The methods used by Duffy *et al.*[31] to arrive at their monstrously exaggerated estimate were inappropriate. They cherry-picked the Two-County trial, and used a 38% reduction in breast cancer mortality, which is 2.5 times higher than our estimate based on all the trials. They also used data from the UK Breast Screening Programme but misrepresented them. They wrote that they considered the mortality stable in the unscreened age groups, but they contradicted themselves, as they reported a significant 18% decline in breast cancer mortality in women below 50 years of age. The decline in the age group 50–69 years was 27%, but by some obscure method described in a footnote to a table, they nevertheless concluded that screening had reduced breast cancer mortality by 28% compared with other age groups.

Duffy's lack of transparency in his research methods is startling, and his result disagrees starkly with official data. Cancer Research UK writes: 'Between 1989 and 2008 the breast cancer mortality rate fell by 44% in women aged 40–49 years; by 44% in women aged 50–64; by 37% in women aged 65–69; by 39% in women aged 15–39; and by 19% in women over 70.'[32] Thus, there is no sign of a screening effect, as women aged 40–49 years who were never invited to screening had the same decline in mortality as those aged 50–64 years.

In a figure, Duffy *et al.*[31] lumped together data for women under 50 years of age. As deaths from breast cancer before age 30 are extremely rare,[32] and as there are many women and girls in this age group, the graph is close to the x-axis at the bottom of the figure, which conceals the inconvenient truth that there was a huge decline in mortality in young women.

Duffy *et al.*[31] also combined data from the age group 50–64 years with the age group 65–69 years, although screening of the latter group didn't start before 2001. This conceals another inconvenient truth; namely, that breast cancer mortality in the age group 50–64 years began to decline *before* the UK programme started in 1988.

The methods Duffy *et al.*[31] use for estimating overdiagnosis are also flawed and lead to serious underestimation. First, they excluded carcinoma *in situ*, which wasn't stated in their paper. Karsten Juhl Jørgensen asked Duffy on national British radio whether he only included invasive cancer,[33] which Duffy confirmed. It is a serious error to exclude carcinoma *in situ* and it is unacceptable not to state in the paper that this was done. Carcinoma *in situ* constitutes 21% of the diagnoses made through the screening programme, and they are more often treated by mastectomy than invasive breast cancer.[34]

Second, they used an unverified model with incorrect assumptions. It is clearly wrong to assume that essentially all increase in incidence with screening represents earlier diagnosis.

Third, they adjusted for a compensatory decline in breast cancer incidence in UK women no longer screened because of advanced age, which didn't exist for the years they examined.[35] This is clear if one looks at the freely available graphs at Cancer Research UK that show the incidence of invasive breast cancer.[36] More updated numbers show an abrupt *increase* when screening was extended to the age group 65–70 years in 2001 (*see* Figure 16.2), which far exceeds any possible recent compensatory decline.

We estimated 57% overdiagnosis in England and Wales when we included carcinoma *in situ* based on other data.[35] Duffy *et al.*[31] estimated that only 12% of cancers are overdiagnosed.

Their faulty methods led Duffy *et al.*[31] to estimate that 2.3 cases are overdiagnosed per 1000 women after 20 years. However, as five women per 1000 are overdiagnosed already after 10 years according to the trials, and as many additional overdiagnosed cases will accumulate over the next 10 years, their estimate is far too low.

In discussing our data, Duffy *et al.*[31] said the reason for the disagreement partly lay in the fact that their benefit was estimated 'directly from empirical data, and we have been careful to avoid confusing invitation to screening with actually receiving screening'. Thus, Duffy says again that data from randomised trials are not empirical. Furthermore, as I have already explained, it is not important for the ratio between benefits and harms whether one looks at those invited or those attending.

Duffy *et al.*[31] were also selective in their choice of references. They claimed that only 37% of breast cancers are screen-detected, but this was based on a 200-word conference abstract. The abstract mentions an unexplained algorithm to evaluate the West Midlands screening programme[37] and notes that 22% of diagnoses were interval cancers, 11% were detected in non-attenders and 2% were lapsed attenders. An additional 14% were diagnosed before invitations were sent out and should therefore not count. Thus, the sum of the relevant percentages was only 72% (as it was not clear how the remaining 14% were diagnosed). This confusion leads Duffy *et al.*[31] to conclude that our result on overdiagnosis in public screening programmes implies that virtually all screen-detected cancers are overdiagnosed; they then say this is an 'absurd and frankly incredible conclusion'. What is absurd is their cherry-picking of unreliable data and their lack of honesty. It is well known that between half and two-thirds of cancers are detected through screening. For example, 68% of cancers were screen-detected in the United Kingdom in 2006,[34] not 37% as Duffy *et al.*[31] write.

Perhaps I should explain what it is that makes cherry-picking such an unacceptable method in science. It is pretty obvious that you're cheating if you throw a basketball 10 times from a large distance, say 20 m, and hit the basket once, and then ignore the nine failed attempts and use a video of that single fortunate hit as documentation that you are a fantastic basketball player. Duffy has published many papers on the Two-County trial with Tabár (60 hits on PubMed combine the two names), and he may not think he is cherry-picking when he consistently uses that trial to convince people that mammography screening has a substantial effect. He would most likely say that it's only natural to do so, as he has access to the raw data from that trial. Others will nevertheless see it as cherry-picking, compared with using all the trials when deriving estimates.

There was one positive aspect of their paper, though. Duffy *et al.*[31] acknowledged overdiagnosis of invasive breast cancer, which is little short of revolutionary, as Duffy, Tabár and Smith have previously considered this to be a minor problem, and as another co-author, Anne-Helene Olsen, published the study that claimed 'mammography screening can operate without overdiagnosis of breast cancer'.[38]

Duffy and colleagues'[31] choice to publish in the *Journal of Medical Screening* was unfortunate, as doubts can be raised about the impartiality of the review process. It is the journal of the Medical Screening Society, located at the Wolfson Institute of Preventive Medicine. The institute is also the home institution of Duffy and two of his co-authors. Duffy serves on the editorial committee of the journal, together with the director of the NHS Breast Screening Programme, Julietta Patnick. Nicholas Wald is president of the Medical Screening Society, director of the Wolfson Institute and editor of the journal. Malcolm Law is associate editor, and is also a professor at the Wolfson Institute. An arrangement that guarantees a high level of agreement about issues related to breast screening.

Others of Duffy's co-authors, particularly Tabár and Smith, have competing interests, but none were declared in their paper, although the *Journal of Medical Screening* requests a statement from authors.

We first published our critique of Duffy's paper on the *BMJ* website.[39] Two months later, we put our heads into the lion's den and submitted a similar criticism as a full paper to the *Journal of Medical Screening*, partly to inform the readers about the errors, and partly as an experiment to see what happened.

Nicholas Wald asked us to submit a letter to the editor instead and said that our section on competing interests was unwarranted. I wrote back that we believed Wald might have his own conflict of interest when he said we were not allowed to write about conflicts of interest and asked him to reconsider his decision, e.g. in consultation with the journal's ombudsman.

Wald also informed us that he would send our letter for peer review. We responded that we very much wondered why he would do this, as none of the hundreds of letters to the editor we had published earlier that discussed a previous paper in a journal had ever been sent out for peer review. We also noted that the journal's guidelines for authors said nothing about peer-reviewing letters, only about peer-reviewing papers. Therefore, we asked Wald whether his journal sent all letters for peer review, which we doubted, and if not, why our letter should be an exception, particularly as Wald had said that the authors we criticised would be given the opportunity to respond to our criticism. We also explained that the very idea with letters was to allow people to publish their criticism, without any influence from peer reviewers who might be conflicted and might have their own interests to protect. Finally, we noted that the journal complied with the Uniform Requirements for Manuscripts Submitted to Biomedical Journals formulated by the International Committee of Medical Journal Editors, and we quoted from these requirements. The most important parts were:

> Financial relationships are the most easily identifiable conflicts of interest and the most likely to undermine the credibility of the journal, the authors, and of science itself. However, conflicts can occur for other reasons, such as personal relationships, academic competition, and intellectual passion.
>
> Editors should avoid selecting external peer reviewers with obvious potential conflicts of interest – for example, those who work in the same department or institution as any of the authors.
>
> Editors who make final decisions about manuscripts must have no personal, professional, or financial involvement in any of the issues they might judge.

In reply, Wald said, 'Whether a submission, be it an article or a letter to the Editor, is peer reviewed is at the discretion of the Editor and members of the Editorial Board who may be consulted. We will do so in this instance.'

We didn't feel this was a satisfactory answer but we did nothing more. We never saw any peer reviews but we were informed 2 months later that our letter was accepted, without any demands for changes, which was a good outcome of our 'experiment'. The word count for letters is quite limited, and since we needed space to explain the many errors Duffy *et al.*[31] had committed, we deleted all descriptions of conflicts of interest apart from this one:[40]

> We also note that no conflicts of interest were declared. Tabár founded Mammography Education Inc, Arizona in 1980, which still exists,[10] and in 1999, he declared an income of five million SEK in Sweden, which is an extraordinary amount according to Nordic standards. We believe that such an important conflict of interest should be declared.

In their response to our letter, Duffy *et al.*[31] continued to confuse their readers, as they had done in their paper.[41] Most bizarre perhaps was their view on conflicts of interest, which clashes with accepted international definitions:

> No communication from Professor Gøtzsche would be complete without the customary accusation of a conflict of interest. We do not propose to join in undignified finger-pointing. We would say that it is no secret that Professor Tabar makes his living by practising and teaching breast radiology. Indeed, it is a point of pride that he has trained 20,000 radiologists in breast imaging, students who in turn proved to be able to achieve substantial reductions in breast cancer mortality by early detection.[7] He will continue to do so regardless of publication or otherwise of our research results. Thus it does not constitute a conflict of interest.

The exaggerations finally backfire

Scientific debates can be very frustrating when those you criticise have disregard for the evidence. It isn't sufficient to demonstrate that your opponents have used wrong numbers, performed erroneous calculations and manipulated the data beyond belief. I have often observed that replies to criticism can be so skilfully deceptive that the editors cannot make a proper judgement about which side is right and which is wrong.

Another fundamental problem in medical science is that researchers tend to praise papers that support their beliefs and criticise those that don't. One might think it would be difficult to criticise studies that have been very well done, but it isn't. In that case, the critics discuss trivial or irrelevant problems, magnify dots to make them look like hand grenades, invent problems, misrepresent the methods or, if all else fails, lie. Both readers and editors often lack the content expertise or methodological expertise, or both, needed to see through the tricks, particularly when the tricksters hide what they have done in an impenetrable cloud of statistical mumbo jumbo. Psychological research has shown that people have greater respect for what they don't understand than for what they do understand. This is one of the reasons why religions are so popular, and it also means that tricksters often win intellectual battles with truth-seekers.

However, everything has its limits. After our most recent papers in the *BMJ* and subsequent endless debates with Duffy, Wald and Law, plus accusations from the screening advocates that the *BMJ* had taken sides, its editors had finally had enough. They wrote that, being 'unable to see sufficient light amidst the heat of this debate', they 'asked a highly trusted observer of preventive health strategies, Klim McPherson, to take a look and come to a view'.[42]

McPherson's paper was unusually frank.[43] He asked whether the time had come for a serious scientific rethink of the benefits of the NHS screening programme in the context of cost-effective care. The *BMJ*'s editor-in-chief, Fiona Godlee, took the unusual step of drawing her own conclusions after having looked at the evidence.[42] She said that 'those who argue that screening may be almost as harmful as it is beneficial come out on top'. She also sensed measured outrage in McPherson's paper, which ended:

> We all need to understand better how a national programme of such importance could exist for so long with so many unanswered questions. Maybe the breast screening service exists on its face validity plus concomitant scientific polarisation in the face of uncertainty? That would be irresponsible.

McPherson's criticism of Duffy's methods and results was devastating. He noted, for example, that Duffy's ratio of benefit versus harm[31] was 10 times more positive than that offered by the Malmö investigators (even though their estimate was also too positive).

The press in the United Kingdom covered the story extensively. The *Independent* published an editorial,[44] and in an interview Godlee said:[45]

> The screening lobby thinks the *BMJ* has got a bee in its bonnet about screening. That is not the case – we follow the evidence. The Danish team [from The Nordic Cochrane Centre] do good work which is very thorough and of good quality. It is fair to say that we have not had the same quality of submissions from the other side. We would be delighted if someone came forward with a robust defence of the screening programme – I don't think they have done that.

It was outrageous to read the next day what Professor Dame Valerie Beral, chair of the Department of Health's Advisory Committee on Breast Screening, had to say.[46] We heard again about the 1400 lives saved each year; Beral said, 'What Klim McPherson and other critics have done is used old data from the US and Scandinavia, largely from the 1970s and 1980s', to which McPherson replied, 'The idea that this is old data is neither here nor there: it is real data.' Even worse, Beral claimed that 'the majority' of an untransparent 2006 report from the NHS Breast Screening Programme[47] had dealt with the harms, and she added: 'In the old days women had mastectomies for breast cancer – now they don't [in cases where the tumour is small enough] so the harms have reduced', and 'there are claims that cancer is over-diagnosed – but it's a misnomer. We don't know there are some cancers that won't progress – it is an unanswerable question.'

This is outright nonsense. Beral's denial of overdiagnosis reinforces Godlee's statement that much more honesty from the NHS screening programme is needed.[42]

The ultimate exaggeration

I had often joked about when we would see the ultimate exaggeration – that screening reduces breast cancer mortality by 100% and therefore saves everybody – but I had not expected it would ever happen. It did happen. In the *BMJ* News section, a headline in 2008 ran: 'Survival of women treated for early breast cancer detected by screening is same as in general population, audit shows'.[48] I was interviewed for the news piece and I noted that it was not the least surprising that women who had a small breast cancer diagnosed at screening and who were judged to have 'a good or excellent prognosis' actually had a good or excellent prognosis.[48] If these lesions were detected 5 years earlier than they would otherwise have been, the 5-year survival rate would be similar to that in the general population. The audit data came from the Association of Breast Surgery and the 'usual suspects', the NHS Breast Screening Programme. My interpretation of this was that the programme had most likely fed the *BMJ* with a misleading press release.

The ultimate exaggeration had already been produced by the Tabár/Duffy/Smith trio and colleagues in 2002 in the *Journal of Medical Screening*, at least indirectly.[49] They predicted that when a screening programme had been established for some time, one could expect a reduction of 3%–4% in total mortality. The lifetime risk of dying from breast cancer is 3% in the United Kingdom[28,29] and it was 3%–4% in many countries before screening was introduced. One cannot, therefore, achieve a 3%–4% reduction in total mortality with screening without avoiding all breast cancer deaths. If Tabár, Duffy and Smith continue their line of research for other diseases, they may find the recipe for eternal life.

In 2007, an extraordinary exaggeration of overdiagnosis was published by Christiane Kuhl and colleagues[50] in the *Lancet*, which they ascribed to us. These authors had published a paper about diagnosis of carcinoma *in situ* with magnetic resonance imaging to which Mangesh Thorat and Hazel Thornton responded, drawing attention to the problem of overdiagnosis with screening, citing our Cochrane review. Thorat and Thornton published another letter where they noted that they were disturbed by the misrepresentation of facts by the authors in their reply, but this just made matters worse. In their second reply, Kuhl and colleagues[50] argued:

> Thorat and Thornton's calculation of the number needed to treat implies that

> 10 of 11 cancers diagnosed by screening would, if left undiagnosed, never become a threat to a woman's life, corresponding to an overdiagnosis rate of 91%. This view, and others in the 2006 Cochrane review,[1] has to be regarded as a hypothesis, is based on calculations (not empirical data), and is certainly not commonly held. Empirical data on the issue of overdiagnosis do exist and suggest a very different proportion.

Thorat, Thornton and I have never implied anything as absurd as an overdiagnosis rate of 91%, and our numbers cannot be used to arrive at this percentage.

References

1 Rennie D. Guarding the guardians: a conference on editorial peer review. *JAMA*. 1986; **256**(17): 2391–2.

2 Thornton H. Inappropriate use of evidence? *BMJ*. 2002 Aug 24. Available at: http://bmj.com/cgi/eletters/325/7361/418#24972 (accessed 22 May 2011).

3 Jørgensen KJ, Klahn A, Gøtzsche PC. Are benefits and harms in mammography screening given equal attention in scientific articles? A cross-sectional study. *BMC Med*. 2007; **5**: 12.

4 Raffle AE. Information about screening: is it to achieve high uptake or to ensure informed choice? *Health Expect*. 2001; **4**(2): 92–8.

5 Jørgensen KJ, Gøtzsche PC. Content of invitations to publicly funded screening mammography. *BMJ*. 2006; **332**(7540): 538–41.

6 Møller H, Davies E. Over-diagnosis in breast cancer screening. *BMJ*. 2006; **332**(7543): 691–2.

7 Gøtzsche PC, Jørgensen KJ. Estimate of harm/benefit ratio of mammography screening was five times too optimistic. *BMJ*. 2006 Mar 27. Available at: http://bmj.bmjjournals.com/cgi/eletters/332/7543/691 (accessed 22 May 2011).

8 Nyström L, Rutqvist LE, Wall S, *et al*. Breast cancer screening with mammography: overview of Swedish randomised trials. *Lancet*. 1993; **341**(8851): 973–8.

9 Gøtzsche PC, Nielsen M. Screening for breast cancer with mammography. *Cochrane Database Syst Rev*. 2006; (4): CD001877.

10 Humphrey LL, Helfand M, Chan BK, *et al*. Breast cancer screening: a summary of the evidence for the U.S. Preventive Services Task Force. *Ann Intern Med*. 2002; **137**(5 Pt. 1): 347–60.

11 Zahl P-H, Mæhlen J, Welch HG. The natural history of invasive breast cancers detected by screening mammography. *Arch Intern Med*. 2008; **168**(21): 2311–16.

12 Smith RA, Duffy SW, Gabe R, *et al*. The randomized trials of breast cancer screening: what have we learned? *Radiol Clin North Am*. 2004; **42**(5): 793–806.

13 Gøtzsche PC, Nielsen M. Screening for breast cancer with mammography. *Cochrane Database Syst Rev*. 2009; (4): CD001877.

14 Wald NJ, Law MR. Response to Gotzsche. *BMJ*. 2009 Feb 27. Available at: www.bmj.com/cgi/eletters/338/jan27_2/b86 (accessed 22 May 2011).

15 Gøtzsche PC, Hartling OJ, Nielsen M, *et al*. Estimate of breast screening benefit was

6 times too large. *BMJ*. 2009. Available at: www.bmj.com/cgi/eletters/338/jan27_2/b86 (accessed 22 May 2011).

16 Duffy S. Re: Estimate of breast screening benefit was 6 times too large. *BMJ*. 2009 Mar 29. Available at: www.bmj.com/cgi/eletters/338/jan27_2/b86 (accessed 22 May 2011).

17 Flanders J. Who isn't 'doing the math' right here? *BMJ*. 2000 Apr 23. Available at: www.bmj.com/cgi/eletters/338/jan27_2/b86 (accessed 22 May 2011).

18 Gøtzsche PC, Jørgensen KJ. Stephen Duffy's claims on the benefits and harms of breast screening are seriously wrong. *BMJ*. 2009 May 1. Available at: www.bmj.com/cgi/eletters/338/jan27_2/b86 (accessed 22 May 2011).

19 Duffy SW. Commentary on 'What is the point: will screening mammography save my life?' by Keen and Keen. *BMC Med Inform Decis Mak*. 2009; **9**: 19.

20 Godlee F. Less medicine is more. *BMJ*. 2009; **338**: b2561.

21 Heath I. Life and death: it is not wrong to say no. *BMJ*. 2009; **338**: b2529.

22 Wald NJ, Law MR, Duffy SW. Breast screening saves lives. *BMJ*. 2009; **339**: 188.

23 Jørgensen KJ, Zahl P-H, Gøtzsche PC. Breast cancer mortality in organised mammography screening in Denmark: comparative study. *BMJ*. 2010; **340**: c1241.

24 Nehrlich HH. Primum non nocere. *BMJ*. 2009 Jul 23. Available at: www.bmj.com/cgi/eletters/339/jul21_2/b2922 (accessed 22 May 2011).

25 Bonneux L. Unacceptable answer. *BMJ*. 2009 Jul 24. Available at: www.bmj.com/cgi/eletters/339/jul21_2/b2922 (accessed 22 May 2011).

26 Wald NJ, Law MR, Duffy SW. Lives saved by breast cancer screening. *BMJ*. 2009 Sep 2. Available at: www.bmj.com/cgi/eletters/339/aug25_1/b3359 (accessed 22 May 2011).

27 Jørgensen KJ, Gøtzsche PC. Authors reply: Wald *et al.*'s estimate of the effect of breast screening is about 10 times higher than the most reliable evidence shows. *BMJ*. 2009 Sep 15. Available at: www.bmj.com/cgi/eletters/339/aug25_1/b3359#220390 (accessed 22 May 2011).

28 Jørgensen KJ, Gøtzsche PC. Breast screening: fundamental errors in estimate of lives saved by screening. *BMJ*. 2009; **339**: 474.

29 Office of Population Censuses and Surveys. *Mortality Statistics: cause 1988*. London: HMSO; 1990. (Series DH2 no. 15. Table 2).

30 Oreskes N, Conway EM. *Merchants of Doubt*. New York: Bloomsbury Press; 2010.

31 Duffy SW, Tabár L, Olsen AH, *et al*. Absolute numbers of lives saved and overdiagnosis in breast cancer screening, from a randomised trial and from the breast screening programme in England. *J Med Screen*. 2010; **17**(1): 25–30.

32 Cancer Research UK. *Breast Cancer: UK mortality statistics*. Available at: http://info.cancerresearchuk.org/cancerstats/types/breast/mortality (accessed 7 April 2010).

33 BBC Today. *Breast Screening 'Saves Lives'* [debate]. 2010 March 31. Available at: http://news.bbc.co.uk/today/hi/today/newsid_8596000/8596225.stm (accessed 31 March 2010).

34 Patnick J, editor. *NHS Breast Screening Programme Annual Review 2008: Saving Lives through Screening*. Available at: www.cancerscreening.nhs.uk/breastscreen/publications/2008review.html (accessed 4 March 2009).

35 Jørgensen KJ, Gøtzsche PC. Overdiagnosis in publicly organised mammography screening programmes: systematic review of incidence trends. *BMJ*. 2009; **339**: b2587.

36 Cancer Research UK. *Breast Cancer: UK incidence statistics*. Available at: http://info.cancerresearchuk.org/cancerstats/types/breast/incidence/?a=5441 (accessed 7 April 2010).

37 Hudson J, Lawrence GM, Kearins O, *et al*. West Midlands screening histories project: methodology and use as an audit tool. *Breast Cancer Res*. 2004; **6**(Suppl. 1): 26–7.
38 Olsen AH, Jensen A, Njor S, *et al*. Breast cancer incidence after the start of mammography screening in Denmark. *Br J Cancer*. 2003; **88**(3): 362–5.
39 Jørgensen KJ, Gøtzsche PC. Mammography screening hasn't lived up to expectations. *BMJ*. 2010 Apr 15. Available at: www.bmj.com/cgi/eletters/340/mar23_1/c1241 (accessed 22 May 2011).
40 Gøtzsche PC, Jørgensen KJ, Zahl P-H. Breast screening: why estimates differ by a factor of 20–25. *J Med Screen*. 2010; **17**(3): 158–9.
41 Duffy SW, Tabár L, Olsen AH, *et al*. Cancer mortality in the 50–69 year age group before and after screening. *J Med Screen*. 2010; **17**: 159–60.
42 Godlee F. Breast screening and other fights. *BMJ*. 2010; **341**: c4096.
43 McPherson K. Should we screen for breast cancer? *BMJ*. 2010; **341**: 233–5.
44 Time for a fresh look at cancer screening. *Independent*. 2010 Aug 4.
45 Laurance J. Review puts merits of breast cancer screening under the microscope. *Independent*. 2010 Aug 4.
46 Laurance J. Cancer specialists insist criticism of breast-screening is 'out of date'. *Independent*. 2010 Aug 5.
47 Advisory Committee on Breast Cancer Screening. *Screening for Breast Cancer in England: past and future*. NHSBSP publication no. 61. Sheffield: NHS Cancer Screening Programmes; 2006. Available at: www.cancerscreening.nhs.uk/breastscreen/publications/nhsbsp61.pdf (accessed 27 February 2006).
48 Mayor S. Survival of women treated for early breast cancer detected by screening is same as in general population, audit shows. *BMJ*. 2008; **336**(7658): 1398–9.
49 Tabár L, Duffy SW, Yen M-F, *et al*. All-cause mortality among breast cancer patients in a screening trial: support for breast cancer mortality as an end point. *J Med Screen*. 2002; **9**(4): 159–62.
50 Kuhl C, Nieling HB, Wardelmann E, *et al*. MRI breast screening. *Lancet*. 2008; **371**: 1416.

21

Tabár threatens the *BMJ* with litigation

Truth should not be decided by those with greatest wealth using bullying and threats to make a scientist retract what he or she knows is true.

Peter Wilmshurst[1]

ON 15 APRIL 2010, THE NORDIC COCHRANE CENTRE POSTED A comment on the *BMJ* website[2] on the 25-fold exaggeration Duffy *et al.* had published in the *Journal of Medical Screening.*[3] The very next day, László Tabár emailed the *BMJ* and asked the editor to bring his letter to the attention of the legal adviser of the British Medical Association. Tabár complained about these two sentences of our comment on the Two-County trial:

> Assessment of cause of death was not blinded in this trial, and the investigators reported an effect of 24% in one of the counties when the official cause-of-death register only showed a 10% effect (11). We will probably never know what happened in the other county, as Tabár has denied other researchers – even the other Swedish mammography trialists (14) – access to his data.

Tabár argued, 'these allegations concerning my scientific integrity amount to defamation of character. I am certain that the authors are aware of the attached publication by Holmberg *et al.* in the *Journal of Medical Screening.*'

Tabár said this article clearly explained exactly why the 2002 meta-analysis of the Swedish trials reported other results than those reported by the trialists. He remarked, 'This provides a clear example of why individual investigators, and especially journals, should be cautious about implying scientific misconduct without proof, or as in this case, without an understanding of the actual situation.' He continued:

> Civility has never been valued by Jorgensen, Gotzsche and others associated with the Nordic Cochrane Center, but we expect more from the editors of the BMJ, who have turned a blind eye to their caustic, slanderous remarks. The publication of the article by Holmberg *et al.*, which is based on a thorough review of each of the individual patient charts in both the W and E counties, disproves the libelous claim according to which 'Tabár has denied other researchers – even the other Swedish mammography trialists access to his data.'
>
> Contrary to Jørgensen and Gøtzsche's libelous allegations against me personally, published online by the BMJ, the leaders of the W-E trial worked for many years to ensure that the errors presented in the 2002 *Lancet* article would be rectified in a joint effort with all authors reviewing the data available in the Swedish Cancer and Death Registries and compared with the individual patient charts in the archives of the W-E trial. This collaborative effort included Lennarth Nyström and Jan Frisell, two of the authors of the *Lancet* 2002 article. Publication of this joint project (Holmberg 2009) serves as a good example of resolution of methodological disputes by constructive collaboration.
>
> Given these facts, Karsten J. Jørgensen and Peter C. Gøtzsche must take responsibility for their libelous allegations, as must the BMJ for allowing them to be published.

In contrast to Tabár's assertion, we were not aware of the paper by Holmberg and colleagues,[4] which had been published less than a year earlier. It was said to be 'a complete audit of breast cancer cases and deaths' in the Two-County trial, but it is not convincing. First of all, it is *not* an independent audit. This is illustrated by the list of authors – Holmberg, Duffy, Yen, Tabár, Vitak, Nyström and Frisell – and a search on PubMed for the many papers they have published together.

Second, the Two-County trialists were directly involved with resolving disagreements between their own publications and those in the 2002 meta-analysis, and they were also members of a Joint Review Committee, which determined the reasons for the disagreements and arrived at its own estimates of the effect of screening in the two counties.

Third, 'where necessary, clinical records were retrieved.' Thus, there was no attempt at producing a new data set based on the clinical records that could have been assessed independently from what had taken place in the past. This must have influenced what was reported not only by the Two-County trialists in their publications but also what was reported to the cancer registry and the cause-of-death registry.

Fourth, *there was no description of any attempt at blinding the provision of the data or the assessments*, which could have ensured that no one knew whether a woman belonged to the screened group or to the control group when they agreed on the cause of death. This fatal and inexcusable flaw in the study is remarkable, as independent observers have ascribed the very positive results that have been published for the Two-County trial to lack of blinding in the cause-of-death assessments. Assessment of cause of death can be very difficult, indeed sometimes impossible, and to do this in an unbiased fashion requires blinded recording of cause of death, blinded selection of data for review, and blinded review.

I am not impressed by such methodology. And I am not surprised that after the Joint Review Committee had done its work, its estimates were very similar to those published by the Two-County trialists originally. To me, the study looks like window dressing, aimed at rehabilitating the Two-County trial, which it failed to do because of poor methodology. In that respect, the study resembles the Two-County trial itself.

I wrote to the *BMJ* that even though Tabár had shared his data now, this in no way compromised our statement that he has previously denied access to others. I couldn't see any basis for defamation of character or for libel, as what we had written was well known, also by the other Swedish trialists.[5] I documented this in email messages to the editors and suggested they invite Tabár to publish his views as a contribution to the scientific debate, but it took 2½ months and negotiations between the lawyers from either side before Tabár accepted the offer.

The *BMJ* editors are obliged by their insurance to follow their lawyer's advice, and they deleted the two sentences Tabár didn't like. I cannot describe the lawyer's reasoning, or discuss Tabár's American lawyer's arguments, as this was sent to me marked 'Private and Confidential; legally priviledged'. This is a shame, as the deliberations are very interesting for scientists, like voices from another planet. We don't hire lawyers to go carefully through every word we use when we write papers. I reported back to the *BMJ* that Tabár's American lawyer muddled the issues and that I had found many errors in his statements, which I explained over five pages.

The result of the legal interference with our work was that our comment became preceded by: 'This rapid response was amended on 22 April 2010 by David Payne, bmj.com editor, on legal advice, and then again by Tony Delamothe, deputy editor, on 23 April 2010.' Furthermore, the first of the two deleted sentences was reinstated, with an additional explanation, which I show in italics:

> Assessment of cause of death was not blinded *by the investigators' own reports of* this trial, and the investigators reported an effect of 24% in one of the counties when the official cause of death register showed only a 10% effect.[11]

This change is pretty ridiculous in my view. It was already clear from the text we originally published that the lack of blinding was related to the 24% effect in the next sentence.

The second sentence, about lack of data access, remains deleted, but we wonder why Tabár was so eager to have it removed when he wrote essentially the same in his published reply that starts thus: 'Jørgensen and Gøtzsche have claimed in their recent Rapid Response on the *BMJ* website that "Tabar has denied other researchers – even the other Swedish mammography trialists – access to his data" (1).'[6]

Tabár then claimed, 'This is untrue' and said, 'It is to be welcomed that the *BMJ* removed this false claim from the Rapid Response website.' Tabár didn't explain that the *BMJ* did this after legal pressure exerted by himself and that the *BMJ* has not acknowledged that it made any errors by publishing what Tabár calls a 'false claim'. Later, Stephen Duffy added insult to injury when he stated in the *BMJ* that 'one claim made by Jorgensen and Gotzsche in the correspondence was withdrawn by the editors on legal advice'.[7] Duffy didn't explain how foolish all this was and he therefore conveyed the impression that we had done something wrong, just as Tabár did.

This looked like bullying the *BMJ*, using a lawyer as the 'gorilla' and a pyrrhic victory for Tabár. But the hair-splitting continued because of the *BMJ*'s fear of litigation. Luc Bonneux informed us that the *BMJ* removed his whole comment from its website and he wrote that, as far as he could tell, his text was legally very innocent. Bonneux had merely described the discrepant results reported for the Two-County trial and had noted, 'The data from Kopparberg have not been made available for independent scrutiny and reclassification', with reference to Nyström's 2002 meta-analysis. I believe this is absolutely true, even after the Holmberg paper, as I do not regard the Holmberg team an independent group.

After having seen Tabár's lengthy comment on the *BMJ* website, which may give the erroneous impression that there really aren't any problems with getting access to his data,[6] Cornelia Baines submitted a letter that the *BMJ* didn't dare publish. Its handling editor explained, 'There is a legal history to the response from Dr Tabar, and our lawyer has advised us that we should not publish the part of your response about combining/sharing data. However, we have published a shortened version making your second point (below).' What Baines submitted was this:

> Dr. Tabar tells us he has been very collaboratively inclined although according to his own information not between 1998 and 2005. However I distinctly remember participating in a meeting convened by the US National Cancer Institute January 18 and 19, 1994: the NCI Working Group on Breast Cancer Screening Meta/Overview-analyses in Rockville, Maryland.
>
> Obviously it had been hoped that the trialists would agree to submit their data so that analyses of combined raw data could be done by year rather than by quinquennieum. I so clearly remember Dr. Tabar disdaining to meld his data with data from other inferior trials. I so clearly remember the trialist beside me saying: If the women who participated in all the screening trials heard this they would be outraged.
>
> Additionally I remain sceptical about the amazing muddle of crucial numbers in his trial outcomes should not require such interminable exegesis. And when it comes to determining outcomes such as deaths from breast cancer, regrettably I just cannot be persuaded to give more credence to decisions by selected specialists compared to data from Cancer and Death Registries.
>
> But then I have had occasion to disagree with much Dr. Tabar has to say about screening evidence.

What the *BMJ* published was this:[8]

> I remain skeptical about the amazing muddle of crucial numbers (participants and breast cancer deaths) in the Two-County trial that should not require interminable exegesis 24 years after the trial results were first published in 1985. And when it comes to validating causes of death, I just cannot be persuaded to lend more credence to decisions by selected 'specialists' compared to data from Cancer and Death Registries.

It is unacceptable that threats of libel can be used to prevent inconvenient truths to be published. This is not in the best interest of science, and not in the best interest of the patients and citizens, whom we all are expected to serve the best we can. Zahl and colleagues[9] reported in 2001 that when they found that the tumour data in the Two-County trial were inconsistent, their requests for access to the data were refused.

I believe the *BMJ* acted in a rational fashion in an irrational, absurd and unjust system. The archaic UK libel laws protect perpetrators and punish whistle-blowers; they stifle the academic debate and may intimidate scientific writers into not writing what they know are facts. In 2008, Simon Singh wrote in the *Guardian*:[10]

> You might think that modern chiropractors restrict themselves to treating back problems, but in fact they still possess some quite wacky ideas. The fundamentalists argue that they can cure anything. And even the more moderate chiropractors have ideas above their station. The British Chiropractic Association claims that their members can help treat children with colic, sleeping and feeding problems, frequent ear infections, asthma and prolonged crying, even though there is not a jot of evidence. This organisation is the respectable face of the chiropractic profession and yet it happily promotes bogus treatments.

That seems a pretty fair comment to me, reflecting the facts, but Singh was sued for libel by the British Chiropractic Association. The judge held that using the phrase 'happily promotes bogus treatments' meant that Singh was stating, as a matter of fact, that the association was being consciously dishonest in promoting chiropractic for treating the children's ailments in question.

That was an awfully bad judgement and, fortunately, the Court of Appeal overruled it, saying that Singh's staments were fair comment. In its decisions,[11] the court said that it would respectfully adopt what Judge Easterbrook, now chief judge of the US Seventh Circuit Court of Appeals, said in a libel action over a scientific controversy in 1994:

> [Plaintiffs] cannot, by simply filing suit and crying 'character assassination!', silence those who hold divergent views, no matter how adverse those views may be to plaintiffs' interests. Scientific controversies must be settled by the methods of science rather than by the methods of litigation. . . . More papers, more discussion, better data, and more satisfactory models – not larger awards of damages – mark the path towards superior understanding of the world around us.

The charity Sense About Science launched a campaign to draw attention to Singh's case. It issued a statement entitled 'The English law of libel has no place in scientific disputes about evidence'. The campaign drew more than 50 000 signatures from all over the world and it worked. Prior to general elections in 2010, all three major political parties in the United Kingdom declared they were committed to libel law reform. This will hopefully put an end to libel tourism, with exorbitant fees to lawyers, which is not something for a country to be proud of. Simon Singh wrote that a survey found that fighting actions in London cost 140 times the average of the rest of Europe.[12] It is not a printing error. *One hundred and forty times!* Singh mentioned that the United Nations had condemned the judges' practice of welcoming rich libel tourists from across the world to their hospitable courts and urged Britain to allow free speech on matters of public interest. The US Congress has now passed a law that guarantees that English libel judgements have no validity in America.

In May 2010, Lord Lester published a Private Members' Defamation Bill to reform the laws, which includes a statutory defence for responsible publication on a matter of public interest, and which will also:

- require claimants to provide evidence their reputation was damaged by an alleged libel before they can bring a case forward and make corporations prove financial damage before they can sue.
- address the problems introduced by the rise of the Internet and the culture of online publication, including the multiple publication rule that makes each download a fresh instance of libel, and alter the responsibility of forum hosts for what is posted on their sites.
- encourage the speedy settlement of disputes without parties having to bring in costly lawyers.
- promote the speedy settlement of disputes without recourse to the courts.

Screening advocates have threatened litigation several times before, but people are reluctant to talk about it. They seem to be afraid of the deep pockets of some of those who earn a living from mammography screening. I have mentioned above the threat against the *European Journal of Cancer*, which caused the editor to commit editorial misconduct by retracting our published paper (*see* Chapter 13).

I consider it intellectual bankruptcy when a researcher whose work is being criticised hires lawyers. It is anti-science. I could have filed many libel suits, and indeed for very good reasons, but I prefer to fight with the pen. This is what science is about, and free debates advance science.

References

1 Peter Wilmshurst. The effects of the libel laws on science: a personal experience. *Radical Statistics*. 2011; (104): 13–23.

2 Jørgensen KJ, Gøtzsche PC. Mammography screening hasn't lived up to expectations. *BMJ*. 2010 Apr 15. Available at: www.bmj.com/cgi/eletters/340/mar23_1/c1241 (accessed 22 May 2011).

3 Duffy SW, Tabár L, Olsen AH, *et al*. Cancer mortality in the 50–69 year age group before and after screening. *J Med Screen*. 2010; **17**: 159–60.

4 Holmberg L, Duffy SW, Yen AM, *et al*. Differences in endpoints between the Swedish W-E (two county) trial of mammographic screening and the Swedish overview: methodological consequences. *J Med Screen*. 2009; **16**(2): 73–80.

5 Nyström L, Andersson I, Bjurstam N, *et al*. Long-term effects of mammography screening: updated overview of the Swedish randomised trials. *Lancet*. 2002; **359**(9310): 909–19.

6 Tabár LK. To individuals with an interest in breast cancer screening. *BMJ*. 2010 Jun 29. Available at: www.bmj.com/cgi/eletters/340/mar23_1/c1241 (accessed 22 May 2011).

7 Duffy SW. Response to: 'Should we screen for breast cancer' by Klim McPherson. *BMJ*. 2010 Sep 9. Available at: www.bmj.com/content/340/bmj.c3106.extract/reply#bmj_el_241378 (accessed 22 May 2011).

8 Baines CJ. Comment. *BMJ*. 2010 Jul 21. Available at: www.bmj.com/cgi/eletters/340/mar23_1/c1241 (accessed 21 July 2010).

9 Zahl P, Kopjar B, Mæhlen J. [Mammography trials] [Norwegian]. *Tidsskr Nor Lægeforen*. 2001; 121: 2636.

10 Wikipedia. *Simon Singh*. Available at: http://en.wikipedia.org/wiki/Simon_Singh (accessed 17 June 2010).

11 British and Irish Legal Information Institute. *England and Wales Court of Appeal (Civil Division) Decisions*. Available at: www.bailii.org/ew/cases/EWCA/Civ/2010/350.html (accessed 17 June 2010).

12 Singh S. BCA v Singh: the story so far. *Sense About Science*. 2009 Jun 3. Available at: www.senseaboutscience.org/pages/bca-v-singh-the-story-so-far-3-june-2009.html (accessed 7 June 2009).

22

Falsehoods and perceived censorship in Sweden

THE NORDIC COCHRANE CENTRE'S 2009 *BMJ* PAPERS ON THE UK screening leaflet and on overdiagnosis elicited reactions also in Sweden. But very sad ones. Our opponents had nothing to offer other than distasteful personal attacks, which began with the first title, 'Scare campaign about mammography'.[1] The title suggested that our motives were to scare women from attending screening, but the authors, oncologist Sven Törnberg and epidemiologist Lennart Nyström, couldn't know of course what our motives were. Our aim is to get as close to the truth as we can. And the truth is the opposite of what the title implies: women have been scared into getting screened.[2]

Törnberg and Nyström were not reluctant to reveal their own motives. They considered it frivolous to publish scare campaigns, which reduce confidence in healthcare and attendance to screening. We have not published a scare campaign, and we argued that it is shocking for a country guarding the rights and autonomy of its women in a tradition that goes back to the Vikings that its women are deprived of access to the information they need to make their own decision.[2] We also encouraged the women to read our leaflet, which exists in Swedish (*see* www.cochrane.dk and Appendix 2).

As usual with screening advocates, Törnberg and Nyström manipulated numbers. They used the relative risk for benefit so that it looked big (30% reduction in breast cancer mortality) and absolute risk for overdiagnosis so that it looked small (0.1%, which is wrong by a factor of 5, since, according to the trials, there is not one but five overdiagnosed women per 1000). The semantics was also misleading, as they described overdiagnosis as a 'negative side effect'. This term could also be used about temporary itching after a drug. They even argued it is a scare campaign when we talk about harms and also call them harms, which we are obliged to do according to the CONSORT guidelines for good reporting of randomised trials.[3]

Törnberg and Nyström also spread doubt about what overdiagnosis is and asked how one should distinguish between a cancer that is overdiagnosed and one that is not. This is sheer nonsense. The very problem with overdiagnosis is that this is *not* possible, which is why all detected cancers are treated! Finally, they mentioned the misleading 10% estimate of overdiagnosis from the extended follow-up of the Malmö trial.

As always, when you show your opponents wrong, their style deteriorates. The title of their second letter was: 'Is anxiety related to the investigation worse than premature death from breast cancer?'[4] We have never contrasted these two effects, and we showed in our title what Törnberg and Nyström had denied: 'Overdiagnosis with mammography screening is a serious problem'.[5] Törnberg and Nyström's *ad hominem* attacks were unscrupulous and untruthful. They claimed we didn't share their view that the problem was that women died prematurely from breast cancer. Of course this is a problem, but it is also a problem that healthy women women get treated for a disease they don't have.

They continued to ascribe views to us that we have never had nor expressed. Their paper ran to just over one page. I haven't seen so many untrue statements in so little space before. Here are seven examples:

1. We are unscientific or have deliberately misled the readers with false numbers.
2. We have clearly forgotten how we once calculated (we calculate in the same way each time, don't forget, and document our calculations).
3. 'In our extrapolations . . .' (there are no extrapolations anywhere).
4. Our goal is clearly not to be objective (it is to give the women honest information).
5. Clearly, our aim is to scare women into not attending screening, which we also admit in the rest of our article (we do not have such an aim and have not admitted this).
6. Our prior belief (no prior belief; we are researchers and rely on evidence).
7. We have called all incidence increase for overdiagnosis and would not accept that there are several causes for incidence increases (quite the contrary, we have discussed this at length in our papers).

Törnberg and Nyström argued that our estimate on overdiagnosis is not 'theoretically possible', but it is not theory, it is empirical data. They manipulated numbers again, exactly as in their first paper, by estimating the number of overdiagnosed women for only one screening round, while they noted the effect on mortality after several rounds. This is like complaining about paying too much income tax by totalling the tax over 10 years, but the income over just 1 year.

We were also disappointed by the way we were being treated by the journal's editor-in-chief, Jan Lind. We were not aware of Törnberg and Nyström's first article, but after Swedish colleagues had informed us about it, we submitted an unsolicited reply. We wrote to Jan Lind that if he allowed Törnberg and Nyström to reply in the same issue, we would like to get the same opportunity, to reply to their reply also in the same issue, as we had not had this opportunity when they published their first article, although it contained *ad hominem* attacks.

When we submitted a revised, shorter version, we reminded Jan Lind of our request. As he didn't say anything about our request in his replies, we interpreted it as acceptance. We usually trust people who don't have conflicts of interest and couldn't imagine what was in store for us. Lind later sent us Törnberg and Nyström's second article 'for information'. Although we believed it was full of lies, Lind noted that it was the final comment and that no more debate would be accepted.

We were very distressed by this, which we interpreted as undue censorship that denied us the possibility of defending our reputation. We wrote to Lind that his position was unacceptable for many reasons that we outlined. We also noted that Lind and I were colleagues and that I had raised issues about publication ethics and conflicts of interest in my capacity as editor on the listserve of the World Association of Medical Editors on several occasions due to my interest in these subjects. I gave compelling reasons why he should publish our reply and remarked that there had been far too little debate about mammography screening in Sweden. Lind should therefore take the opportunity, in particular as the much-needed debate was ongoing elsewhere, e.g. in *JAMA*,[6] and as the *Läkartidningen* should not contribute to stopping it in Sweden.

I also explained that I had received many email messages after our first comment from Swedish doctors who were very happy that, finally, there would be a debate in Sweden, and I quoted one of them:

> 'A big THANKS for your achievements in this matter, which for so long has been completely impossible to lift the tiniest bit here in Sweden. For my own part, I have not had enough knowledge to be able to say or do anything, but I will now write to the Board of Health and attach your papers, the information leaflet and the article from JAMA in order to press the need for a change in the invitation to screening.'

I also quoted an email from a Norwegian colleague:

> 'You address an interesting phenomenon: Why is Sweden a country with so much (self)censorship and political correctness? I do not have a good answer to this, but can report that my colleague [name removed by me] also travelled and worked in Sweden at the same time as Peter [Peter Gøtzsche] (in the beginning of the 1970s). He went there as a social democrat with left-radical views, but came back as a right-winger (a very thoughtful and humanistic one). He has explained this shift with his experience of a lack of freedom of thought, the self-inflicted correctness, which was so oppressive that he "converted". The Swedish foreign minister once said that Norway was the last Sovjet state. I think several of us compete for such a status! I hope that the reply you have written to TN [Törnberg and Nyström] will be published. Anything else would be completely unacceptable.'

My letter to Lind worked. It would have been difficult for him to deny us a reply, and he might have guessed we didn't intend to let him off the hook. Journals have owners and editors should be held accountable for their actions, just as they hold authors accountable for theirs.

But one question remains. Why do Swedish screening advocates react so violently? Is it because mammography screening is seen as a national treasure and an object of national pride, something Sweden has given to the world, like Volvo, Saab and ABBA? Maybe it is.

Inger Atterstam, from the major Swedish newspaper *Svenska Dagbladet*, described her experiences with freedom of speech in 2001.[7] For 20 years, it had not been possible to have a decent intellectual discussion about positive and negative aspects of mammography screening. Any criticism had been aggressively and emotionally condemned with accusations of the most awful motives and of irresponsible and unscientific behaviour. Despite this, there had been constant rumours about mistakes and flaws in the trials, particularly the one done in Kopparberg. Atterstam had looked at publications from this trial and was upset because of the many obvious violations of established scientific method. She wrote about it, but met hysterical reactions, including personal accusations and persecution. She also remarked that there was a strange anti-intellectual lack of open discussion, and that screening had been presented to the women as a solution to the whole breast cancer tragedy, which was very dishonest. The main comment from the screening advocates had been that she harmed the patients. This was the eternal mantra from the screening defenders. But despite all the intimidations, she had actually met more reactions of gratitude for having the courage to speak up.

The Nestor of Swedish medicine, Professor Lars Werkö, also noted that it was difficult, if not impossible, to have a reasoned debate in Sweden about mammography screening and that the space for critical opinion was minimal.[8]

Screening advocates often give the impression that they have some sort of higher moral authority, because they act on behalf of the women and for their benefit. I believe a Swedish journalist hit the nail on the head when she said: Women prefer people who speak the truth, even when the truth is uncomfortable. Just as men do.

References

1 Törnberg S, Nyström L. [Scaremongering propaganda and mammography] [Swedish]. *Läkartidningen*. 2009; **106**(42): 2664–5.

2 Gøtzsche PC, Jørgensen KJ. [Honest information about mammography screening, please!] [Swedish]. *Läkartidningen*. 2009; **106**(44): 2860–1.

3 Ioannidis JP, Evans SJ, Gøtzsche PC, *et al*. Better reporting of harms in randomized trials: an extension of the CONSORT statement. *Ann Intern Med*. 2004; **141**(10): 781–8.

4 Törnberg S, Nyström L. [Is anxiety related to the investigation worse than premature death from breast cancer?] [Swedish]. *Läkartidningen*. 2009; **106**(45): 3018.

5 Gøtzsche PC, Jørgensen KJ. [Overdiagnosis in mammographic screening is a serious problem] [Swedish]. *Läkartidningen*. 2009; **106**(47): 3180.

6 Esserman L, Shieh Y, Thompson I. Rethinking screening for breast cancer and prostate cancer. *JAMA*. 2009; **302**(15): 1685–92.

7 Atterstam I. Not everyone loves a critical medical journalist. *Nordic Evidence-Based Health Care Newsletter*. 2001; **5**. Available at: www.folkehelsa.no/dok/rapporter/ebhc.html (accessed 15 January 2002).

8 Atterstam I. [Mammography receives severe criticism] [Swedish]. *Svenska Dagbladet*. 2000 Jul 20: 1, 4.

23

Celebrating 20 years of breast screening in the United Kingdom

It is only totalitarian governments that suppress facts. In this country we simply take a democratic decision not to publish them.

Yes Minister (BBC series)

REPORTS FROM THE NHS BREAST SCREENING PROGRAMME ARE NOT scientific papers but glorifications of own achievements that steam with political correctness. The Nordic Cochrane Centre had therefore not paid much attention to them over the years, but when the Annual Review from 2008 celebrated the programme's 20th birthday,[1] we made an exception. It was published by the Department of Health and was a fascinating read, as it so clearly shows – albeit unintentionally – what the main problems are with screening and the way it is being touted to the public. We dissected the review and exposed its innards in January 2010 in the *Journal of the Royal Society of Medicine*.[2]

Twenty years is a long time. One would therefore expect to see data – or at least a reference to such data – demonstrating to which degree screening had lowered breast cancer mortality in the United Kingdom. One would also expect to see a comparison of this benefit with a quantification of the most important harms, as this would allow politicians and others to judge for themselves whether the programme was worth its large cost.

However, this is not what the 26-page review does, although it should have been easy to demonstrate the expected 30% reduction in breast cancer mortality, which was the basis for the introduction of the screening programme. The review celebrates the anniversary, calls it a 'momentous occasion', exaggerates the benefit, omits the harms, and looks like propaganda aimed at persuasion, wrapped in a beautiful layout that would pride any marketing department if it had been a sales brochure for a drug. The first words on the cover page are 'Saving lives through screening', and the symbolism is strong with a picture of a delicate rose in the distinctive pink colour that has become iconic for the fight against breast cancer (*see* Figure 23.1). The rose is transparent, symbolising the scientific illumination and radiological technique through which the programme operates.

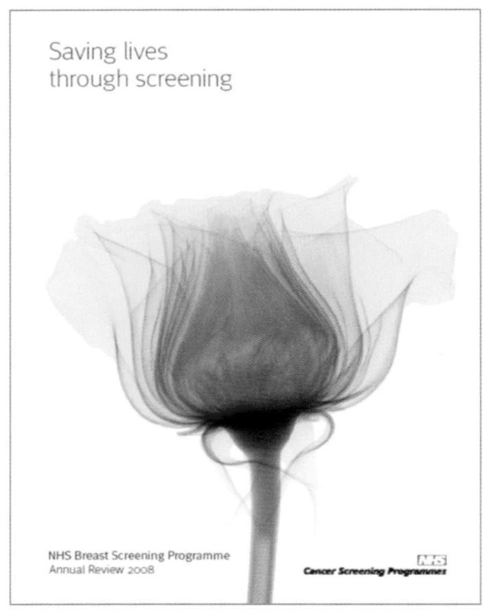

FIGURE 23.1 The cover page from the NHS Breast Screening Programme Annual Review 2008

The report states that the 'NHS Breast Screening Programme is now estimated to save 1400 lives each year.' As already noted, this message pops up as a knee-jerk reaction in the media whenever the programme's scientific or ethical basis is criticised. The 1400 lives saved are called a 'key fact', and one would therefore think it had a scientific basis, but we were unable to find any despite intensive detective work backwards in time. The reference offered in its support is to another NHS report, which states that 'the totality of the evidence from randomised trials shows that regular mammographic screening commencing at ages 50–69 years reduces mortality from breast cancer by about 35%'.[3] There is no explanation in the report how the 35% estimate was derived either, but it states elsewhere that breast cancer mortality is reduced 'from 8.0 to 5.2 per 1000 women in the target age range if they are regularly screened over a 10-year period'. The origin of these rates is also obscure, but the reduction equates to 35%.

If this were a crime case, I think the police detective would be convinced that the suspects were deliberately concealing essential evidence. As I have explained in earlier chapters, it is impossible to save three women (8.0 – 5.2 is about three) out of 1000 from dying from breast cancer through 10 years of screening.

The programme cannot have saved anywhere near 1400 lives each year. There were only 3500 annual deaths from breast cancer in the relevant age range in 2003, and the study by Blanks and colleagues[4] that was published in the *BMJ* in 2000 credited screening for only a 6% reduction in breast cancer mortality in England and Wales. *These authors estimated that the number of lives saved was 320.*

In 2002, the programme's website noted that at least 300 lives are saved per year, with reference to Blanks's study.[5] But the next sentence read: 'That figure is set to rise to 1,250 by 2010.' Set to rise? By whom? Julietta Patnick? There was no explanation how this miracle would be achieved. The next sentence was even more astonishing. Screening, improved treatment and other factors 'could result in a halving of the breast cancer death rate in women aged 55–69 from that seen in 1990'. The reference to this statement in the reference list was: 'Dr Roger Blanks, The Institute of Cancer Research'. Having passed 2010, we know that Blanks's look into the crystal ball hasn't come true. Few scientists would be willing to multiply their result by a factor of 4 (320 times 4 is 1280) by looking into the future, and I wonder what pressure was put on Blanks to come up with such a rosy prophecy that provided a fig leaf for the Department of Health to carry on with the programme, rather than to pause and think.

Elsewhere in the material I downloaded from the programme's website in 2002, the prophecy of 1250 lives saved in 2010 had already come true – overnight, it seemed. Julietta Patnick declared, 'We estimate that screening is now saving on average 1250 lives a year. On October 31st 2001, we will publish the NHS Breast Screening Programme's annual review.' That was only 1 year after Blanks's estimate of 320 lives! If this isn't dishonest, I don't know what it is.

'Screening saves lives' is an emotive and very efficient way to promote screening, but screening cannot save anyone from dying, only prolong life, at best. Furthermore, the claim assumes that one can equate avoided breast cancer deaths with saved lives, and this is also wrong. Screening kills healthy women through overdiagnosis and overtreatment.

Unsurprisingly, overdiagnosis and overtreatment were not mentioned in the glossy report. We estimated about 7000 unnecessary breast cancer diagnoses per year in the United Kingdom in the invited age group.[2] The review not only ignores this harm, it converts it into something positive:

> A huge number of breast cancers, over 100,000, have been detected since 1988, highlighting the importance of the screening programme in the early detection of breast cancer in England.

It cannot be the purpose of screening to detect many cancers. In fact, screening detects *far too many* cancers. This is an example of 'the popularity paradox'. The more harm through overdiagnosis, the more efficient screening is described to be, and the more people will think screening saved their life.[6]

The other major harm of screening, the false positive findings, wasn't mentioned either. We calculated that about 70 000 women experience a false positive recall every year in the United Kingdom.[2] The report downplayed this risk by describing it for a single screening session and not as the accumulated risk over 20 years of screening, which is about 20% in the United Kingdom.[7]

Other essential information was also concealed. Biopsies, for example, can be either needle biopsies or surgical excisions (which are much worse, as they remove the whole lesion from the breast), but the review is not specific about this. Again, we had to do detective work and found out from another report that 3% of those recalled will have a surgical excision. *Based on that information, we deduced that what the report – with a euphemism that downplays this harm – lists as 1676 'benign biopsies' must be 1676 surgical excisions.* We believe that, although a lesion may look benign for the pathologist, it is not benign for the woman who undergoes a surgical excision on a false suspicion of cancer. This harm was further downplayed as affecting 0.1% of those screened per year. For comparison, we calculated that the exaggerated mortality benefit mentioned in the review also amounts to 0.1% of those screened, but in this case over 10 years.

The number of needle biopsies wasn't presented either, but we calculated from the report that 28 000 unnecessary needle biopsies are made per year.

It is far worse than needle biopsies or surgical excisions to lose a whole breast because of overdiagnosis. The report presented no data on the absolute number of mastectomies, although this number increased by 36% for invasive cancer and by 422% for carcinoma *in situ* from 1990 to 2001 in the United Kingdom.[8]

The review also contained misleading survival statistics. A quote from Stephen Duffy is highlighted in the review: 'The 10-year fatality of screen-detected tumours is 50% lower than that of symptomatic tumours.' This headline comes with no caveats, although such information is extremely misleading. This was recognised already in the Forrest report in 1986 that paved the way for screening in the United Kingdom, and it is also mentioned in the book on screening by Angela Raffle and Muir Gray:[6]

> The kind of people who come for screening, and the kind of disease that is easy to find with screening, add up to a highly selected group with regard to both the overall health and longevity of the individuals and to the benign natural course of the uncovered pathology. The combined effect is a very favourable prognosis. Outcomes in screened people will therefore be very good, whether or not screening makes a difference.

The review from the NHS Breast Cancer Screening Programme was edited by its director, Julietta Patnick. It is embarrassing if Duffy and Patnick, in their positions as professors working with screening, were not aware of this fundamental bias, and even worse if they were aware of it but misled their readers by being quiet about it.

In the opening statement of the review, its authors 'look forward to the future developments that will deliver even greater benefits to thousands of women in the years to come.' This marketing speak is wrong. It says nothing about the thousands of women that will be harmed. Furthermore, because of improvements in therapy we will likely see *fewer* benefits of screening in future, not more. Increased sensitivity will lead to more overdiagnosis,[9] and the balance between benefit and harms will become less favourable by the extension of the programme to include women aged 47–73 years, as announced in the review.

Digital mammography was described as being the best technology for detecting abnormalities in the breast tissue of premenopausal women, but there are no randomised trials of this screening tool, which could lead to more false positives, more biopsies and more overdiagnosis. It is impressive that '£100m will be invested in digital mammography equipment in 2008' when so little is known about it.

The review is full of old-fashioned 'don't-ask questions', paternalism and a patronising attitude to the women. For example,

> The aim is to increase the level of invitation acceptance in target populations, by continuing to support women to make the right choice for them.

This aim goes directly against a decision in the National Screening Committee that 'the purpose of information about screening is to allow individuals to make an informed choice about whether to participate.'[6] Julietta Patnick writes she is worried that the attendance at screening has decreased slightly, but this may simply indicate that more women are making informed choices because of the public debate and despite the attempts by Patnick and her colleagues to decide for the women what is 'the right choice for them'.

A statement that the NHS should provide material that allows the decision to be 'based on balanced factual information', is what Frankfurt would have called 'bullshit!'[10] The review furthermore sells screening with an old marketing trick, the loyal and satisfied customer. This is an effective sales strategy, as few would wish to be a non-preferred customer. I once checked in at a Sheraton hotel in the United States and described myself as one of those customers the hotel would rather not like to see. Amazed, the clerk asked me what I meant by this. I pointed at a huge signboard that hung over the desk next to me that said 'Preferred customers', and I explained that since I had no platinum card, or whatever passport was needed to differentiate between the Chosen People and the rest of us, I must be a non-preferred customer.

A happy and faithful customer named Dorothy Adams said: 'I know how important it is to have regular checks and to make sure you accept your invitations or make your appointment', and she had even continued to request screening beyond the invited age range (and beyond what is supported by evidence). We are told that 'Women like Dorothy . . . have attended without fail for decades', which means that not accepting the invitation is a failure, like being a non-preferred customer. The omission of Dorothy's surname is another marketing trick that conveys a sense of familiarity and a sense of belonging to the regular customers' executive club. We are also told that, 'now a grandmother, Dorothy is passing on her knowledge and experience to her daughter and granddaughter to help them make decisions about screening when the time comes.' When the time comes. Sounds like picking the right husband. Not a trace of doubt about what the 'right' decision will be for Dorothy's offspring.

I came to think of a popular type of advertising that runs somewhat like this: 'Fifty thousand happy customers cannot be wrong.' Oh yes, they can: when the customers don't know what they are doing and why and no one wants to tell them.

Unlike Sheraton hotels, where the directors can be held personally accountable for shortcomings and omissions in their annual report to tax authorities and shareholders, it is unclear who is accountable for an annual review of a public health programme where the costs are much greater than just monetary.

The media took an interest in our critique of the report, and Thornton's prediction that those who selectively present inadequate evidence to support a belief will ultimately lose the trust of the public at large[11] came true, as the responses and comments to pieces in the press and on blogs showed there was a considerable loss of trust in the programme.

David Rose from *The Times* reported that thousands of women are wrongly told that they have life-threatening cancer and undergo unnecessary treatment each year.[12] He also wrote that doctors warned that continuing disputes over the value of breast screening could cause confusion among women and could lead to dangerous diseases being missed. I wonder whether we will ever get rid of the unsolicited paternalism and 'doctors know best' when the issue is cancer screening.

Margaret McCartney from the *Financial Times* felt we deserved a medal because we have published, unwaveringly over the years, what our research has shown.[13] She also noted that the problem with breast screening is that it seems to contain an enormous amount of emotional investment, and that the only parallel she could think of was alternative medicine.

Another female journalist, Zoe Williams from the *Guardian*, found it fascinating to get insight into the grey areas of screening and surprising that people whose intent is good could be so much at odds with one another.[14] She ended on an amusing note: 'Out of respect for their collected expertise, I'm going to have one breast screened, and the other left alone. It'll be my very own randomised control trial.' Less amusingly, she quoted Stephen Duffy for saying that our data points were misleading, although the mortality graphs we had published for the United Kingdom speak for themselves (*see* Chapter 15); it is not necessary to select any data points to see this. More disturbingly, Duffy referred to his own analysis and is quoted as saying: 'It's a shame my paper isn't published till March', and he added that the mortality went down in the screened ages 28% more than all other ages combined.

Williams explained that Duffy's paper would be peer-reviewed in due course, but there are three problems. First, how can a paper be accepted, with a publication date, *before* it has been peer-reviewed? Perhaps because it was published in the favourite journal of screening lovers, the *Journal of Medical Screening*. Second, it is regarded as deplorable for a scientist to publish his results in the press before they have been peer-reviewed and published in a scientific journal. Third, the paper is flawed to an incomprehensible degree (*see* Chapter 20, Extraordinary exaggerations).

Duffy had another surprising remark:[14] 'When you're a child, you don't want an injection to protect you from this or that disease. That bit of discomfort can sometimes be worthwhile.' It is shocking that Duffy likens the serious harms that result from screening to the discomfort of an injection. Furthermore, vaccinations are used to prevent disease from occurring. Screening doesn't prevent breast cancer from occurring; it detects it, and it detects too much of it. In a way, one could therefore say that screening *causes* breast cancer. To compare that with vaccination is far out.

Patnick's remark was also surprising:[14] 'I know it's not for everybody. We all make decisions that would run contrary to good advice all the time, that's part of the richness of human life.' So, it's part of the richness of human life that some women are so stupid that they decide not to attend screening, contrary to the good advice offered by Patnick and her colleagues.

The 2009 report from the NHS Breast Screening Programme is equally dishonest as the 2008 anniversary report we dissected.[15] It says on the first page:

> Recent statistics show that the number of women in the UK dying from breast cancer has fallen to its lowest level in almost 40 years. This decline in breast cancer mortality rates is proof of the real improvements in our cancer services and a tribute to the continued progress made by the NHS Breast Cancer Screening Programme.

The reference to this is to official mortality statistics, but these statistics tell you that there is *no visible effect of the screening programme* (*see* Figure 19.5).[16] Nonetheless, the programme extended its invitations to women aged 47 to 49 and a named woman appeared as a happy customer who had her cancer detected when she was 48. This happy customer will never know if she had all the reason in the world to be unhappy because her cancer was overdiagnosed!

The 2009 report quoted our two recent papers about the UK screening leaflet and overdiagnosis:[17,18]

> The NHS Breast Screening Programme has strongly rebutted the claims made by Gøtzsche, believing his papers to be highly selective in the statistics used.

This sentence is shameless. The programme (which really means Stephen Duffy, I suspect) hasn't rebutted our findings, we are not selective but systematic in our research and the facts we have communicated are there to see for everyone. They don't go away by shooting the messenger, and statistics are not needed to see that our 'claim' about substantial overdiagnosis is correct.

The misleading information continued unabated: 'Survival rates for all screen-detected cancers are still 85% at 15 years and the screening programme has proved vital in saving thousands of women's lives.'

There is one interesting piece of information in this 2009 report, though: 'Just over a quarter of women diagnosed with invasive breast cancer receive a mastectomy, while the figure is slightly higher for *in situ* and micro-invasive disease.' Considering an overdiagnosis of about 50% that also involves many invasive cancers,[18] this comes close to an admission by the programme that screening leads to a substantial increase in mastectomies. It is a shame, then, that the report wasn't more transparent and showed the trend for mastectomies over time, starting before screening was introduced in 1988.

References

1 Patnick J, editor. *Saving Lives through Screening: Breast Screening Programme; annual review 2008*. Available at: www.cancerscreening.nhs.uk/breastscreen/publications/2008review.html (accessed 4 March 2009).

2 Jørgensen KJ, Gøtzsche PC. Who evaluates public health programmes? A review of the NHS Breast Screening Programme. *J R Soc Med*. 2010; **103**(1): 14–20.

3 Advisory Committee on Breast Cancer Screening. *Screening for Breast Cancer in England: past and future*. February 2006. Available at: www.cancerscreening.nhs.uk/breastscreen/publications/nhsbsp61.pdf (accessed 4 March 2009).

4 Blanks RG, Moss SM, McGahan CE, *et al*. Effect of NHS Breast Screening Programme on mortality from breast cancer in England and Wales, 1990–98: comparison of observed with predicted mortality. *BMJ*. 2000; **321**(7262): 665–9.

5 NHS Breast Screening Programme. *Does Breast Screening Save Lives?* Available at: www.cancerscreening.nhs.uk/breastscreen/index.html (accessed 2 October 2002).

6 Raffle A, Gray M. *Screening: evidence and practice*. Oxford: Oxford University Press; 2007.

7 Smith-Bindman R, Ballard-Barbash R, Miglioretti DL, *et al*. Comparing the performance of mammography screening in the USA and the UK. *J Med Screen*. 2005; **12**(1): 50–4.

8 Douek M, Baum M. Mass breast screening: is there a hidden cost? *Br J Surg*. 2003; **90**(Suppl. 1): (Abstract Breast 14).

9 Morrell S, Barratt A, Irwig L, *et al*. Estimates of overdiagnosis of invasive breast cancer associated with screening mammography. *Cancer Causes Control*. 2010; **21**(2): 275–82.

10 Frankfurt H. *On Bullshit*. Princeton, NJ: Princeton University Press; 2005.

11 Thornton H. Inappropriate use of evidence? *BMJ*. 2002 Aug 24. Available at: http://bmj.com/cgi/eletters/325/7361/418#24972 (accessed 22 May 2011).

12 Rose D. Benefits of breast screening 'are a myth'. *The Times*. 2010 Jan 19.

13 McCartney M. Effectiveness of breast screening requires more objective analysis. *Financial Times*. 2010. Available at: http://blogs.ft.com/healthblog/2010/01/18/effectiveness-of-breast-screening-requires-more-objective-analysis (accessed 22 May 2011).

14 Williams Z. Memo to medics: it's about emotions as well as tumours. *Guardian*. 2010 Jan 20. Available at: www.guardian.co.uk/commentisfree/2010/jan/20/emotions-tumours-breast-cancer-screening (accessed 22 May 2011).

15 Patnick J, editor. *Expanding Our Reach: NHS Breast Screening Programme: annual review 2009*. Available at: www.cancerscreening.nhs.uk/breastscreen/publications/nhsbsp-annualreview2009.pdf (accessed 22 May 2011).

16 Jørgensen KJ, Brodersen J, Nielsen M, *et al*. Fall in breast cancer deaths: a cause for celebration, and caution. *BMJ*. 2009; **338**: b2126.

17 Gøtzsche P, Hartling OJ, Nielsen M, *et al*. Breast screening: the facts – or maybe not. *BMJ*. 2009; **338**: 446–8.

18 Jørgensen KJ, Gøtzsche PC. Overdiagnosis in publicly organised mammography screening programmes: systematic review of incidence trends. *BMJ*. 2009; **339**: b2587.

24

Can screening work?

When medical scientists disagree about the effectiveness of an intervention, it almost always means that whatever effect may be present is small.

Suzanne Fletcher[1]

Plausible effect based on tumour sizes in the trials

Breast cancer is a heterogeneous disease, with widely varying growth rates and metastatic potential. The growth rate for the individual cancer is usually constant for long periods of time, and can therefore be described as the doubling time, which is the time it takes to double the number of malignant cells. The range of doubling times for breast cancers is very large. A big study from Heidelberg found that 95% of the doubling times were between 65 and 627 days.[2] An even bigger US study estimated that 90% of the doubling times were between 69 and 1622 days.[3] It complicates the issue, though, that spontaneous death of cancer cells is common and may increase with tumour size.[4] This means that the growth rate may decrease, which is often seen when the cancer becomes large. The growth may also stop altogether,[3] and many screen-detected breast cancers are harmless, as their normal fate is to regress and disappear (*see* Chapters 2 and 16).

If we assume that the observed doubling times are valid until the tumour becomes detectable, it means that the average woman has harboured the cancer for 21 years before it acquires a size of 10 mm, which is when it becomes detectable at breast screening.[3] Further, screening is more likely to pick up slow-growing tumours (length bias), i.e. those that are oldest. Therefore, it is misleading to say that cancers are caught 'early' with screening. They are caught very late, even though our assumption was too simple, as cancers likely grow faster in the beginning.

Fortunately, it isn't necessary to know much about the intricacies of tumour biology in order to understand whether screening can work and what a plausible effect might be. The easiest way to take us there is to look at the randomised trials to see how big the cancers were, on average, in the group invited to screening and in the control group.

That is what I did and I tabulated all the data I could find.[4] There are useful data on tumour size from five trials (Table 24.1):[5–8]

TABLE 24.1 Average size of invasive breast cancers in the randomised trials

Trial	Invited group (mm)	Control group (mm)
Canadian trials	16	19
Malmö trial	14	19
Stockholm trial	14	19
Two-County trial	18	25
Mean of all trials	*16*	*21*

These data refer to invasive cancers (I shall discuss carcinoma *in situ* shortly). The average tumour size was 16 mm in the screened groups and 21 mm in the control groups. Using the formula for the volume of a sphere, we can see that a cancer of 16 mm will grow to 20 mm after only one more cell division. The window of opportunity for mammography screening to work is therefore about one cell division, after the malignant cells have already divided more than 30 times. For mammography screening to have more than a marginal effect, quite a few cancers would need to metastasise in this little time window.

This isn't plausible and it doesn't happen. Some cancers never metastasise, and some grow so slowly that it doesn't matter that they would ultimately have metastasised, as the women would have long been dead from other causes. Most importantly, many cancers metastasise early, before they can be detected on a mammogram. A German study of 12 423 patients found a linear correlation between tumour size and the existence of one or more positive lymph nodes,[9] and I calculated that tumours with a diameter of 16 mm have metastasised in 35% of the cases. This is a conservative estimate, as many metastases are overlooked. For example, a US study of 24 740 cases showed that nearly 25% of the node-negative patients eventually develop distant metastasis.[10]

As screening is supposed to work by detecting cancers before they have metastasised, we can convert the tumour sizes into an expected effect of screening. The German study showed that tumours of sizes 16 and 21 mm are node-positive in 35% and 42% of cases, respectively, whereas the US study showed a difference of only 4% in node-positive tumours for a size difference of 5 mm. The weighted average of the two studies is 5%. If we assume for simplicity that all patients with metastases will die from breast cancer, and those without will not, the expected effect of screening is a relative risk of (42% – 5%)/42% = 0.88, or a 12% reduction in breast cancer mortality.

> *This is very close to what the most reliable trials have shown. After 13 years, these trials showed a 10% reduction in breast cancer mortality.*[11]

This is reassuring, considering that the tumour size difference of 5 mm has been somewhat overestimated because of overdiagnosis in the screened groups. Overdiagnosed tumours are generally smaller than other tumours, as they grow more slowly (length bias). Therefore, if an overdiagnosed tumour was missed at one screening session by a small margin, it would not be much larger when detected at the next screening.

What is missing in the calculations is carcinoma *in situ*. Carcinoma *in situ* is mainly detected at screening. As these lesions are often multifocal, it is difficult to understand how they can be precursors to small single tumours, as is generally stated, unless we assume that the vast majority of these lesions regress. They are often treated by mastectomy, and treatment with anti-hormone therapy also reduces the risk of new tumours occurring.[12] These prophylactic treatments would only be expected to lower breast cancer mortality marginally, e.g. cancer can still arise in the remaining breast.

The tumour data tell us that it is misleading to say to a woman that she has been cured from breast cancer. The cancer may come back at any time, e.g after 5, 20 or 40 years, and there is no upper limit as to when it could happen. It is understandable, however, that clinicians say to their patients that they are cured if, for example, there are no signs of recurrence of the cancer after 5 years. It feels good for the clinician and it gives the women the chance of living a more normal life without thinking too often whether the cancer might come back. But I am still in doubt whether this white lie is a good idea. We shall all die, and we all know it, but that doesn't prevent us from living happy lives. And most people have heard about cancers that came back after 10 or 20 years. Then why not be honest with the patients? In northern Europe we tell patients they have cancer, whereas it is common in southern and eastern Europe to tell only the relatives.[13]

There was also a time when we didn't tell the patient in northern Europe. But this can lead to a lack of trust between the patient and her doctor.

Lead time

The data on tumour size raise interesting questions about published estimates of lead time, which is the average time screening brings the diagnosis forwards. There are only 2.3 times as many cells in a tumour of size 21 mm as in one of size 16 mm, which means that the average lead time for invasive cancer is only a little more than the doubling time.

In the literature, estimates of lead time have generally varied between 2 and 5 years.[14,15] This cannot be reconciled with the tumour data and with our knowledge of doubling times. The mean doubling time in the study from Heidelberg was 212 days,[2] and the median in the bigger US study was 260 days. As these doubling times were derived from tumour sizes in the relevant growth intervals where tumours can be detected clinically or on a mammogram, it means that the lead time should be less than a year.

Epidemiological data also tell us that lead-time estimates of 2 or more years cannot be correct. With such long lead times, the large and persistent increase in breast cancer incidence rates that occur when screening is introduced must be followed by a huge incidence drop when women are no longer screened due to advanced age.[14] But studies have shown that a drop either doesn't occur or is very small.[16,17]

Carcinoma *in situ* is a special case, as most of these lesions never progress to invasive cancer (*see* Chapter 16). They can therefore be said to have an infinite lead time. The same is true for regressing overdiagnosed cancers. We cannot calculate averages based on numbers that include infinity, and it would also be meaningless to use hypothetical truncated numbers, e.g. the estimated remaining lifespan of women with carcinoma *in situ* that does not progress.

I believe it is a dubious approach to adjust statistical analyses for lead-time estimates when studying overdiagnosis. However, this is commonly done, and by using too-high estimates of lead time and statistical models, some researchers have spuriously 'adjusted away' virtually all overdiagnosis (*see* Chapter 16). We should stick to the raw data, which tell us a very different story.

Plausible effect based on tumour stages in the trials

For the reasons just explained, screening cannot result in anything near a 30% reduction in breast cancer mortality, as screening advocates claim. It is entirely implausible that the smaller size of the tumours or lower stages of the tumours detected at screening can explain such a large effect, although Tabár, Duffy and Day have claimed this for the Two-County trial.[18,19] Tabár has also claimed a 25% reduction in the rate of advanced breast cancers (stage II or more) in the group invited to screening.[20]

I believe none of this is possible and will show why by turning our attention from the relative risks researchers usually report to risk differences. The difference in tumour size in the Two-County trial was 7 mm, which is only slightly larger than the average of 5 mm for all the trials. Further, data from the Two-County trial presented in a graph show that after 10 years, 6% of women with cancers between 10 and 14 mm in size have died, whereas 11% of those with cancers between 15 and 19 mm have died.[18] Thus, a difference in size of 5 mm corresponded to a difference in breast cancer deaths of only 5%, which, moreover, is in agreement with the difference of 5% in tumours with metastases as calculated earlier. However, as I have shown, this corresponds to only a 12% reduction in mortality from breast cancer, and not 31% as Tabár *et al.* reported.

For cancers somewhat bigger, between 20 and 29 mm, no less than 34% of women in the Two-County trial had died after 10 years.[18] This is far too many, considering the linear relationship between tumour size and risk of metastasis. In Table 24.2, I show the percentage of women with metastases for the same tumour size categories as those published for the Two-County trial. As there were

TABLE 24.2 Tumour size as a predictor of metastases and death in breast cancer: the three tumour sizes in the German study correspond to those reported for the Two-County trial

Study	Tumour size (mm)	Metastases or death in breast cancer (%)
German study	12	29% metastases
	17	36% metastases
	24.5	46% metastases
Two-County trial	10–14	6% died
	15–19	11% died
	20–29	34% died

as many as 39 cancers at the first screen in the Two-County trial with a tumour size between 20 and 29 mm, the sudden increase in mortality when tumour size increased by only 7.5 mm cannot be explained by random variation. This discrepancy suggests that tumour data, assessment of cause of death, or both, are not reliable in the Two-County trial.

Another unfortunate example of misleading research in this area is a letter to the editor in the *Lancet* by Tabár, Duffy and Smith.[21] The authors showed a table with results from the screening trials and claimed that those trials that lowered the rate of node-positive cancers also lowered the rate of breast cancer deaths. This relationship would be expected if screening worked, but the authors did not perform a statistical analysis. Further, they only included women in the age group 40–49 years, which was curious, as the effect of screening is considered controversial in young women. Finally, important findings should not be published in a correspondence about something else, namely Nyström's 2002 meta-analysis, but in a full, peer-reviewed paper that allows the readers to judge whether the study's methods are adequate.

I tried to reproduce their findings, using explicit methods and data for the whole age range of women that were included in the trials.[22] Since the purpose of screening is to advance the time of diagnosis (thereby reducing the occurrence of cancers with metastases), the trials that found many cancers, compared with the unscreened control group, would be expected to have the largest effect on breast cancer mortality, but there was no such relation.

For cancers in stage II and above, and also for node-positive cancers, there was a significant relation in the expected direction, but the linear relation between advanced cancers and breast cancer mortality was in the wrong place. A screening effectiveness of zero (which means that the rate of node-positive cancers is the same in the screened group as in the control group) corresponded to a significant 16% reduction in breast cancer mortality (95% confidence interval: 9% to 23% reduction) (*see* Figure 24.1; when log relative risk (RR) = 0.00 for number of cancers, then log RR for breast cancer mortality is −0.18, and RR for breast cancer mortality is 0.84). This could only happen if there is bias. Further analyses uncovered evidence that assessment of cause of death and of the number of cancers in advanced stages were both biased. Since the size of the bias, 16%, was similar to the estimated effect of screening,[11,23] this result suggests that screening is ineffective.

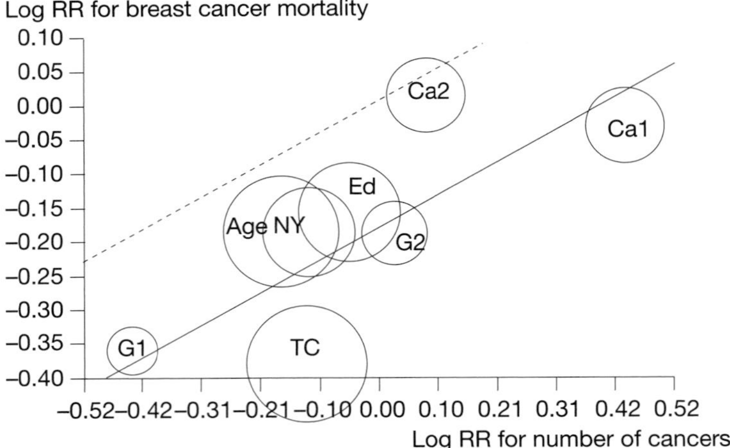

Trial abbreviations: Ca1 (Canada, 40–49 yr); Ca2 (Canada, 50–59 yr); TC (Two-County, 40–74 yr); G1 (Göteborg, 40–49 yr); G2 (Göteborg, 50–59 yr); NY (New York, 40–64 yr); Ed (Edinburgh, 45–64 yr); Age (UK Age Trial, 39–41 yr).

FIGURE 24.1 Relation between detection of node-positive breast cancer and the risk of dying from breast cancer in the randomised trials after 13 years of follow-up. Fewer node-positive cancers in the screened group are associated with fewer breast cancer deaths (lower left corner). Circle areas are proportional to the weights in the regression analysis.

The hatched line represents an unbiased regression line that goes through (0,0) and has the same slope as the calculated regression line

No decrease in advanced cancers

Before screening was introduced in the United States, the age-adjusted incidence of breast cancer was rather constant. When screening spread in the 1980s, there was a sharp rise in cases of carcinoma *in situ*. This would be expected to be followed by a decrease in the incidence of early-stage invasive breast cancer later on, but as this also increased,[24] it indicated substantial overdiagnosis of harmless invasive cancers. More recent US data have shown that the incidence of cancers with metastases has changed very little.[25,26]

Since the fundamental idea with screening is to decrease the number of cancers that have metastasised, this suggests that the theoretical rationale for screening is wrong and that screening doesn't work in today's setting.

Using methods other than those I've just shown, Zahl and colleagues[27] showed in 2001 that a 31% reduction in breast cancer mortality was impossible, considering the tumour stages in the Swedish mammography trials. Their study was criticised by Rutqvist[28] who declared it 'lacked scientific merit'. This seems to be a preferred terminology screening advocates use for results they don't like, e.g. both Peter Dean and Nicholas Wald used this phrase when they criticised our first *Lancet* review.[29,30] However, in my opinion, the study was well done and is very convincing. Furthermore, the criticism – which was inappropriate – was refuted by the authors.[31]

The leader of the Norwegian screening programme, Steinar Thoresen, made himself look ridiculous[32] when he complained that the authors had not cited Tabár's first 'beyond reason' study[33] and furthermore remarked that the Zahl study should not have been accepted in a scientific journal. He ended his wrath by saying he didn't know the motives of the Institute of Public Health (where two of the authors worked) for the 'very unscientific battle it conducted against mammography screening' and he feared that its credibility also in other areas would suffer. The authors replied to this harassment that they – in contrast to Thoresen – didn't have any economic interests in screening.[34]

Tabár didn't threaten with litigation on this occasion, but it would also have been futile, as the paper had already appeared in print and therefore couldn't be removed from the public record.

Zahl had other important data at hand. The Norwegian Cancer Registry is the only Nordic registry that records clinical stage at diagnosis, and he sent me data that showed that the whole incidence increase after the prevalence screening in Norway when screening started was for localised cancers. The rates of cancers with regional or distant metastases were unaffected by screening.

This means that screening cannot work. Similar findings were reported in 2006 by researchers from the Norwegian Cancer Registry and the Institute for Population-Based Cancer Research for counties that started screening early, in 1995 and 1996.[35] However, the researchers didn't discuss their results accurately, but resorted to wishful thinking when they said that their findings indicated that the programme worked as intended. Two years later, they showed that the total number of advanced cancers (those that had metastasised) *increased* when screening started and remained higher than before screening even 8 years later.[36] That result was even more convincing, but the authors concluded otherwise: 'Breast cancer diagnosed in the screening period had prognostically favorable tumor characteristics compared to breast cancer diagnosed in the prescreening period.' This is completely misleading. Overdiagnosed cancers have favourable tumour characteristics of course, and it is therefore wrong to look at percentages.

The error they made is very common, but inexcusable. For example, if 60 of 100 cancers in a group without screening are advanced, and the only thing screening does is to overdiagnose another 30 localised cancers (which agree fairly well with data from the Malmö trial),[6] then the *percentage* of advanced cancers is 60/(100 + 30) = 46% in the screened group and 60/100 = 60% in the control group. Thus, although the *absolute* rate of advanced cancers was not reduced with screening, and although screening didn't work in Malmö (relative risk: 0.96),[6] there were *relatively* fewer advanced cancers with screening. One needs to look at *total* numbers of advanced cancers, not percentages.

Screening enthusiasts from other countries have also misled their readers. Zahl drew my attention to a particularly egregious example published by Harry de Koning and others involved with the Dutch screening programme.[37] The programme did not reduce the incidence of cancers with metastases, but the researchers concealed this fact by splitting the cancers with metastases in two groups, above and below 2 cm in size. This makes no sense, but what immediately catches the eye in their figure is a graph with metastasised cancers bigger than 2 cm that appears to go down over time. The split of the data is misused in the abstract, which only mentions the larger cancers and notes that their incidence declined significantly. When I added the data from the graphs, I found that there was *no* reduction in incidence of cancers with metastases, in fact the combined incidence was identical for the first year reported, 1989, and for the last year, 1997.

The authors concluded, 'It is evident that breast cancer screening contributes to a reduction in advanced breast cancers and breast cancer mortality.' This is not what their study showed, and there are no data on breast cancer mortality in the paper. The dishonesty continued in the discussion section: 'It is important to realise that the initial increase does not signify overdiagnosis, but that it is the result of the necessary downstaging of breast cancer diagnoses, if screening will be effective. Several authors concluded that overdiagnosis might be limited to a few percent.' *There was no downstaging to cancers that had not metastasised.*

What the study really showed was that screening is ineffective in the Netherlands and that it leads to a huge amount of overdiagnosis (as the incidence of localised cancers doubled, with no sign of a decrease). But the authors wrote exactly the opposite of what they found on both counts.

Researchers from Australia also misled their readers, in a similar fashion. They wrote in the abstract that the incidence of large breast cancers (3 cm or larger) fell by 20% in those 50–69 years of age.[38] However, when we stage tumours, we don't use 3 cm as cutoff, we use 2 cm, and the incidence of cancers size 2 cm or larger did not fall, it increased!

A systematic review from 2010 that included several countries and regions from the United States, Europe and Australia found that, on average, the rates of advanced cancers, defined as those larger than 20 mm, were not affected by screening.[39]

References

1 Fletcher SW. Whither scientific deliberation in health policy recommendations? Alice in the Wonderland of breast-cancer screening. *N Engl J Med*. 1997; **336**(16): 1180–3.

2 Von Fournier D, Weber E, Hoeffken W, *et al*. Growth rate of 147 mammary carcinomas. *Cancer*. 1980; **45**(8): 2198–207.

3 Spratt JS, Meyer JS, Spratt JA. Rates of growth of human neoplasms: Part II. *J Surg Oncol*. 1996; **61**(1): 68–83.

4 Gøtzsche PC, Jørgensen KJ, Zahl P-H, *et al*. Why mammography screening has not lived up to expectations from the randomised trials. *Cancer Causes Control*. 2012; **23**: 15–21.

5 Narod SA. On being the right size: a reappraisal of mammography trials in Canada and Sweden. *Lancet*. 1997; **349**(9068): 1846.

6 Andersson I, Aspegren K, Janzon L, *et al*. Mammographic screening and mortality from breast cancer: the Malmö mammographic screening trial. *BMJ*. 1988; **297**(6654): 943–8.

7 Frisell J, Eklund G, Hellström L, *et al*. Analysis of interval breast carcinomas in a randomized screening trial in Stockholm. *Breast Cancer Res Treat*. 1987; **9**(3): 219–25.

8 Tabár L, Fagerberg G, Chen HH, *et al*. Tumour development, histology and grade of breast cancers: prognosis and progression. *Int J Cancer*. 1996; **66**(4): 413–19.

9 Engel J, Eckel R, Kerr J, *et al*. The process of metastasisation for breast cancer. *Eur J Cancer*. 2003; **39**(12): 1794–806.

10 Carter CL, Allen C, Henson DE. Relation of tumor size, lymph node status, and survival in 24,740 breast cancer cases. *Cancer*. 1989; **63**(1): 181–7.

11 Gøtzsche PC, Nielsen M. Screening for breast cancer with mammography. *Cochrane Database Syst Rev*. 2009; (4): CD001877.

12 Cuzick J, Sestak I, Pinder SE, *et al*. Effect of tamoxifen and radiotherapy in women with locally excised ductal carcinoma in situ: long-term results from the UK/ANZ DCIS trial *Lancet Oncol*. 2011; **12**(1): 21–9.

13 Thomsen OO, Wulff HR, Martin A, *et al*. What do gastroenterologists in Europe tell cancer patients? *Lancet*. 1993; **341**(8843): 473–6.

14 Boer R, Warmerdam P, de Koning H, *et al*. Extra incidence caused by mammographic screening. *Lancet*. 1994; **343**(8903): 979.

15 Tabár L, Duffy SW, Yen MF, *et al*. All-cause mortality among breast cancer patients in a screening trial: support for breast cancer mortality as an end point. *J Med Screen*. 2002; **9**(4): 159–62.

16 Jørgensen KJ, Gøtzsche PC. Overdiagnosis in publicly organised mammography screening programmes: systematic review of incidence trends. *BMJ*. 2009; **339**: b2587.

17 Jørgensen KJ, Zahl PH, Gøtzsche PC. Overdiagnosis in organised mammography screening in Denmark: a comparative study. *BMC Womens Health*. 2009; **9**: 36.

18 Tabár L, Fagerberg G, Duffy SW, *et al*. Update of the Swedish two-county program of mammographic screening for breast cancer. *Radiol Clin North Am*. 1992; **30**(1): 187–210.

19 Tabár L, Fagerberg CJG, Day NE. The results of periodic one-view mammographic screening in Sweden: Part 2. Evaluation of the results. In: Day NE, Miller AB, editors. *Screening for Breast Cancer*. Toronto: Hans Huber; 1988. pp. 39–44.

20 Tabár L, Fagerberg CJG, Gad A, *et al*. Reduction in mortality from breast cancer after mass screening with mammography: randomised trial from the Breast Cancer Screening

Working Group of the Swedish National Board of Health and Welfare. *Lancet*. 1985; **1**(8433): 829–32.

21 Tabár L, Smith RA, Duffy SW. Update on effects of screening mammography. *Lancet*. 2002; **360**(9329): 337.

22 Gøtzsche PC. Relation between breast cancer mortality and screening effectiveness: systematic review of the mammography trials. *Dan Med Bull*. 2011; **58**(3): A4246.

23 Humphrey LL, Helfand M, Chan BK, *et al*. Breast cancer screening: a summary of the evidence for the U.S. Preventive Services Task Force. *Ann Intern Med*. 2002; **137**(5 Pt. 1): 347–60.

24 Fletcher SW, Elmore JG. Clinical practice: mammographic screening for breast cancer. *N Engl J Med*. 2003; **348**(17): 1672–80.

25 Esserman L, Shieh Y, Thompson I. Rethinking screening for breast cancer and prostate cancer. *JAMA*. 2009; **302**(15): 1685–92.

26 Jørgensen KJ, Keen JD, Gøtzsche PC. Is mammographic screening justifiable considering its substantial overdiagnosis rate and minor effect on mortality? *Radiology*. 2011; **260**(3): 621–7.

27 Zahl P-H, Kopjar B, Mæhlen J. [Norwegian breast cancer mortality rates and validity of Swedish mammographic studies] [Norwegian]. *Tidsskr Nor Lægeforen*. 2001; **121**(16): 1928–31.

28 Rutqvist LE. [Mammography trials] [Norwegian]. *Tidsskr Nor Lægeforen*. 2001; **121**(22): 2636–7.

29 Dean P. Final comment: the articles by Gøtzsche and Olsen are not official Cochrane reviews and lack scientific merit. *Läkartidningen*. 2000; **97**(25): 3106.

30 Wald N. Populist instead of professional. *J Med Screen*. 2000; **7**(1): 1.

31 Zahl P, Kopjar B, Mæhlen J. [Mammography trials] [Norwegian]. *Tidsskr Nor Lægeforen*. 2001; **121**: 2636.

32 Thoresen SØ. [Mammography screening saves lives] [Norwegian]. *Tidsskr Nor Lægeforen*. 2001; **121**(25): 2995.

33 Tabár L, Vitak B, Chen HH, *et al*. Beyond randomized controlled trials: organized mammographic screening substantially reduces breast carcinoma mortality. *Cancer*. 2001; **91**(9): 1724–31.

34 Strand B, Zahl P-H. [Mammography screening saves lives] [Norwegian]. *Tidsskr Nor Lægeforen*. 2001; **121**: 2995.

35 Hofvind S, Sørum R, Haldorsen T, *et al*. [Incidence of breast cancer before and after implementation of mammography screening] [Norwegian]. *Tidsskr Nor Laegeforen*. 2006; **126**(22): 2935–8.

36 Hofvind S, Sørum R, Thoresen S. Incidence and tumor characteristics of breast cancer diagnosed before and after implementation of a population-based screening-program. *Acta Oncol*. 2008; **47**(2): 225–31.

37 Fracheboud J, Otto SJ, van Dijck JA, *et al*. Decreased rates of advanced breast cancer due to mammography screening in the Netherlands. *Br J Cancer*. 2004; **91**(5): 861–7.

38 Kricker A, Farac K, Smith D, *et al*. Breast cancer in New South Wales in 1972–1995: tumor size and the impact of mammographic screening. Int J Cancer 1999; **81**: 877–80.

39 Autier P, Boniol M, Middleton R, *et al*. Advanced breast cancer incidence following population-based mammographic screening. *Ann Oncol*. Epub 2011 Jan 20.

25

Where is screening at today?

AS EXPLAINED IN EARLIER CHAPTERS, THE EFFECT OF SCREENING must have been much overestimated in the randomised trials. For example, the tumour data suggest that the true effect cannot have been more than a 12% reduction in breast cancer mortality. Much has happened since the trials were carried out and it is not likely that screening is effective today. There are several compelling reasons for this.

First, when screening doesn't reduce the occurrence of advanced cancers, it cannot work.

Second, the treatments are far better today. When the old trials were done, the women didn't receive much adjuvant therapy, such as chemotherapy and hormonal treatment. For example, there was almost no use of hormonal treatment in the Two-County trial,[1] although tamoxifen is highly effective, as is polychemotherapy, and these effects are largely independent of nodal status and other tumour characteristics.[2] Thus, the treatments work whether or nor the cancer is detected 'early'.

Third, the amount of overdiagnosis seems to have increased since the trials were performed, as evidenced by recent data from New South Wales (*see* Chapter 16),[3] and with more overdiagnosis comes increased mortality from the harms of radiotherapy and chemotherapy.

Fourth, greater breast cancer awareness seems to have played a role. Breast cancer awareness is different from regular breast self-exams, as it means being aware of changes in the breasts, e.g. detected during a shower, and consulting with a doctor without delay when such changes are noted. In Denmark, the average size of the tumours was 33 mm in 1978–79, which decreased to 24 mm in 1988–89.[4] This change occurred before screening started, and it is therefore a doubtful argument when screening advocates say screening has led to greater breast cancer awareness. Breast cancer awareness started *before* screening and it was clearly beneficial, as it did not lead to overdiagnosis.[5] Further, the difference of 9 mm is much greater than the average difference between the screened and the control groups in the old trials, which was only 5 mm. This suggests that breast cancer awareness has been more important than screening for the decrease in breast cancer mortality that has been observed in many countries, although the contribution of breast cancer awareness has likely been small compared to the contribution of improved adjuvant therapy.[2]

Fifth, the decrease in breast cancer mortality has consistently been larger in young age groups that were not screened than in the screened age groups (*see* Chapters 5 and 15).

Sixth, it is well known that effects seen in randomised trials can rarely be reproduced in clinical practice. For mammography screening, an important reason is problems with reading mammograms, which I shall discuss next.

Seventh, it hasn't been possible to see an effect of screening on breast cancer mortality in Denmark or in other European countries (*see* Chapter 15).

Problems with reading mammograms

In the randomised trials, those who read the films were highly motivated, as they hoped to show that screening worked. In contrast, it is very difficult in everyday practice to attract top-level doctors to something as boring as looking at mammograms, day in and day out, for a whole career. Furthermore, even dedicated people will have difficulty maintaining concentration and carefulness when by far most of the readings are negative. It is so easy to overlook the occasional cancer; in fact, it is regarded as one of the most difficult tasks in radiology to spot cancers on mammograms. Failure to diagnose breast cancer is the most common cause of medical malpractice litigation in the United States, and *half of the cases resulting in payment to the claimant had negative mammograms*, which is difficult to understand, as nothing appeared to have been missed.[6] Finally, the quicker the reader is, the more money will be earned, and there is a scarcity of doctors for the job.

These facts invite big trouble. Radiologists miss many breast cancers and the level of agreement when two or more observers evaluate the same mammograms independently is poor.[7–10] Some of this research was described in a long article by Michael Moss in the *New York Times* in 2002.[11]

The US government holds the doctors to only minimum standards, which are set by the American College of Radiology. Little training is required, and only

480 readings a year are needed to stay sharp, which many experts say is so low as to be virtually meaningless. In Canada, the number required is 2500.[12] When increased demands and regular skills tests were suggested, this was met with fierce resistance from doctors and their allies. Therefore, the existing rules deal primarily with technical specifications, while doctors keep on regulating themselves.

Surveys have shown that average doctors missed more than 25% of the cancers, and that some clinics missed nearly 40%. Essentially nothing happens even when it is known that particular doctors perform very poorly; they just go on missing cancers. Moss reported that more than 40% of the clinics had been cited for violating one or more federal rules every year.

Recall rates for further investigations because of a suspicion of breast cancer are about twice as high in the United States as in the United Kingdom, although cancer rates are similar.[13] Open surgical biopsies that don't result in a cancer diagnosis are also twice as high. Another study found that the recall rate in 31 US practices varied from 2% to 13%, which again suggested serious problems with reading the mammograms.[14]

Thus, the situation is far better in Canada and in Europe than in the United States. In Europe, there are national government-led programmes with quality control, and the readers generally don't increase their salaries by being quick and superficial. However, as we cannot see an effect of screening in Europe, even carefully regulated systems don't pay off.

The US aggressiveness, coupled with fear of litigation, much more frequent testing and the lack of a nationally organised programme with quality assurance measures in place, causes tremendous and unnecessary harm to US women, far above what women experience elsewhere. Yet, former president George W Bush declared that the US healthcare system is the best in the world. I wonder by what measures this system supersedes other systems, except for its high costs, which are second to none.[15] Even so, the United States consistently underperforms on most dimensions of performance, relative to other countries.[15,16] Healthcare should not be regulated by market forces.

False promises

The overselling of screening has been global, and the denial of the essential and indisputable facts has been equally global. The screening literature has been polluted to an extraordinary degree by statistical modelling of the raw data, often combined with wishful thinking and the use of favourable, but unrealistic assumptions for variables that cannot be measured. This has helped conceal inconvenient facts and has yielded results people wanted to see.

In 1999, Harry de Koning and colleagues[17] published rosy screening forecasts in the core journal for screening zealots, the *Journal of Medical Screening*. Using modelling, they predicted that screening would reduce breast cancer mortality by 18% in the relevant age groups 10 years after screening started in the United Kingdom and the Netherlands (which is in 1998 and 1999, respectively), and by 24% and 29%, respectively, in the long term.

Jan Hendriks, who developed the Dutch screening programme, remarked a year later in an interview that if the mortality from breast cancer had not been dramatically reduced by 2003, the nationwide screening programme should be stopped.[18]

It hasn't been possible to see *any* effect of screening in national mortality data that goes up to 2007 and 2006, respectively, in the two countries.[19,20] However, such sobering facts haven't had any visible effect on Harry de Koning, who wrote in 2003 that evaluation of breast cancer mortality during the next 5 years would be crucial.[21] Furthermore, he remarked: 'There seems to be no reason to change or to halt the current screening programmes, for example in The Netherlands. Nor is there any justifiable reason for negative reports towards women or professionals.' We are now past these 5 'crucial' years, which were conveniently added when no effect was seen at the earliest 'crucial' years in 1998–99, or at the next 'crucial' year, 2003, but de Koning still seems unaffected by the facts. It is somewhat like those religious people who predict the world will go under at a certain date, and when it doesn't, the doomsday prophets come up with a new date.

In the United Kingdom, it was expected that screening would reduce breast cancer mortality by about 25% by the year 2000 in the population invited to screening.[22,23] In her foreword to the report of the NHS Breast Screening Programme for the year 2000, Yvette Cooper, under-secretary of state (Commons), said: 'Breast cancer mortality in England and Wales decreased by 21.3% between 1990 to 1998, and it is estimated that 30% of this reduction was due to breast screening.'[24] That was pretty smart PR – in fact, an amazing example of political spin. Most decision-makers are busy people who read fast, and they may only notice that the numbers they see are big, which is what they expect. Hazel Thornton explained that 30% of 21.3% is 6%.[25] It would have been more informative, transparent and honest to tell the citizens that screening had been a disappointment, as it had reduced breast cancer mortality by only 6%. But that wouldn't have sold tickets and earned knighthoods.

In 2006, when our updated Cochrane review with data on overdiagnosis had just come out, Michael Baum suggested that the National Institute for Health and Clinical Excellence (NICE) should evaluate the screening programme, but a spokesman from the Department of Health said it would not be appropriate, as mammography screening was an accepted, evidence-based technology.[26] One of the things NICE does is to evaluate the cost for saving one life, and it is pretty clear that such an assessment would come out with thumbs down for mammography screening. Therefore, the Department of Health will not allow NICE to touch the holy cow.

In 1999, the expert on mammography at the Swedish National Board of Health, Ingvar Andersson, the primary investigator for the Malmö trial, expressed disappointment that it was still not possible to see any notable change in breast cancer mortality in Sweden.[27] He felt it was necessary to wait another couple of years. Eleven years later, it is still not possible to see any effect of screening in Sweden,[19] but this hasn't led to the slightest official reaction.

In Norway, people from the Cancer Registry remarked in 2000 that screening would reduce breast cancer mortality by 50%.[28] A pretty amazing forecast, considering that screening doesn't reduce the amount of advanced cancers in Norway.

The Ig Noble Prize for the most surrealistic promises should be given to the American Cancer Society. In 1996, the society set goals for cancer screening,[29] which still appear in its 2009 Strategic Plan Progress Report.[30] Its nationwide objectives were, by 2015, to:

- reduce the age-adjusted incidence of breast cancer by 15%
- reduce the age-adjusted mortality rate of breast cancer by 50%
- increase to 90% the proportion of women aged 40 and older who have breast screening consistent with ACS guidelines.

These objectives are insane. Screening has increased the incidence of breast cancer in the United States dramatically over the last 20 years, and it is therefore difficult to understand how the society can have an objective about *reduced* incidence.

It is equally misguided to expect the mortality rate of breast cancer to decrease by 50%, which begs the question why a cancer society would publish objectives that are far beyond what is biologically possible? If I had similar disregard for facts, I might equally well come up with the objective that by 2020, the lifespan of the average Dane should be 120 years. Is it all about getting money to the society by promising people what insiders know is too good to be true? Somewhat like the financial scandals and fraud we have seen recently where, for example, Bernard Madoff promised totally unrealistic returns on investments and was sentenced to 150 years in jail, the maximum allowed, in 2009.

The society seems to have known from the outset that the goal for mortality was unrealistic,[29] and, needless to say, it is also highly problematic from an ethical perspective to have a goal of almost all women turning up for screening, as it wouldn't be achievable if the women were honestly informed about the benefits and harms of screening.

For prostate cancer, the society's goals were even more far out. Although screening has exploded the incidence (*see* Figure 25.1),[30] the goal is by 2015 to reduce the age-adjusted incidence by 15%.

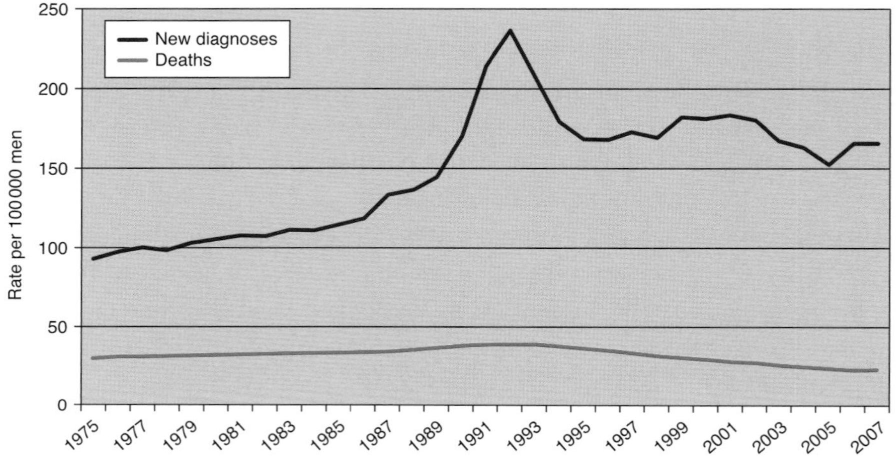

FIGURE 25.1 Age-adjusted incidence and mortality rates of prostate cancer in the United States 1975–2007. Data from http://seer.cancer.gov (accessed 15 April 2011)

It is also totally unrealistic to expect a reduction in the age-adjusted mortality rate of prostate cancer by 50%.[31] Such dream scenarios, completely detached from evidence, suggest that it all has to do with fundraising.

Important information is being ignored

There has been too little focus on how small the effect of screening is. In the most recent trial, the UK age trial, which randomised women aged 39–41 years, the 10-year risk of dying from breast cancer in the control group was only 0.2%.[1] As a commentator pointed out, a 10-year risk of dying from cardiovascular disease of 1% is considered very low, even for women, and unless being dead of breast cancer is far worse than being dead of stroke or myocardial infarction, it doesn't seem reasonable that we focus so much on screening for breast cancer as we do.[32]

We have also heard far too many exaggerations and rosy forecasts, and far too little about what it means to be a cancer patient. This is a serious omission, as screening turns so many healthy women into cancer patients unnecessarily.

A patient described her experience in the *Sunday Times* in 2009.[33] She had been diagnosed with carcinoma *in situ* 4 years earlier and noted what the reality of this diagnosis had been:

> I expect that I have been classified as a screening success. Yet, everything about my experience tells me the opposite. Screening has caused me considerable and lasting harm . . . Two wide excisions, one partial mutilation (sorry, mastectomy), one reconstruction, five weeks' radiotherapy, chronic infection, four bouts of cellulitis (a bacterial skin infection), several general anaesthetics, and more than a year off work.

In the same article, the UK Department of Health mentioned that it didn't agree with the numbers we had provided and said, 'The majority of international experts on breast screening would agree with us.' Very odd. Who shouts the loudest? As our numbers come from the trials, it is not a question of agreeing or disagreeing. It's a question of facts and whether one wishes to be evidence-based or not, which the Department of Health obviously will not. And who are the 'majority of experts'? No doubt most of them have conflicts of interest and turf and money to defend. Eight days earlier, the *Lancet* had published an editorial, 'The trouble with screening', that described our leaflet and our numbers, without any reservations, and also quoted us for saying that the responsibility for the information provided should be kept separate from that for the screening programme.[34] Where were we without independent journals? If only departments of health would listen.

Getting a cancer diagnosis – or just being told that it could be cancer and that additional investigations are needed – can impact importantly on people's lives (*see* Chapter 19). Suicides have been reported, and in one case the woman wrote her suicide note on her recall letter.[35] The strongest increase in suicide rate among cancer patients is seen in the first years after diagnosis: 16-fold in the first year and 7-fold in the second and third years; for women with breast cancer the overall rate is increased by 40%.[36] In absolute numbers, this is a small problem. However, when a cancer diagnosis can increase suicide rates, it may also increase mortality from other forms of self-destructive behaviour, e.g. drinking and smoking, which are quantitatively far more important. A woman who thinks she will die from breast cancer may not be particularly motivated to give up smoking.

What we have also heard too little about, and which has not been described in any of the leaflets I've seen, is how often women suffer from chronic pain after surgery. I was shocked when I read a 2009 paper about this.[37] Two to three years after breast cancer treatment, 47% of the women reported pain, usually several times a week.[37] Only half of those with pain reported that it was of light intensity. The pain was equally common among those who had had breast-conserving surgery as among those with a mastectomy, and pain was more common when the women had received radiotherapy. Thus, half of all women – including all the overdiagnosed ones who were healthy before they got screened – will suffer from chronic pain, presumably for the rest of their lives.

Beliefs warp evidence at conferences

The basic issues in cancer screening are generally little understood. To most clinicians, it seems, a cancer is a cancer. They often don't realise that the disease has changed radically, now that we have screening, and that much of it isn't even a disease. When cancers are detected clinically because patients present with symptoms, the situation is completely different. Treatments are often available that reduce both cancer-specific mortality and all-cause mortality substantially.

After I had given a lecture on breast screening at a hospital in 2009 and had carefully explained about overdiagnosis and that screening might not have any effect on all-cause mortality, several clinicians argued that even if this were correct, it would still be an advantage to have screening, as early detection meant less aggressive treatment. I had shown during my lecture that screening leads to more mastectomies and I had explained why, but even so, the clinicians failed to realise:

- the patients they see today are very different from those they saw before screening
- there are many more of them and many of them are healthy citizens rendered patients unnecessarily
- the sum total is therefore *more* use of aggressive treatment, not *less*.

Unfortunately, many of those who are responsible for screening don't understand these issues either. Although I rarely go to conferences, I accepted an invitation to speak at a pro and con session on mammography screening at a German cancer congress with 10 000 participants in February 2010. It was an interesting experience, as it recapitulates much of what I have written about in this book.

On my arrival, the chairman said that it had been difficult to persuade the organisers to invite me. People had been afraid that I would somehow leave the upcoming German screening programme in ruins. I was amused by this, as was the chairman, who said I didn't look dangerous to him.

The pro speaker was Karin Bock, who is responsible for the breast screening programme in south-west Germany. She made three errors in her talk that are typical of screening advocates. First, she claimed that screening leads to less extensive surgery, as it finds tumours that are smaller than without screening. Second, she showed data indicating that relatively more cancers are found in early stages than without screening. Such data are misleading, as they don't take overdiagnosed cancers into account. Third, she noted that screening saves one life for every 200 women who are screened for 20 years, which is impossible.

Someone handed me a mammography screening leaflet from the Ministry of Health[38] after the meeting and said it was evidence-based. It repeated the error that screening leads to less surgery and stated that most experts agreed that for every death prevented, one woman was overdiagnosed, an error of 10 times. It dutifully added that many thought there was more overdiagnosis than this, but it is not a thought in people's minds like a doomsday date for when the world will end; it is fact. There were only four references, which is very few for a publication of 23 pages that purports to be evidence-based, and they showed that the leaflet was *not* evidence-based: an unpublished German report about how it went when screening was introduced in a selected part of the country; a paper in German that the authors themselves called a 'selective literature review'; an editorial in the *BMJ*; and an observational study from the Netherlands[39] published in a journal I have never heard of, *Seminars in Breast Diseases*. It is not indexed by PubMed, it seems to have become extinct and we don't have access to the fossils at our university library.

Following my presentation, one clinician remarked about mastectomies that screening didn't lead to more mastectomies because he didn't see mastectomies any longer. This cannot be correct, and it is similar to saying there are no tigers in India, since I didn't see any when I was there.

I was also told that the reason the decrease in breast cancer mortality in Denmark was larger in young women who are not screened than in those who are screened[19] was that young women go to Germany to get screened. This ridiculous argument is not true of course, which can be seen from the very low rate of carcinoma *in situ* in these women.

When I said that the perceptions women had of screening were seriously distorted because of the propaganda, I was told that *I* was making propaganda because I talked about others making propaganda. Does this mean that if a judge says a person accused of murder is a killer, the judge is himself a killer?

A clinician asked me if I wasn't happy I had airbags in my car, as if this should somehow be the ultimate proof of the value of screening. Worst of all, a rather vocal person argued repeatedly that overdiagnosis was only a hypothesis. It didn't impress him in the least that I had just explained it is mathematically impossible to avoid overdiagnosis and that this has been empirically demonstrated, both in trials and in national screening programmes. It is not a hypothesis, not even a theory; it is fact.

After all these years – with all of our publications on screening and those of others that have explained the issues time and again – it escapes me how such well-educated people who work with cancer can be so oblivious to evidence. I will think twice before I accept an invitation to speak at a congress about mammography screening again.

Does breast screening make women live longer?

If screening increases mortality from other causes to the same degree as it decreases breast cancer mortality, it may not have any effect. Already when the Two-County trial was published in 1985, Swedish colleagues remarked that it was necessary to look also at total mortality (also called all-cause mortality).[40] The Project Group for the trial and the Swedish National Board of Health replied that an account of total mortality would be irrelevant and without basis in scientific practice and that it was an absurd idea that screening could have caused increased mortality.[41] Eleven years after these surprising remarks from the highest authority on health in the country, the Swedish trialists admitted that 'the total cumulative mortality would seem to be the most objective measure'.[42] Michael Baum noted in 2004 that, 'the bland assumption that the process of diagnosis and treatment of screen-detected lesions in the population at large, some of which might never have expressed a malignant potential in the woman's natural lifetime, is totally free of risk to life, is breathtaking in its arrogance.'[43]

It is disingenuous to suggest that total mortality is irrelevant, as screening inevitably increases mortality from causes other than breast cancer, e.g. because of the harms of radiotherapy and chemotherapy inflicted on overdiagnosed healthy women.[44] These deaths are not coded as breast cancer deaths. Furthermore, assessment of cause of death is unreliable and biased in favour of screening.[1]

These well-known facts didn't temper the arrogance in Swedish power circles. When Ole Olsen and I published our review in the *Lancet* in 2000 and noted there was no reliable evidence that screening reduced the mortality from breast cancer, Måns Rosén from the Swedish National Board of Health declared on Danish television that our criticism was absurd.

We knew from the beginning that total mortality was important and therefore we reported it in our assessment of the trials to the Danish National Board of Health in 1999. From 2001, we also reported on total cancer mortality.[45–47]

Screening doesn't reduce total cancer mortality. This is one of our most important findings, as a reduction is expected if screening were effective. We explained this in some detail, both in 2004[48] and in our updated Cochrane review from 2006.[49] We estimated that the relative risk for total cancer mortality in screened women would be 0.95 compared with controls if in fact a 29% reduction in breast cancer mortality had occurred as claimed. But what was reported in the same trials was a relative risk for total cancer mortality of 1.00 (95% confidence interval: 0.96 to 1.05), which is significantly higher than what was expected ($p = 0.02$). This leads to the inevitable conclusion that ascertainment of cause of cancer death was biased in favour of screening.

It can be particularly difficult to determine the cause of death when the patient harbours more than one malignant disease. In the Malmö trial, which had a high autopsy rate, 21% of the women with breast cancer who died had two or three types of different cancers.[1] Many of these cancers were rather harmless, e.g. some skin cancers, but some presented real difficulties when determining the cause of death.

The implicit premise for using cancer-specific mortality as outcome in screening trials is that an effect of screening translates into a proportional effect on all-cause mortality. It is clear that this premise doesn't hold for breast cancer.

Even the use of blinded end-point committees or official cause-of-death registries cannot avoid the problem that breast cancer mortality is biased in favour of screening.[1] Biased cause-of-death assessment has also been shown to occur for prostate cancer.[50] Belief in the effectiveness of an intervention may influence the decision on which type of cancer caused the patient's death,[50] and lethal complications of cancer treatments are often ascribed to other causes. The size of this misclassification is 37% for cancer generally and 9% for breast cancer.[51]

All-cause mortality is the only unbiased mortality outcome. Screening advocates either say that breast cancer mortality is a reliable outcome, which is definitely false, or say that it would require an unrealistically large sample size to show an effect on total mortality, which is not a scientific but a practical issue.

The conclusion of all this and of the preceding chapters is that it hasn't been shown that screening makes women live longer. In fact, it is highly likely that it doesn't.

Let us assume, however, that the reported effect of screening on breast cancer mortality in the randomised trials *could* be translated into a similar effect on total mortality. Then each woman's life would have been extended by 1 day, on average, after 10 years of screening.[1] From this, we need to subtract the time it takes for the woman to travel and attend the screening sessions and the time used by staff members and other people, e.g. her general practitioner. This is probably more than 1 day in 10 years, and the overall effect is therefore negative. For comparison, women with node-positive breast cancer obtain a life extension of 6 months, on average, when they are treated with tamoxifen for 10 years,[52] which, in addition, is very cheap. Donald Berry has compared the effect of screening with mishaps in life and noted that the same increment in expected additional life could be obtained by losing an ounce of body weight or wearing a helmet for 10 hours of bicycling.[53]

However, throughout all these years, repeated editorials written by screening advocates have countered criticisms with the mantra 'time to move on'.[54,55] Which means that it is no longer relevant to question screening, as the criticism has been responded to, and as it is clear that screening does more good than harm.

To me, it is the opposite. It seems clear that breast screening does far more harm than good. It is a lottery where there are many losers and very few winners, if any. Screening should increase the sum total of human happiness, and if it fails to do this, it should be abandoned.[56] It is not so easy to 'calculate' human happiness and there are philosophical problems. However, if one tries, and attaches utilities to the various outcomes of screening, it seems that screening is harmful. Happiness is usually called quality of life in research papers, and the typical method of assigning utilities gives a maximum of one if a person is alive and well, and zero if she is dead. Anything else lies in between.

This can be examined using Cochrane estimates of benefits and harms. After 10 years of screening, one woman out of 2000 will be alive who would have died without screening. It is reasonable to assume that on average, this life extension will have happened somewhere near the middle of the 10-year interval; assuming she is well, this therefore gives a utility of $1 \times 0.5 = 0.5$. There will be 10 overdiagnosed and overtreated women. We don't know what their utility is but it will be somewhat reduced, compared with being healthy. I have asked women with breast cancer, who replied that it bothered them and that their self-reported utility was about 0.9. Thus, the 10 women have lost $0.1 \times 10 \times 0.5 = 0.5$ in utility. Then there are 200 false positives. If we assume, just for the sake of the example, that their utility is 0.99, they will have lost $0.01 \times 200 \times 0.5 = 1.0$ in utility. Adding these up, we get a net loss of 1.0 in utility. In the United States, there are about twice as many false positives as in Europe, which gives a net loss of 2.0 in utility.

This was a crude exercise and the results should not be taken for more than they are. However, the net utility is likely more negative than in the exercise because the true effect of screening today is likely much smaller than 15%, if any, and the overdiagnosis is likely greater than 30%.

It follows that one shouldn't pay any attention to reports of health economic assessments that purport to have shown that breast screening is cost-effective because the cost of saving one life is within the usually accepted range. We pay for screening, and what we get out of this is a decrease in happiness. But even if we assumed there *were* a true 15% reduction in breast cancer mortality with screening – and a corresponding reduction in total mortality, which is an untenable assumption – the cost of extending one life was recently estimated at US$329 000.[57]

Studies on Quality Adjusted Life Years (QALYs) can be illuminating, and by the end of 2011 one such study was accepted for publication in the *BMJ*.[58] This study was much more refined than my primitive exercise above but arrived at similar conclusions. The authors found that screening could be causing more harm than good after 10 years. After 20 years, it looked better for screening, but the 20-year data involved extrapolations and assumptions and also built on a 15% reduction in breast cancer mortality, which we know is unlikely to be true today.

It is rather clear that if mammography screening was subjected to a health technology assessment today, the recommendation would be to stop screening.

References

1 Gøtzsche PC, Nielsen M. Screening for breast cancer with mammography. *Cochrane Database Syst Rev*. 2009; (4):CD001877.

2 Early Breast Cancer Trialists' Collaborative Group (EBCTCG). Effects of chemotherapy and hormonal therapy for early breast cancer on recurrence and 15-year survival: an overview of the randomised trials. *Lancet*. 2005; **365**(9472): 1687–717.

3 Morrell S, Barratt A, Irwig L, *et al*. Estimates of overdiagnosis of invasive breast cancer associated with screening mammography. *Cancer Causes Control*. 2010; **21**(2): 275–82.

4 Rostgaard K, Vaeth M, Rootzén H, *et al*. Why did the breast cancer lymph node status distribution improve in Denmark in the pre-mammography screening period of 1978–1994? *Acta Oncol*. 2010; **49**(3): 313–21.

5 Jørgensen KJ, Zahl PH, Gøtzsche PC. Overdiagnosis in organised mammography screening in Denmark: a comparative study. *BMC Womens Health*. 2009; **9**: 36.

6 MedNews. *Screening Statement for Health Professionals: screening for breast cancer*. National Cancer Institute; 2003 Oct 24. Available at: www.meb.uni-bonn.de/cancer.gov/CDR0000062751.html (accessed 18 December 2003).

7 Kerlikowske K, Grady D, Barclay J, *et al*. Variability and accuracy in mammographic interpretation using the American College of Radiology Breast Imaging Reporting and Data System. *J Natl Cancer Inst*. 1998; **90**(23): 1801–9.

8 Beam CA, Layde PM, Sullivan DC. Variability in the interpretation of screening mammograms by US radiologists: findings from a national sample. *Arch Intern Med*. 1996; **156**(2): 209–13.

9 Poplack SP, Tosteson AN, Grove MR, *et al*. Mammography in 53,803 women from the New Hampshire mammography network. *Radiology*. 2000; **217**(3): 832–40.

10 Sickles EA, Wolverton DE, Dee KE. Performance parameters for screening and diagnostic mammography: specialist and general radiologists. *Radiology*. 2002; **224**(3): 861–9.

11 Moss M. Spotting breast cancer: doctors are weak link. *New York Times*. 2002 Jun 27.
12 Baines CJ. The Canadian National Breast Screening Study: science meets controversy. In: Temple NJ, Thompson A, editors. *Exce$$ive Medical $pending*. Oxford: Radcliffe Publishing; 2007. Chapter 12. Available at: www.radcliffe-oxford.com/medicalspending (accessed 22 May 2011).
13 Smith-Bindman R, Chu PW, Miglioretti DL, *et al*. Comparison of screening mammography in the United States and the United kingdom. *JAMA*. 2003; **290**(16): 2129–37.
14 Yankaskas BC, Cleveland RJ, Schell MJ, *et al*. Association of recall rates with sensitivity and positive predictive values of screening mammography. *AJR Am J Roentgenol*. 2001; **177**(3): 543–9.
15 Nolte E, McKee CM. Measuring the health of nations: updating an earlier analysis. *Health Aff (Millwood)*. 2008: **27**(1): 58–71.
16 Davis K, Schoen C, Stremikis K. *Mirror, Mirror on the Wall: how the performance of the U.S. health care system compares internationally, 2010 update*. 2010 Jun 23. Available at: www.commonwealthfund.org/Content/Publications/Fund-Reports/2010/Jun/Mirror-Mirror-Update.aspx (accessed 22 May 2011).
17 Van den Akker-van Marle E, de Koning H, Boer R, *et al*. Reduction in breast cancer mortality due to the introduction of mass screening in the Netherlands: comparison with the United Kingdom. *J Med Screen*. 1999; **6**(1): 30–4.
18 Schindele E, Stollorz V. [Be careful, care!] [German]. *Die Woche*. 2000 Mar 3: 28–9.
19 Jørgensen KJ, Zahl PH, Gøtzsche PC. Breast cancer mortality in organised mammography screening in Denmark: comparative study. *BMJ*. 2010; **340**: c1241.
20 Bonneux L. [Advantages and disadvantages of breast cancer screening: time for evidence-based information] [Dutch]. *Ned Tijdschr Geneeskd*. 2009; **153**: A887.
21 De Koning HJ. Mammographic screening: evidence from randomised controlled trials. *Ann Oncol*. 2003; **14**(8): 1185–9.
22 Austoker J. Screening and self examination for breast cancer. *BMJ*. 1994; **309**(6948): 168–74.
23 Department of Health. *The Health of the Nation: a strategy for health in England*. London: HMSO; 1992.
24 Department of Health. *NHS Cancer Screening Report: reducing the risk; breast screening programme*. London: Department of Health; 2000.
25 Thornton H. Mammographic screening: belief or evidence driven? *BMJ*. 2001 Nov 4. Available at: www.bmj.com/cgi/eletters/323/7319/956#17310 (accessed 22 May 2011).
26 Breast screen 'wrong care' fears. *BBC News*. 2006 Oct 18.
27 Atterstam I. [Mass X-ray does not decrease mortality] [Swedish]. *Svenska Dagbladet*. 1999 Jul 22: 1, 4.
28 Skogstrøm L. [Scepticism towards breast cancer screening] [Norwegian]. *Aftenposten*. 2000 Nov 23: 1, 3.
29 Byers T, Mouchawar J, Marks J, *et al*. The American Cancer Society challenge goals: how far can cancer rates decline in the U.S. by the year 2015? *Cancer*. 1999; **86**(4): 715–27.
30 American Cancer Society. Strategic plan progress report: American Cancer Society 2009. Available at: www.cancer.org/downloads/AA/2009_Strategic_Plan_Progress_Report.pdf (accessed 18 December 2009).
31 Jemal A, Siegel R, Ward E, *et al*. Cancer statistics, 2009. *CA Cancer J Clin*. 2009; **59**(4): 225–49.
32 Bonneux L. Mammographic screening from age 40 years. *Lancet*. 2007; **369**(9563): 737.

33 Templeton S-K. Anger at 'needless' breast ops. *Sunday Times*. 2009 Apr 19: 8.
34 The trouble with screening. *Lancet*. 2009; **373**(9671): 1223.
35 Weil JG, Hawker JI. Positive findings of mammography may lead to suicide. *BMJ*. 1997; **314**(7082): 754–5.
36 Allebeck P, Bolund C, Ringbäck G. Increased suicide rate in cancer patients: a cohort study based on the Swedish Cancer-Environment Register. *J Clin Epidemiol*. 1989; **42**(7): 611–16.
37 Gärtner R, Jensen MB, Nielsen J, *et al*. Prevalence of and factors associated with persistent pain following breast cancer surgery. *JAMA*. 2009; **302**(18): 1985–92.
38 [Mammography screening. Early detection of breast cancer. What you should know] [German]. *Bundesministerium für Gesundheit*; 2009. pp. 1–23.
39 Fracheboud J, Groenewoud JH, de Koning HJ. Fifteen years of population-based breast cancer screening in the Netherlands. *Semin Breast Dis*. 2007; **10**: 72–82.
40 Isacsson S-O, Larsson L-G, Janzon L. [Is the documentation really sufficient? Don't promote screening without debate] [Swedish]. *Läkartidningen*. 1985; **82**: 2672–3.
41 [Project group for the WE study in Kopparberg and Östergötland counties and the National Board of Health's working group for the WE project. Reply about mammography.] *Läkartidningen*. 1985; **82**: 2674.
42 Larsson LG, Nyström L, Wall S, *et al*. The Swedish randomised mammography screening trials: analysis of their effect on the breast cancer related excess mortality. *J Med Screen*. 1996; **3**(3): 129–32.
43 Baum M. Commentary: false premises, false promises and false positives; the case against mammographic screening for breast cancer. *Int J Epidemiol*. 2004; **33**(1): 66–7.
44 Darby SC, McGale P, Taylor CW, *et al*. Long-term mortality from heart disease and lung cancer after radiotherapy for early breast cancer: prospective cohort study of about 300,000 women in US SEER cancer registries. *Lancet Oncol*. 2005; **6**(8): 557–65.
45 Olsen O, Gøtzsche PC. Cochrane review on screening for breast cancer with mammography. *Lancet*. 2001; **358**(9290): 1340–2.
46 Olsen O, Gøtzsche PC. Systematic review of screening for breast cancer with mammography. *Lancet*. 2001. Available at: http://image.thelancet.com/extras/fullreport.pdf (accessed 5 May 2010).
47 Olsen O, Gøtzsche PC. Screening for breast cancer with mammography. *Cochrane Database Syst Rev*. 2001; (4): CD001877.
48 Gøtzsche PC. On the benefits and harms of screening for breast cancer. *Int J Epidemiol*. 2004; **33**(1): 56–64.
49 Gøtzsche PC, Nielsen M. Screening for breast cancer with mammography. *Cochrane Database Syst Rev*. 2006; (4):CD001877.
50 Newschaffer CJ, Otani K, McDonald MK, *et al*. Causes of death in elderly prostate cancer patients and in a comparison nonprostate cancer cohort. *J Natl Cancer Inst*. 2000; **92**(8): 613–21.
51 Brown BW, Brauner C, Minnotte MC. Noncancer deaths in white adult cancer patients. *J Natl Cancer Inst*. 1993; **85**(12): 979–87.
52 Early Breast Cancer Trialists' Collaborative Group. Tamoxifen for early breast cancer: an overview of the randomised trials. *Lancet*. 1998; **351**(9114): 1451–67.
53 Berry D. Commentary: screening mammographic; a decision analysis. *Int J Epidemiol*. 2004; **33**(1): 68.
54 Dixon JM. Screening for breast cancer: time to accept that, despite limitations, it does save lives. *BMJ*. 2006; **332**(7540): 499–500.

55 Duffy SW. The controversy over breast cancer screening. *Hosp Med*. 2002; **63**(12): 708–9.
56 Tindall G. Behind the screens. *Time*. 1994 Oct 8.
57 Wainer H. How should we screen for breast cancer? *Significance*. 2011 March: 28–30.
58 Raftery J, Chorozoglou M. Possible net harms of breast cancer screening: updated modelling of Forrest Report. *BMJ*. 2011; **343**: d7627.

26

Where next?

Promoting screening irrespective of the evidence may garner votes but will not create healthier voters. It may do the opposite.

Steven Woloshin and Lisa Schwartz[1]

MAMMOGRAPHY SCREENING HAS BEEN TOUTED WITH TWO SIMPLE messages: it saves lives and it saves breasts. The messages are the same as they were 25 years ago, but the facts have changed. The first message is probably wrong, and the second is definitely wrong. More and more people realise that screening for breast cancer is a doubtful enterprise, and despite stubborn opposition for decades, these people now also include some who work with screening.

One saw it very early. Maureen Roberts, the clinical director of the Edinburgh Breast Screening Programme, wrote a paper shortly before she died of breast cancer in 1989 that was published posthumously.[2] She felt the decision to introduce screening was political, in an election year. Furthermore, she noted that there was an air of evangelism about screening and she expressed the hope that pressure was not put on women to attend. She said:

> We all know that mammography is an unsuitable screening test: it is technologically difficult to perform, the pictures are difficult to interpret, it has a high false positive rate, and we don't know how often to carry it out. We can no longer ignore the possibility that screening may not reduce mortality in women of any age, however disappointing this may be.
>
> Are we brainwashing ourselves into thinking that we are making a dramatic impact on a serious disease before we brainwash the public?

> The decision must be theirs, and a truthful account of the facts must be made available to the public and the individual patient. It will not be what they want to hear . . . the currently expressed or strongly implied statement that if women attend for screening everything will be all right is not acceptable.

Roberts concluded that she believed a rethink was required before the programme went much further. More than 20 years on, we haven't seen a rethink, and the programme has gone further, which includes inviting a much broader age group, 47–73 years.[3]

It is very rare to see such an honest account from anyone involved with a screening programme, and the reasons are rather obvious. Several colleagues doing independent research on cancer screening have told me silverbacks in their home country with influence in funding committees at cancer charities have threatened them. They have also said that they have modified their papers out of fear of losing funding. Cornelia Baines has reported that politicians can be equally nasty. After the US consensus conference in 1997 about screening women aged 40–49 years, Senator Arlen Specter wrote to the directors of the US National Institutes of Health and the National Cancer Institute that until they had announced that mammography saves lives, budget approval would be withheld![4]

The American College of Radiology and the Society of Breast Imaging published new recommendations on breast screening in 2010, authored by Daniel Kopans and Stephen Feig, among others.[5] What we can learn from these recommendations, most of which are not evidence-based, is that one shouldn't get advice from people with a financial conflict of interest related to the advice. If these recommendations were to be followed, they would ensure a lucrative income for those society members who work with screening. The guidelines quote two of Tabár and Duffy's 'beyond reason' papers[6,7] and mention that these authors estimated that three-quarters of the reduction in breast cancer mortality was due to mammographic screening.

Women are recommended to start screening at age 40, and by age 30 (but not before age 25) if they have more than a 20% lifetime risk of developing breast cancer or if a mother or a sister has premenopausal breast cancer. Women with biopsy-proven lobular carcinoma *in situ*, atypical lobular hyperplasia, atypical ductal hyperplasia and ductal carcinoma *in situ* should be screened yearly from time of diagnosis, regardless of age. As very many women have such lesions, which are usually totally harmless, the detection of them in women in their thirties who get a mammogram because they worry about cancer would lead to about 50 mammograms, which carries a non-negligible risk of radiation-induced breast cancer.

The harmful consequences of these recommendations don't stop there. Magnetic resonance imaging is also recommended, although it is very expensive and hasn't been tested in randomised trials. And yet again, women should start at age 30 with annual screens if their lifetime risk is more than 20%.

A section called 'At what age should breast cancer screening end?' would have been amusing if it had been a joke. But as it is real, it is tragic. The authors say there is no reason to expect that mammographic screening would be any less effective among older women and recommend screening for as long as the life expectancy is 5 years or more. As it is close to impossible to judge whether an elderly woman's life expectancy is 1, 5 or 9 years, this opens the door to screening women till they die. And there is not a word about overdiagnosis, which increases tremendously with age.

These recommendations remind me of my childhood where we fabricated our own money, which, however, didn't harm anyone.

After we had shown that one in three breast cancers are overdiagnosed,[8] the US Center for Medical Consumers reported on this result with the telling title: 'Reduce your risk of breast cancer: avoid mammograms'.[9] I am sure many people will regard this as polemic, but it isn't. It deserves to be repeated and quantified (*see* Chapter 16):

> ***If we wish to reduce the incidence of breast cancer, there is nothing as effective as avoiding getting mammograms. It reduces the risk of getting breast cancer by one-third.***

Epidemiologist Klim McPherson said almost the same in his 2010 *BMJ* review, although indirectly. In his strong criticism of the NHS Breast Screening Programme he noted that 'reducing incidence must be the primary goal, with reducing mortality an important but secondary end point.'[10] Since screening became a holy cow, I have never seen this being the primary goal for our fight against breast cancer. *But it should be our primary goal for any cancer to reduce its occurrence.* Everything else must be secondary to this.

It was once said that the only thing we can learn from history is that we cannot learn from history. The logic doesn't hold, of course. If we cannot learn from history then we cannot learn from history that we cannot learn from history. This is a classical example of philosophical reasoning.

But it is true that we don't learn much from history. We have had devastating epidemics of hysterectomies and tonsillectomies and we currently have an epidemic of Caesarean sections, although these operations may lead to substantial harm. We also have epidemics of mastectomies and prostatectomies because people seem to be more worried about dying than they are interested in living. As one of my colleagues recently wrote: 'Why the obsession with trying to root out diseases before they are actually there?' Europeans have difficulty understanding the popularity of prostate cancer screening in the United States. Most men become permanently impotent after the operation,[11] and 30 years without sex is a high price to pay for preventing a non-disease from not killing us (as the disease would most likely never have arrived; even in men in their thirties who died from something else, prostate cancer has been detected in 30% at autopsy).[12]

This leads me to paraphrase a famous Danish humourist, Robert Storm Petersen:

> 'Doctor, if you remove my prostate, can you then promise me that I will live longer?'
> 'No, but I can promise you it will *feel* longer!'

I think most men are more interested in their sex lives than in their prostates. But the Americans are very aggressive and passionate about it. Two editors of a US medical journal wrote an opinion piece in the *San Francisco Chronicle* in January 2002 arguing that screening for prostate cancer may cause more harm than good.[13] Within hours of the piece being published, advocates of PSA testing sent a joint email alert to urologists, national prostate cancer support groups and charities around the country. These groups bombarded the two editors with email accusing them of having the deaths of hundreds of thousands of men on their hands. A member of a prostate cancer email discussion group urged other members to write to the editors' bosses: 'Tell them to fire these imposters. Tell them these folks should be silenced.' These bosses, who included the dean of University of California, were overwhelmed with letters demanding that the university take disciplinary action. One of the editors noted that there is an extremely powerful pro-screening lobby, which has a major financial stake in diagnosing and treating prostate cancer in the United States. Meanwhile, neither Canada nor the United Kingdom recommended screening. So perhaps the US passion is just a question about money.

The uncritical attitude to screening in the United States is also apparent among elderly women. Half of women aged 80 and older had received a screening mammogram within the past 2 years, and 42% were at least 85 years old,[14] although the harms vastly outweigh any benefit in this age group. In 2001, the US Preventive Services Task Force recommended screening cease at age 70 years, but the American Geriatrics Society recommended possible discontinuation of screening at age 85 years, while the American Cancer Society had no age limit.[15]

A study of screening for cervical cancer found that two-thirds of women who no longer had a cervix because of previous hysterectomy continued to have smears. This proportion didn't even change after the US Preventive Services Task Force recommended against screening these women.[16] There seems to be a large, untapped market for screening people for a disease they cannot get. What about screening *women* for prostate cancer? Just in case someone had an unrecognised hermaphroditism.

Is screening a religion?

The screening advocates have created a world of their own where they share ideas, beliefs and rituals. They also have a mantra – '30% reduction in breast cancer mortality' – and share the idea that screening isn't harmful. Doubts and questions are not acceptable and can lead to excommunication and vilification, as happened for Michael Baum in the United Kingdom and Mette Kalager in Norway. These hostile attitudes are very harmful to the progress of science, in fact a form of reverse evolution: those who think differently are selected away, and only the biased researchers remain.

Richard Dawkins wrote in his book *The God Delusion*[17] that Martin Luther was well aware that reason was religion's arch-enemy and had said, 'Reason is the greatest enemy that faith has.' Petr Skrabanek made a similar point when he, in his 1985 *Lancet* review 'False premises and false promises of breast cancer screening', noted that, 'in the published work, wishful thinking abounds.'[18] There has been a lot of false evidence that purported to show that the effect of screening was large. Researchers who have shown what the errors were have often been met with fierce *ad hominem* reactions, like some people react against alleged blasphemy.

I cannot help wonder why many people just shrug their shoulders when they learn of scientific misconduct, and why many scientists don't care that they deceive their readers repeatedly and betray the confidence society has bestowed on them, whether for a political gain, for fame, for money, for getting research funding, or for any other reason. People may keep on being dishonest, may get away with it and may publish in the same journals time and again, to the hurrahs of like-minded people who are often editors of the same journals.

They also often succeed in suppressing unwelcome news. My book is full of examples of this and the next section outlines the most recent one.

A press release from *Radiology* that wasn't

By the end of 2010, the editor of the US journal *Radiology*, Herbert Kressel, invited The Nordic Cochrane Centre to write a paper in the Controversies in Radiology series and noted that Daniel Kopans had agreed to take the opposing view. We requested that none of the parties should be allowed to see the other's contribution before publication, which was granted.

In our piece, we explain why screening cannot have more than a trivial effect today, if any, whereas the harms are substantial.[19] Kopans's paper, which has Robert Smith of the American Cancer Society and Stephen Duffy as co-authors, is very different.[20] The authors cherry-pick fatally flawed studies such as Tabár's 'beyond reason' studies (*see* Chapter 14), supporting their views of a large effect of screening and an overdiagnosis of only 1%, and they misrepresent the facts, ignoring even serious errors that have been pointed out to them previously. Kopans *et al.*'s criticism of our *BMJ* meta-analysis of overdiagnosis (*see* Chapter 16) is an example of using the 'if you can't beat them, lie about them' trick. We *did not* assume a stable underlying incidence, but took account of increasing trends; we *did not* base our estimate on a single year after screening, but on many years; we *did not* assume that all carcinoma *in situ* is overdiagnosed; we *did* take lead time into account (by adjusting for a fall in incidence in elderly, previously screened women when it occurred); we *did not* assume that all additional incidences after the initiation of screening were overdiagnosed, and our follow-up *was* long enough (by a wide margin).

We submitted a letter to *Radiology* explaining Kopans's many errors, but Kressel refused to publish it. We then sent a letter to the blog on the journal's website where it was published as an E-letter,[21] which few people will find, as E-letters are not indexed on PubMed.

That issue of *Radiology* also contained a 29-year update of the Two-County trial that wasn't particularly interesting.[22]

Radiology prepared a press release about the two controversy papers to which Kopans and we contributed. A few days before the papers came out, we were informed that the press release had been cancelled because of 'last minute issues with our coordinating process' and because 'we occasionally have issues come up that require us to make the difficult decision to cancel the distribution of a press release and, unfortunately, this has been the case here'.

We explained that we were disappointed that there would not be a press release to increase attention to the papers, which we felt were very important for the screening debate. The editor seemed to agree, as he had found our paper thought-provoking, which would 'certainly generate a good deal of conversation among our readers'. We also called for an explanation and urged the journal to reconsider its decision.

We were then told that 'because this was a two-sided news release, we needed to have full participation from the authors of both sides. We strive to provide fair and balanced news to the media and it was at the last minute that we found out not all of the authors agreed to participate and we needed to respect their wishes and cancel distribution.'

I participated in a podcast recording with Smith and Kressel 2 weeks before our papers came out, and as both sides had shared their papers for the purpose of the podcast, our opponents knew what was coming. Our co-author, US radiologist John Keen, suspected there might have been political pressure from the American Cancer Society. The society was probably really concerned about Autier's papers that showed screening didn't work (*see* Chapter 15) and which we had cited. Therefore, it was not only Cochrane and the US Preventive Services Task Force the society was up against. Further, they very likely did not want to publicise a paper where we looked a lot better than Kopans.

It would have been very easy for *Radiology* to issue the press release. The editor could have allowed Kopans to withdraw his statements that he had previously approved and made a note about this, or he could have stated that Kopans refused to comment. The editor might have been under considerable pressure when he abstained from doing the obvious.

It is unfortunate that people or institutions with vested interests can suppress press releases and it also shows that they put their own interests above those of the American women whose interests they otherwise constantly remind us they take care of.

I hope many people will take notice of the two papers, even without the press release, which is shown in Appendix 3, as they are so telling, and I think they will. Many US radiologists subscribe to the news service AuntMinnie, which mentioned the papers and had quotes from Kopans.[23] It is clear from the blogs on the website that the readers generally felt Kopans's arguments had no credibility. We described the untruthful statements he had made to the news service about our research.[24]

Has all my struggle achieved anything?

Although being newcomers to the field, it took us just a couple of weeks in 1999 to find out that the benefit of mammography screening is very small, if any; that the harms are substantial; and that most of the trials were quite problematic.

However, I spent the next 10 years trying to get these simple facts through before they finally started to become more generally accepted, and it was often extremely difficult. Both the *Lancet* and the *BMJ* were instrumental in accomplishing a change in people's beliefs about breast scrreening, which is a tribute to the free press. The house of cards of screening began to tremble when we published a devastating criticism of the United Kingdom screening leaflet in the *BMJ* in February 2009.[25] It is very difficult to get papers into the *BMJ*, which accepts only about 2% of submitted manuscripts, but to our surprise this paper, which wasn't revolutionary in any respect and just discussed one information leaflet, was accepted without problems.

We feel that our two most important papers after 2001 are our systematic review on overdiagnosis in countries with organised screening programmes from July 2009[8] and the paper showing screening doesn't work in Denmark from March 2010.[26] These papers were very threatening to the screening advocates, which is probably why the peer reviews were generally hostile and unfair. The *BMJ* rejected both papers, but after we had appealed, they were accepted.

In the first case, we demonstrated to the *BMJ* that the two peer reviewers it had selected had huge conflicts of interest. One of them had previously published an estimate of overdiagnosis close to zero using statistical modelling, although the raw data unambiguously showed considerable overdiagnosis. The other belonged to the Danish research group that had claimed that it is possible to screen without overdiagnosis. We ended our letter of appeal thus:

> We can provide an extensive rebuttal of the criticisms raised by the peer reviewers. We therefore feel the rejection of our paper is unfair and may reflect abuse on part of the peer reviewers. We therefore ask, whether *BMJ* would be willing to consider our review again, with our rebuttals. Or whether our review was rejected because of lack of interest, which we doubt, as a systematic review on overdiagnosis has never been published (probably because all those with a conflict of interest would rather like to continue claiming that there is no problem; this is an important reason for the rather poor quality of much of the data that were available to us).

Our overdiagnosis paper was sent for peer review again and this time the selected peer reviewers had the same interest as us, to get as close to the truth as possible.

In the second case, both peer reviewers had extensive knowledge of screening and had co-authored reports on screening trials. The *BMJ*'s statistician praised the 'rigour with which the study was conducted'. In line with this, the first reviewer wrote, 'It is a pleasure to read this well-designed and appropriate analysis refuting a previously published and less than compelling report on breast screening benefits in Copenhagen'; the same reviewer also wrote that our methods were appropriate, that 'the rationale for critiquing the study by Olsen *et al.*[27] are persuasive' and that our paper was 'fascinating and important'.

In contrast, the second reviewer wrote that there were 'a number of problems with the analysis and interpretation' and that 'the authors' assertion that the previous analysis by Olsen and colleagues has methodological weaknesses should not appear in the abstract and is in any case highly contentious.' You might have guessed who the reviewers were. The first reviewer was Cornelia Baines and the second was Stephen Duffy. To our surprise, the *BMJ* rejected our paper, not because of its methods, but because 'we do not think that this paper is clinically helpful for our general readers. It is of interest to those who are interested in the effects of breast screening, some of whom read the *BMJ*, but not relevant to the majority of our readers' clinical practice.' We disagreed and we were pleased the *BMJ* allowed us to appeal and to reply to the two peer reviewers and to a new one. We explained that the second reviewer contradicted himself, misquoted and misrepresented our paper, and maintained positions that we could show were false or irrelevant. For example, he accepted that Olsen found that the full effect of screening appeared after only 3 years, whereas he claimed that our follow-up period of 13–16 years – with a contemporary unscreened control group, in a study with more power than Olsen's study, as we included the whole country – was too short to find an effect!

As of September 2011, I had published 34 papers and book chapters on mammography screening and 75 correspondences. My reward for this was a lot of trouble and enemies. Curiously, although many of those who publish on mammography screening are females, all the fierce *ad hominem* attacks I have been exposed to have exclusively involved males, the only exception being Ilse Vejborg from my own hospital, but she was always in male company when she charged. Perhaps it is just the eternal problem of males being unable to control their testosterone-related aggressiveness; some end up in jail and others become professors.

The research I undertook with Karsten Juhl Jørgensen was unfunded. We tried to get funds but didn't succeed, although we published our research in the world's most prestigious journals, and I therefore paid his salary out of my budget.

This illustrates an important issue in medical research. We constantly hear that competition is good, and researchers spend considerable time writing funding applications. It can certainly be helpful to be forced to think carefully about what one wants to do, how and why. The process of writing this down in a detailed application can sharpen the mind and improve the research.

However, the system can stifle innovative ideas and impede controversial research, which are likely to be shot down by peer reviewers who guard their own interests. Many top researchers have therefore argued that it would be better to give them a load of money, with no strings attached, as this would be much more efficient.

I believe the pendulum has swung too far away from core funding of research groups and institutions towards competition during the last decades. Many university departments are forced to collaborate with the drug industry to survive, which is harmful not only for basic research but also for clinical practice. Most of our breakthroughs in healthcare have come from publicly funded basic research, not from the drug industry, which, however, usually takes all the credit when new substances from innovative public research are handed over to it.[28–30] Another unfortunate development is the politicians' increasing interference with research, often in the form of earmarked research programmes they have chosen. Such initiatives are usually shortsighted, whereas the big breakthroughs often require many years of investment, far beyond the election periods.

When I opened The Nordic Cochrane Centre in 1993, I worked half-time with research and development for the hospital and half-time for Cochrane, supported by small funds from the hospital and the Ministry of Health that allowed me to employ a half-time secretary. I acquired funding for various research projects and my staff grew, but it became more and more difficult to sustain the infrastructure for important Cochrane work that was not research. My funding opportunities started to dry up in 1999; therefore, I informed the ministry that if they weren't able to help, I would need to start firing my key personnel within the next 6 months. I would then conclude that, despite all the moral support I had received over the years, the Danish government didn't feel our centre was important enough to fund it, and I would go back to internal medicine.

The ministry was responsive, and 2 years later, the government provided permanent funding for my centre and the three Cochrane review groups I had helped establish in Denmark the Cochrane Hepato-Biliary Group, the Cochrane Colorectal Cancer Group and the Cochrane Anaesthesia Group. This core funding made it possible for me to continue not only my Cochrane work but also my research on mammography screening.

So, have my efforts improved the understanding of screening? I think they have. And I believe that, without my privileges, we wouldn't have been where we are now, close to a tipping point where people may realise that mass screening with mammography hasn't delivered what it promised and should therefore be abandoned.

It has been a bit frustrating of course that The Nordic Cochrane Centre needed to devote so much time to breast screening before people woke up. But it wasn't the only thing we did. During these years, I have published papers in very different disciplines, including liver disease, asthma, arthritis, skin disease, cystic fibrosis, inherited enzyme deficiency, placebo, acupuncture, antifungal agents, drug trials, research methodology, bias, publication ethics and scientific misconduct. Above all, we have published many papers on statistical issues, which have shown that the medical research literature is generally not very reliable. It has been fun.

Why has so much evidence about screening been distorted?

I have witnessed so much deception about mammography screening in scientific papers, in the media and at the few meetings I have attended, that I will turn Martin Luther's argument around and say: 'Faith is the greatest enemy science has.'

Faith is closely related to authority and depends on it. Children trust their parents, churchgoers trust their priest and patients trust their doctor. The problem with mammography screening is that those who should know most about it, and have a lot of formal authority, cannot be trusted. As I have shown in this book, there are good reasons to distrust national boards of health, people responsible for screening programmes, people earning a living from screening, cancer charities and, more broadly, most people publishing research on screening.

By deceiving the public, these authorities do science a great disservice. They also do women a great disservice, although they constantly remind us that what they do, they do on behalf of the women. In reality, the women have been patronised by them.

This isn't new. In his book *The Breast Cancer Wars*, Barron Lerner tells the story of male surgeons who continued to perform mutilating radical mastectomies in the United States, long after less radical operations had been introduced in Europe, and the contempt they showed for women who asked for less surgery.[31] A paper in *Cancer* from 1980 also illustrates the arrogance.[32] A male surgeon discusses what one should do with the remaining breast after having performed surgery on the other. He writes that 'some authorities' feel that the remaining breast has strong psychological and physical support for many women who regard it as a badge of motherhood, as a sign of feminity and as an important psychosexual symbol. These authorities are famous surgeons, it seems; we are not told what the women think about it, although they have authority over their own breasts. Later, he writes that the remaining breast 'remains as a useless and largely non-functioning organ serving at best as a questionable psycho-sexual symbol'. I wonder whether one could say that the penis of a male rendered permanently impotent as a consequence of prostate surgery could also be removed, as it is 'a useless and largely non-functioning organ serving at best as a questionable psycho-sexual symbol'.

The Two-County trial has also been authoritative. It is the trial that has been by far most influential in starting screening programmes, but also in this case, the authority was undeserved. Already in 1999, Lars Erik Rutqvist from the Swedish Cancer Foundation's expert group said that his only explanation for the problems was that the Tabár group in its first paper wouldn't reveal what had happened, as it could reduce the value of the information, and that it was forced to continue concealing the truth after this.[33]

Time to stop breast cancer screening

Will mass breast cancer screening with mammography be abandoned? I think it will, but it could take some time. In Denmark, it took 20 years after tuberculosis was eradicated before we got rid of the tuberculosis stations, and before it was no longer mandatory, e.g. for newly employed workers at the Carlsberg breweries, to get screened with a chest X-ray as a condition for getting the job. In all those years, the screening was unequivocally harmful, as X-rays carry a small risk of inducing cancer.

By willingly accepting all the hype, and contributing substantially to it themselves, the politicians have put themselves in a catch-22 situation. People have been brainwashed into believing that screening is good for them and saves many lives, so it is not easy to take this privilege away from the voters without running a risk of losing the next election.

In October 2011, Susan Bewley, professor of complex obstetrics, published an open letter in the *BMJ* to England's 'Cancer Tsar,' Sir Mike Richards, calling for an independent review of the NHS breast screening programme.[34] She had compared the NHS and Nordic Cochrane Centre leaflets and found that the NHS leaflets exaggerated benefits and did not spell out the risks. She also criticised Richards for having said that, 'the large majority of experts in this country disagrees with the methodology used in the Cochrane Centre reviews of breast screening' and she noted that simply disagreeing with the open, highly defensible, peer-reviewed Cochrane methodology was not enough. One needed to know what the vested interests were for the experts disagreeing, how they came to their conclusions and why they disagreed.

Richards replied that an independent review of the randomised trials and the observational studies was under way and that the leaflet (which was only one year old) would be rewritten.[35] I wonder what he meant by this, as he also said in February 2009 that a formal review was in progress and would be tested against the best available evidence (*see* Chapter 19). What was the fate of that review, and what is the relation between the 2009 review and the newly promised one? Richards noted that, 'We are seeking independent advisers for this review who have never previously published on the topic of breast cancer screening.' This is also interesting. Shouldn't independent advisers who *had* published in the area be preferred over those who had not? But of course, it would then be rather difficult to argue why The Nordic Cochrane Centre would not be invited, as we have published more about mammography screening than any other independent institution, as far as I know.

A flood of well-argued rapid responses on the *BMJ*'s website followed the two papers and a concomitant editorial,[36] and people generally did not believe that the review would be independent.

Richards was put in charge of the independent review by the Ministry of Health, together with Harpal Kumar, chief executive at Cancer Research UK. It is clear that neither of them are independent but are powerful people favouring screening. Kumar has stated that, 'Screening saves lives, so it's extremely worrying to see that the percentage of women going for breast screening is dropping.'[37] We noted that Richards's bias was apparent from his paper, where he offered three references.[38] The first is the 2002 IARC working group report, which is cited for a 35% effect of breast screening among those attending screening, ignoring that such estimates are flawed, as those who turn up for screening are healthier than those who don't.

The second reference is the programme's 2006 report, and Richards writes that 400 women need to be screened regularly over a 10-year period to save one woman from dying of breast cancer. This estimate is wrong by a factor of five because 2000 women need to be screened, according to the estimate derived directly from the randomised trials of screening, as described by The Nordic Cochrane Centre and the US Preventive Services Task Force, both of which are independent institutions.

Richards's third reference is a study performed by 'eight leading international scientists,' headed by Professor Stephen Duffy. Richards conveyed their estimate of 2–2.5 lives saved by screening for every one women overdiagnosed. As I have explained in Chapter 20, this estimate is monstrously wrong by a factor of 20–25.

We therefore recommended Richards to change his advisors, as they so obviously provide him with wildly exaggerated estimates of the benefits of screening.

Like others, we also suggested that the National Institute for Health and Clinical Excellence (NICE) should be in charge of the review, which would eliminate the risk of whitewash or hiding behind experts with vested interests.

Michael Baum recently suggested a way out of this dilemma, using a risk-based approach that limits screening to women who are at particularly high risk of developing breast cancer.[39] Politically, this may be a sensible first step, and in the United Kingdom, even screening advocates have started to discuss this possibility.

But who will be the first to stop screening altogether? The Canadians? In late 2011, the *Canadian Medical Association Journal* allowed me to publish an editorial to accompany new guidelines for breast screening with the title: 'Time to stop mammography screening?'[40]

I think the Americans and the Swedes will be last. That is where it all started and where the enthusiasm is greatest. In 2007, László Tabár declared in an interview that mammography was the best thing that had happened for women during the last 3000 years and added, 'There are still people who don't like mammography. Presumably they don't like women.'[41]

I see it differently. People who like women, and the women themselves, should no longer accept the pervasive misinformation they have consistently been exposed to. The collective denial and misrepresentation of facts about overdiagnosis and the little benefit there is of screening, if any, coupled with the disregard of the principles for informed consent and national laws, may be the biggest ethical scandal ever in healthcare. Hundreds of millions of women have been seduced into attending screening without knowing it could harm them. This violation of their human rights is the main reason we have done so much research on mammography screening and also why I have written this book.

> *What I have always found troubling is the refusal of my doctors over the last 18 years to explain to me that there are any risks at all associated with mammograms. I can live with uncertainty. I do not wish to live with dishonesty.*
>
> Diane Palacios[42]

> *Having cancer treatment when it is necessary is tragedy enough. Having it unnecessarily is a tragedy of an altogether different kind. Continuing to recommend screening in the current state of knowledge without ensuring informed consent to the known dangers is not just a tragedy, it is a crime.*
>
> Miriam Pryke[43]

References

1 Woloshin S, Schwartz LM. The benefits and harms of mammography screening: understanding the trade-offs. *JAMA*. 2010; **303**(2): 164–5.
2 Roberts MM. Breast screening: time for a rethink? *BMJ*. 1989; **299**(6708): 1153–5.
3 Jørgensen KJ, Gøtzsche PC. Who evaluates public health programmes? A review of the NHS Breast Screening Programme. *J R Soc Med*. 2010; **103**(1): 14–20.
4 Baines C. Breast practices. *Medical Post*. 2002 Jun 25: 11.
5 Lee CH, Dershaw DD, Kopans D, *et al*. Breast cancer screening with imaging: recommendations from the Society of Breast Imaging and the ACR on the use of mammography, breast MRI, breast ultrasound, and other technologies for the detection of clinically occult breast cancer. *J Am Coll Radiol*. 2010; **7**(1): 18–27.
6 Tabár L, Vitak B, Chen HH, *et al*. Beyond randomized controlled trials: organized mammographic screening substantially reduces breast carcinoma mortality. *Cancer*. 2001; **91**(9): 1724–31.
7 Duffy SW, Tabár L, Chen HH, *et al*. The impact of organized mammography service screening on breast carcinoma mortality in seven Swedish counties. *Cancer*. 2002; **95**(3): 458–69.
8 Jørgensen KJ, Gøtzsche PC. Overdiagnosis in publicly organised mammography screening programmes: systematic review of incidence trends. *BMJ*. 2009; **339**: b2587.
9 Napoli M. Reduce your risk of breast cancer: avoid mammograms. 2009 July 14. Available at: http://medicalconsumers.org/2009/07/14/cut-your-risk-of-breast-cancer-avoid-mammograms (accessed 5 September 2009).
10 McPherson K. Should we screen for breast cancer? *BMJ*. 2010; **341**: 233–5.
11 Stanford JL, Feng Z, Hamilton AS, *et al*. Urinary and sexual function after radical prostatectomy for clinically localized prostate cancer: the Prostate Cancer Outcomes Study. *JAMA*. 2000; **283**(3): 354–60.
12 Welch HG, Schwartz L, Woloshin S. *Overdiagnosed: making people sick in the pursuit of health*. Boston, MA: Beacon Press; 2011.
13 Ferriman A. Advocates of PSA testing campaign to silence critics. *BMJ*. 2002; **324**(7332): 255.
14 Schonberg MA, McCarthy EP, Davis RB, *et al*. Breast cancer screening in women aged 80 and older: results from a national survey. *J Am Geriatr Soc*. 2004; **52**(10): 1688–95.
15 Walter LC, Covinsky KE. Cancer screening in elderly patients: a framework for individualized decision making. *JAMA*. 2001; **285**(21): 2750–6.
16 Sirovich BE, Welch HG. Cervical cancer screening among women without a cervix. *JAMA*. 2004; **291**(24): 2990–3.
17 Dawkins R. *The God Delusion*. Boston, MA: Houghton Mifflin; 2008.
18 Skrabanek P. False premises and false promises of breast cancer screening. *Lancet*. 1985; **2**(8450): 316–20.
19 Jørgensen KJ, Keen JD, Gøtzsche PC. Is mammographic screening justifiable considering its substantial overdiagnosis rate and minor effect on mortality? *Radiology*. 2011; **260**(3): 621–7.
20 Kopans DB, Smith RA, Duffy SW. Mammographic screening and 'overdiagnosis'. *Radiology*. 2011; **260**(3): 616–20.
21 Gøtzsche PC, Jørgensen KJ. Kopans, Smith and Duffy misrepresent facts about mammography screening. *Radiology*. 2011; radiology_el; 243781.

22 Tabár L, Vitak B, Chen TH, *et al*. Swedish Two-County trial: impact of mammographic screening on breast cancer mortality during 3 decades. *Radiology*. 2011; **260**(3): 658–63.
23 Yee KM. Mammography debate livens pages of September *Radiology*. 2011 Aug 17. Available at: www.auntminnie.com/index.asp?sec=ser&sub=def&pag=dis&ItemID=96204.
24 Gøtzsche PC. Kopans' arguments are untruthful. 2011 Aug 18. Available at: www.auntminnie.com/index.aspx?sec=log&URL=http%3a%2f%2fwww.auntminnie.com%2findex.aspx%3fsec%3dsup%26sub%3dwom%26pag%3ddis%26ItemID%3d96204 (accessed 1 Sept).
25 Gøtzsche P, Hartling OJ, Nielsen M, *et al*. Breast screening: the facts – or maybe not. *BMJ*. 2009; **338**: 446–8.
26 Jørgensen KJ, Zahl P-H, Gøtzsche PC. Breast cancer mortality in organised mammography screening in Denmark: comparative study. *BMJ*. 2010; **340**: c1241.
27 Olsen AH, Njor SH, Vejborg I, *et al*. Breast cancer mortality in Copenhagen after introduction of mammography screening: cohort study. *BMJ*. 2005; **330**(7485): 220.
28 Angell M. *The Truth About the Drug Companies: how they deceive us and what to do about it*. New York: Random House; 2004.
29 Goozner M. *The $800 Million Pill: the truth behind the cost of new drugs*. Berkeley: University of California Press; 2005.
30 Brody H. *Hooked: ethics, the medical profession, and the pharmaceutical industry*. Plymouth: Rowman & Littlefield; 2007.
31 Lerner BH. *The Breast Cancer Wars*. Oxford: Oxford University Press; 2001.
32 Leis HP Jr. Managing the remaining breast. *Cancer*. 1980; **46**(4 Suppl.): 1026–30.
33 Atterstam I. [Influential cancer study dismissed, dishonest working practices erodes mammography result] [Swedish]. *Svenska Dagbladet*. 1999 Jul 21: 1, 6.
34 Bewley S. The NHS breast screening programme needs independent review. *BMJ* 2011; **343**: d6894.
35 Richards M. An independent review is under way. *BMJ* 2011; **343**: d6843.
36 Hawkes N. New NHS commissioning board gets to work. *BMJ* 2011; **343**: d7078.
37 Kendrick ME. Independent? *BMJ* 2011. www.bmj.com/content/343/bmj.d6843/reply#bmj_el_272056 (accessed 7 Nov 2011).
38 Jørgensen KJ, Gøtzsche PC. The proposed review of breast screening will not be independent without NICE. *BMJ* 2011. www.bmj.com/content/343/bmj.d6843/reply#bmj_el_272056 (accessed 7 Nov 2011).
39 Baum M. Attitudes to screening locked in a time warp. *BMJ*. 2009 Jul 12. Available at: www.bmj.com/cgi/eletters/339/jul09_1/b2587 (accessed 5 May 2010).
40 Gøtzsche PC. Time to stop mammography screening? *CMAJ*. 2011 Nov 21. DOI: 10.1503/cmaj.111721.
41 Gjerding ML. [Breast checks with shock failure] [Norwegian]. *Verdens Gang*. 2007 Oct 27(Suppl.): 18–24.
42 Palacios D. Letter to the editor. *New York Times*. 2000 March 4.
43 Pryke M. Unnecessary patient trauma can be avoided easily pending resolution of academic dispute if screeners pay attention to ethics. *BMJ*. 2010. www.bmj.com/content/340/bmj.c1241?tab=responses (accessed 19 Nov 2011).

Appendix 1

Tabár's explanations in the *Cancer Letter* and our replies

Tabár: Randomization started in W-county in July 1977 and not Oct. 1977 and ended in March 1981 in E-County, not in December 1979, as they state.

Our reply: *The randomization process and the definition of the date of entry have been inconsistently described in various publications (1), and the recent peer review comments (2) we received related to our paper on the missing cancers and deaths in the Two-County trial (3) added to this confusion. However, the crucial assumption for our analyses is not time of randomization but that the average follow-up was 6.0 years as Tabár stated in his initial trial report (4). If the mean time of randomization is later than first published, as Tabár indicates above, our results would still be highly significant, but the mean time of follow-up would then be less than 6.0 years (4).*

Tabár: They claim that the 'trial was closed after the first screening round,' which is simply not true, since the trial was closed after the termination of the first screening round of the control group in each district in succession. This occurred in W-county in Dec 1986 and in E-county even later, in September, 1988.

Our reply: *Tabár's statement that we should have claimed that the trial was closed after the first screening round is entirely misleading. We wrote: 'The trial was closed after the first screening round and new women were not invited' (3). Thus, by closed we referred to the fact that no more women were randomized, which was relevant for our calculations.*

Tabár: Their claim that the trial ended 'at Dec 31st, 1984' is nearly four years in error!

Our reply: *Tabár's statement that we should have claimed that the trial ended 'at Dec 31st, 1984' is seriously misleading and his claim that we should be nearly four years in error is wrong, of course. We wrote: 'the average length of follow-up was 6.0 years [1] December 31st, 1984' (3). Thus, we referred to the date when no more deaths were included in the results, which was relevant for our calculations.*

Tabár: During the trial period, 2,468 breast cancers were diagnosed, as has been repeatedly published but which is totally ignored by Zahl *et al.*

Our reply: *Tabár's claim that the number of breast cancers diagnosed during the trial period was 2468 is misleading. Tabár has described this number in a report with long follow-up (5) but it is completely irrelevant for our results that are based on a shorter time period for which Tabár has published far lower numbers (4).*

Tabár: Most surprisingly, Zahl *et al.*[1] fail to account for the precise method of randomization. The Two-County trial was randomized in stepwise fashion, district by district, from July 1977 through March 1981, as published in 1993.[2] Screening started some weeks after randomisation in study group areas, the first screens taking place in October 1977. When the first district had been randomized and while it was being screened, hundreds of cancers were diagnosed in the remaining districts that had not yet been inducted into the trial. This fact explains why their use of a 'simple and crude method' to assess the incidence and mortality in this trial leads to fatal errors. Twenty-nine years after the initiation of the study and 13 years after publication of the results of the Swedish Cancer Society's independent Overview Committee, Zahl *et al.* chose an arbitrary start date for each county in this trial. Realizing that this strategy was clearly wrong, they attempted to correct it by picking another arbitrary date during the randomization period, guessing the expected incidence from their erroneous first date to their erroneous second date, using prior national incidence data, then, bizarrely, adding this figure to the trial's reported results. This is yet another mistake, since it fails to take time trends in breast cancer incidence into account, further compounding their errors. Thus, the main reason for the difference between the Trial's reported results and the flawed estimates derived by Zahl *et al.* from national registry figures, is their use of an arbitrary single entry date coupled with their naïve attempt to correct for it, instead of using precise data covering the stepwise trial entry design, which was published in 1988 in a book chapter previously cited by Gøtzsche.

Our reply: *Tabár says it is surprising that we did not describe the precise method of randomization. What is surprising is that Tabár has never published it, and that what has been published is inconsistent. We asked Tabár about the method already in 1999 but could not find it in the references he advised us to read. Tabár now mentions a book chapter and claims he has described the randomization method there but does not give a reference to the book. Based on our initial correspondence with Tabár in 1999, we assume it is a book published by Huber (6), but there is no description of the precise randomization method there. Tabár claims we have used arbitrary dates. Not so. We have studied all of his publications carefully, noted discrepancies in the information offered, have estimated what the likely dates must have been, and have calculated several estimates based on different assumptions (2,3).*

Tabár: The effect of these errors is further compounded because the strategy of Zahl *et al.* includes women older and younger than the cut-off ages of 40–74 years at the actual time of randomization in the trial. The surprising phenomenon here is not the existence of a difference between the two figures: the surprise is that supposedly serious researchers ever expected them to be the same. Similar considerations apply to their comparison of breast cancer death, since they have included cases that never belonged to the study.

Our reply: *Tabár says that the effect of our so-called 'errors' is further compounded because we included women older and younger than the cut-off ages of 40–74 years at the actual time of randomization in the trial. This is not true (3). We first recorded cases in the age group 40–74 years in the randomisation period and then recorded new cases among those aged 40–74 years in the remaining period. This method underestimates the number of breast cancers in the screened group, but despite this, we found far more cancers (3) than Tabár reported (4).*

Tabár: Zahl *et al.* also criticize two publications on the basis of different results without noticing that one of them described results from follow-up to 1996 using data from the national death registry[3] while the other used the expert committee's results from follow-up to 1998.[4] When trying to explain any discrepancy, it is important to point out that in 1993 the independent Overview Committee's expert group of the Swedish Cancer Society published results nearly identical to those of the local expert committees. At their second publication, however, when the cause of death was taken from the national death registry, instead of being based on the decision of their own expert committee, a difference is to be expected, since the national registry figures are derived from death certificates while those determined by expert committees are based on each patient's hospital records, including autopsy reports. Again, the surprise is that anyone should expect the results to be identical.

Our reply: *Most importantly, Tabár does not explain how it was possible for him and his colleagues to publish an update of the Two-County trial where they reported a 24% breast cancer mortality reduction for the Östergötland part (5) when an updated overview of the Swedish randomised screening trials that was based on official mortality statistics found only a 10% reduction in breast cancer mortality for the Östergötland part (7) (data were not made available for the Kopparberg part as the Kopparberg trialists – Tabár and colleagues – did not wish to collaborate with the other Swedish investigators) (7). Compared to the overview, Tabár* et al. *reported 10 fewer deaths from breast cancer in the study group in Östergötland despite the fact that the follow-up was slightly longer and the age group was identical, and 23 more deaths in the control group, i.e. all 33 discrepancies were in favour of screening. Such a large difference is extremely unlikely to have happened by chance (p< 0.001). Furthermore, it is not correct when Tabár says that the independent Overview Committee's expert group published results nearly identical to those of the local expert committees. The overview committee reported in 1993, after an average follow-up of 10.0 years, that 481 women in the Two-County trial aged 40–74 years at entry had breast cancer as underlying cause of death and that 496 had breast cancer present at death (8). In contrast, Tabár* et al. *reported only 466 deaths from breast cancer in the same age group, although the average follow-up was 10.8 years, or almost one year longer, which is very surprising, indeed (9).*

Tabár: Perhaps the most egregious error in Zahl *et al.*'s paper is their interpretation and comment that 'the differences in the number of breast cancer deaths between the study and control groups in The Two-County Trial are small.' Can it really have escaped their attention that the study group was more than 30% larger than the control group? Regrettably, Zahl *et al.* imply that deliberate alteration of the data provides the only explanation for their findings, failing to appreciate that their results are merely approximations based on their own flawed estimations and a misreading of the literature.

Our reply: *Tabár's statement, 'Perhaps the most egregious error in Zahl* et al.*'s paper is their interpretation and comment that 'the differences in the number of breast cancer deaths between the study and control groups in*

The Two-County Trial are small.' Can it really have escaped their attention that the study group was more than 30% larger than the control group?' is entirely misleading. We wrote: 'It is of note that the differences in the number of breast cancer deaths between the study and control groups in the Two-County trial are small [1]. The mortality reduction would therefore no longer be statistically significant if only a few more breast cancer deaths were added to the study group' (3). Of course, we were aware that the groups were not of the same size but that is totally irrelevant for our argument. Tabár also says that we should have implied that he deliberately altered the data. This is not correct. We wrote: 'According to an investigator involved with the Two-County trial [9], other Swedish trialists [7], and an IARC/WHO report [10], cause-of-death assessments were not blind. This might be the reason why the cause of death determination by a local endpoint committee [11, 12] in Tabár and colleagues' update [8] appears to be seriously flawed' (3).

Tabár: In view of these elementary errors, sadly, I feel it necessary to make the following observation. If one is asserting that the world has got it wrong about breast screening, and that only a handful of relative newcomers to the subject have the answer, it is surely not too much to ask that these 'instant experts' read the literature carefully and get their facts right. Before showing off one's expertise it is advisable to acquire some. There is one point of agreement between me and Zahl *et al.* They state: 'We have used a simple and crude method . . ..' Indeed.

Our reply: *We believe our methods are adequate to allow us to conclude that many cancers and deaths are missing in reports of the Two-County study. This is supported by other data as well. We conclude that the handling of data was sloppy at best, that the assessment of cause of death was rather subjective in favour of screening, and that the Two-County trial is unreliable.*

Tabár's references

1 Zahl PH, Gøtzsche PC, Andersen JM, Mæhlen J. Results of the Two-County trial of mammography screening are not compatible with contemporaneous official Swedish breast cancer statistics. *Eur J Cancer* 2006 (in press).

2 Nyström L, Rutqvist LE, Wall S, Lindgren A, Lindqvist M, *et al.* Breast cancer screening with mammography: overview of Swedish randomised trials. *Lancet* 1993; **341**: 973–8.

3 Nyström, L, Andresson I, Bjurstam N, Frisell J, Nordenskjöld B, Rutquist LE. Long-term effects of mammography screening: updated overview of the Swedish randomised trials. *Lancet* 2002; **359**: 909–19.

4 Tabár L, Vitak B, Chen HH, *et al.* The Swedish Two-County Trial twenty years later. Updated mortality results and new insights from long-term follow-up. *Radiol Clin North Am* 2000; **38**: 625–51.

Our references

1 Gøtzsche PC, Nielsen M. Screening for breast cancer with mammography. Cochrane Database of Systematic Reviews 2006, Issue 4. Art. No.: CD001877.
2 Gøtzsche PC, Mæhlen J, Zahl P-H. What is publication? *Lancet* 2006; **368**: 1854–5.
3 Zahl P-H, Gøtzsche PC, Andersen JM, Mæhlen J. Results of the Two-County trial of mammography screening are not compatible with contemporaneous official Swedish breast cancer statistics. *Dan Med Bull* 2006; 5**3**: 438–40.
4 Tabár L, Fagerberg CJ, Gad A, Baldetorp L, Holmberg LH, Grontoft O, *et al.* Reduction in mortality from breast cancer after mass screening with mammography. Randomised trial from the Breast Cancer Screening Working Group of the Swedish National Board of Health and Welfare. *Lancet* 1985; **1**(8433): 829–32.
5 Tabár L, Vitak B, Chen HH, *et al.* The Swedish Two-County Trial twenty years later. Updated mortality results and new insights from long-term follow-up. *Radiologic Clinics of North America* 2000; **38**(4): 625–51.
6 Fagerberg CJG, Tabár L. *The results of periodic one-view mammography screening in a randomized, controlled trial in Sweden.* In: DayNE, MillerAB editor(s). Screening for breast cancer. Toronto: Hans Huber, 1988: 33–8.
7 Nyström, L, Andersson I, Bjurstam N, Frisell J, Nordenskjöld B, Rutquist LE. Long-term effects of mammography screening: updated overview of the Swedish randomised trials. *Lancet* 2002; **359**: 909–19.
8 Nyström L, Rutqvist LE, Wall S, Lindgren A, Lindqvist M, Ryden S, *et al.* Breast cancer screening with mammography: overview of Swedish randomised trials. *Lancet* 1993; **341**(8851): 973–8.
9 Tabár L, Fagerberg G, Duffy SW, Day NE, Gad A, Grontoft O. Update of the Swedish two-county program of mammographic screening for breast cancer. *Radiologic Clinics of North America* 1992; **30**(1): 187–210.

Appendix 2

Our 2008 mammography screening leaflet

This leaflet currently exists in 13 languages (www.cochrane.dk): Danish, Icelandic, English, Finnish, French, German, Italian, Norwegian, Polish, Portuguese, Russian, Spanish and Swedish. The English version is reproduced here.

SCREENING FOR BREAST CANCER WITH MAMMOGRAPHY

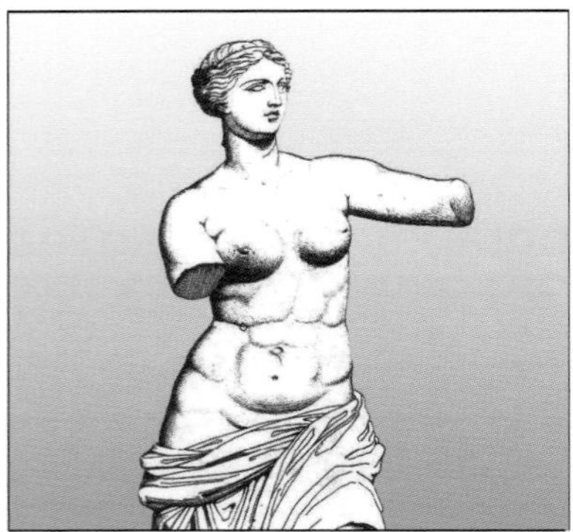

What are the benefits and harms of attending a screening programme?

How many will benefit from being screened, and how many will be harmed?

What is the scientific evidence for this?

1

Contents

Written by:

Peter C. Gøtzsche, chief physician, DrMedSci, director, The Nordic Cochrane Centre, Rigshospitalet, Copenhagen, Denmark.

Ole J. Hartling, chief physician, DrMedSci, chairman, The Ethical Council, Denmark.

Margrethe Nielsen, midwife, MSc, Danish Consumer Council.

John Brodersen, general practitioner, PhD, University of Copenhagen, Denmark.

This leaflet is available at: www.screening.dk and www.cochrane.dk.

January, 2008

2

Summary

It may be reasonable to attend for breast cancer screening with mammography, but it may also be reasonable not to attend, as screening has both benefits and harms.

If 2000 women are screened regularly for 10 years, one will benefit from the screening, as she will avoid dying from breast cancer.

At the same time, 10 healthy women will, as a consequence, become cancer patients and will be treated unnecessarily. These women will have either a part of their breast or the whole breast removed, and they will often receive radiotherapy, and sometimes chemotherapy.

Furthermore, about 200 healthy women will experience a false alarm. The psychological strain until one knows whether or not it was cancer, and even afterwards, can be severe.

3

Why have we written this leaflet?

We have written this leaflet because the information women receive, when they are invited to attend for screening with mammography, is insufficient and one-sided. The letters of invitation emphasize the benefits of screening, but they do not describe how many healthy women will experience the most important harms, overdiagnosis and overtreatment.

When women are invited to screening, the practice often is that, when they receive a letter about mammography screening, they are also given an appointment time for the examination. This procedure puts pressure on women to attend. Because of this, their participation becomes less voluntary.

Women who seek additional information on web sites on the internet are also badly served, as the most important harms are usually not mentioned at all. There are a few exceptions, however, e.g. the National Breast Cancer Coalition (www.stopbreastcancer.org), whose members are mainly women with breast cancer, and the Center for Medical Consumers (www.medicalconsumers.org), both from the USA.

We hope this pamphlet gives sufficient information about the benefits and harms of screening with mammography to enable a woman - together with her family and her doctor - to make a decision on an informed basis whether or not to attend for screening.

The pamphlet is available at www.screening.dk and www.cochrane.dk. We welcome proposals and criticism, at general@cochrane.dk.

What is screening?

Screening means to examine a population group in order to detect disease.

In several countries, women between 50 and 69 years of age are offered an X-ray examination of the breasts – screening with mammography - every second or third year. The purpose of the examination is to find women who have breast cancer in order to offer them earlier treatment.

Screening with mammography has both benefits and harms, and it should be up to the individual woman to weigh the pros and cons. It may be reasonable to attend screening, but it may be equally reasonable not to attend. The examination is not a duty, but an offer that the woman may or may not wish to accept.

It is often claimed that if nothing abnormal is found by screening, it makes the woman feel reassured that she is healthy. But almost all women will feel healthy before they are invited to screening, and the invitation may also cause insecurity. Therefore, one cannot say that screening leads to reassurance. It creates both security and insecurity.

Benefits

Better survival - Regular screening with mammography cannot prevent breast cancer, but it can reduce the risk of dying from breast cancer.

> *If 2000 women are screened regularly for 10 years, one will benefit from screening, as she will avoid dying from breast cancer because the screening detected the cancer early.*

Harms

Overdiagnosis and overtreatment - Some of the cancerous tumours and so-called precursors of cancer that are found by screening grow very slowly, or not at all ("pseudo-cancers"). They would therefore never have developed into a real cancer. Since it is not possible to tell the difference between the dangerous and the harmless cell changes, all of them are treated. Screening therefore results in treatment of many women for a cancer disease they do not have, and that they will not get.

> *If 2000 women are screened regularly for 10 years, 10 healthy women will be turned into cancer patients and will be treated unnecessarily. These women will have either a part*

5

of their breast or the whole breast removed, and they will often receive radiotherapy, and sometimes chemotherapy.

Unfortunately, some of the very early cell changes (which, in medical language, are called carcinoma in situ) are often found in several places in the breast. Therefore, the whole breast is removed in one out of four of these cases, although only a minority of the cell changes would have developed into cancer.

More extensive surgery and aftertreatment - For some women, the operation and aftertreatment may be less extensive when a small "true" cancer was detected by screening, than if it was detected at a later time. However, as screening leads to overdiagnosis and overtreatment of healthy women, more women will lose their breast when there is screening than if there had not been screening. Also, more women will receive radiotherapy.

False alam - If the X-ray shows something that might be cancer, the woman is recalled for additional investigations. In some cases it turns out that what was seen on the X-ray was benign, and that it was therefore a false alarm.

If 2000 women are screened regularly for 10 years, about 200 healthy women will experience a false alarm. The psychological strain until it is known whether or not there is a cancer, can be severe. Many women experience anxiety, worry, despondency, sleeping problems, changes in the relationships with family, friends and acquaintances, and a change in sex drive. This can go on for months, and in the long term some women will feel more vulnerable about disease and will see a doctor more often.

Pain at the examination - The breast is squeezed flat between two plates while an X-ray is taken. It only takes a moment, but about half of the women find it painful.

False reassurance - Not all cancers can be detected by X-ray. It is therefore important that the woman sees a doctor if she finds a lump in her breast, even if she has had a mammogram recently.

Documentation for our facts and figures

The information we have given in this pamphlet is different from the information found in most other materials, e.g. in invitations for screening (1) or from cancer charities and other interest groups (2). We therefore provide the background for our numbers below and explain why other numbers about screening are not equally reliable.

The most reliable results come from trials where the women have been randomized to be screened or not to be screened. About half a million healthy women have participated in such trials (3). Most randomized trials have been carried out in Sweden. A review of the Swedish trials from 1993 showed that screening reduced breast cancer mortality by 29% (4). The review also noted that after 10 years of screening, this reduction in mortality corresponded to saving one woman out of 1000. The benefit of screening is thus very small. The reason for this is that in a period of 10 years only 3 women out of 1000 get breast cancer and die from it. The real reduction in mortality was therefore only 0.1% (1 out of 1000) after 10 years in the Swedish trials. However, in a review of the Swedish trials from 2002, the reduction in mortality was only 15% with one method of calculation, and 20% with another method (5). The two reviews of the Swedish trials have the shortcoming that the researchers did not take into account that some of the trials had been better done - and therefore are more reliable - than others.

The most thorough evaluation of all the randomized trials that exists is a Cochrane review (3). Here, the mortality reduction was 7% in the best trials and 25% in the poorest, and since poor trials usually overestimate the effect, the mortality reduction was estimated to be 15% (3). Another thorough evaluation of the trials has been carried out on behalf of the U.S. Preventive Services Task Force. The researchers found an effect of 16% (6). Hence, these two systematic reviews found an effect on breast cancer mortality that was only half as large as in the first Swedish review from 1993. This means that regular screening of 2000 women for 10 years is necessary to save one of them from dying of breast cancer, i.e. an effect of 0.05%.

An effect of screening on mortality from all causes has not been demonstrated. Thus, it has not been shown that women who attend screening live longer than women who do not attend screening.

The randomized trials showed that screening increased by 30% the number of women who got a breast cancer diagnosis and were treated, compared with the group that was not screened (3). Large population studies from the Nordic countries, United Kingdom, USA and Australia have confirmed that screening results in an overdiagnosis of 30-40% (3,7). The randomized trial that followed the participants the longest showed a 25% rate of overdiagnosis in the mammography-screened women (8) (this calculation took into account the fact that many women in the control group had mammograms, though they had not been invited to be screened).

From the Cochrane review (3) it can be calculated what an overdiagnosis of 30% means for the women. In the trials from Canada and Malmö, either the whole breast or part of it was removed in 1424 women in the screened group and in 1083 women in the control group. Since the control group comprised 66,154 women, the overdiagnosis constituted (1424-1083)/66,154 x 2000 = 10 women per 2000 screened women. Thus, by screening 2000 women, 10 healthy women will get a cancer diagnosis they would not have had if they had not been screened, and they are also treated as if they were cancer patients.

A study of screening for breast cancer in Denmark concluded that it is possible to screen without overdiagnosis (9). However, the study provided no justification for this statement. In another study, co-authored by some of the same investigators, it can be calculated that the number of breast cancer diagnoses increased markedly in Copenhagen after screening was introduced (10). According to data from the National Board of Health on the number of breast cancer diagnoses, screening in Denmark results in substantial overdiagnosis.

The Cochrane review showed that the breast was removed in 20% more women in the screened group than in the control group (3). Other studies have also shown that more breasts are removed when there is screening than when there is no screening (3). Furthermore, in the United Kingdom the whole breast was removed in 29% of those cases where the cancerous lesions were detected in very early stages when they had not spread, although those should have been the very cases where a less extensive operation could have been performed (11).

The psychological strain until it is known whether or not there is a cancer, can be severe (3, 12). In the USA it has been calculated that after 10 rounds of screening, 49% of healthy women will have experienced a false alarm (13). In Norway, 21% will have experienced a false alarm after 10 rounds of screening (14). However, the numbers for Norway and most other countries are too low because recalls due to poor technical quality of the mammogram have usually not been included (14). As the women are just as affected by such recalls as by a real suspicion of cancer (12), they should be counted as false alarms. In Copenhagen, 6% of the women experienced a false alarm at the first screening round (15), and 10% of the women who had turned up for the first 3 rounds experienced a false alarm (16). The researchers have estimated that 10% will have experienced a false alarm in Denmark after 10 years of screening (5 rounds), which corresponds to 200 healthy women for each 2000 women screened regularly for 10 years. This estimate may be a bit too low, however.

We have mentioned earlier that about half of the women experience pain at mammography when the breasts are squeezed flat. This appears from a systematic review of the relevant studies (17).

References

1. Jørgensen KJ, Gøtzsche PC. Content of invitations to publicly funded screening mammography. British Medical Journal 2006; 332:538-41.

2. Jørgensen KJ, Gøtzsche PC. Presentation on websites of possible benefits and harms from screening for breast cancer: cross sectional study. British Medical Journal 2004; 328:148-51.

3. Gøtzsche PC, Nielsen M. Screening for breast cancer with mammography. Cochrane Database of Systematic Reviews 2006, Issue 4. Art. No.: CD001877 (kan også læses på www.cochrane.dk).

4. Nyström L, Rutqvist LE, Wall S, Lindgren A, Lindqvist M, Ryden S, et al. Breast cancer screening with mammography: overview of Swedish randomised trials. Lancet 1993; 341:973–8.

5. Nyström L, Andersson I, Bjurstam N, Frisell J, Nordenskjöld B, Rutqvist LE. Long-termeffects ofmammography screening: updated overview of the Swedish randomised trials. Lancet 2002; 359:909–19.

6. Humphrey LL, Helfand M, Chan BK, Woolf SH. Breast cancer screening: a summary of the evidence for the U.S. Preventive Services Task Force. Annals of Internal Medicine 2002; 137(5 Part 1):347–60.

7. Giles GG, Amos A. Evaluation of the organised mammographic screening programme in Australia. Annals of Oncology 2003; 14:1209-11.

8. Gøtzsche PC, Jørgensen KJ. Estimate of harm/benefit ratio of mammography screening was five times too optimistic. http://bmj.bmjjournals.com/cgi/eletters/332/7543/691, 2006.

9. Olsen AH, Jensen A, Njor SH, Villadsen E, Schwartz W, Vejborg I, Lynge E. Breast cancer incidence after the start of mammography screening in Denmark. British Journal of Cancer 2003; 88:362-5.

10. Törnberg S, Kemetli L, Lynge E, Olsen AH, Hofvind S, Wang H, Anttila A, Hakama M, Nyström L. Breast cancer incidence and mortality in the Nordic capitals, 1970-1998. Trends related to mammography screening programmes. Acta Oncologica 2006; 45:528-5.

11. NHS cancer screening programmes. BASO Breast Audit 1999/2000. www.cancerscreening.nhs.uk/breastscreen/publications.html (accessed Dec 12, 2001).

12. Brodersen J. Measuring psychosocial consequences of false-positive screening results - breast cancer as an example (ph.d.-afhandling). Department of General Practice, Institute of Public Health, Faculty of Health

Sciences, University of Copenhagen. Månedsskrift for Praktisk Lægegerning 2006 (ISBN 87-88638-36-7).

13. Elmore JG, BartonMB,Moceri VM, Polk S, Arena PJ, Fletcher SW. Ten-year risk of false positive screening mammograms and clinical breast examinations. The New England Journal of Medicine 1998; 338:1089–96.

14. Hofvind S, Thoresen S, Tretli S. The cumulative risk of a false-positive recall in the Norwegian Breast Cancer Screening Program. Cancer 2004; 101:1501-7.

15. Vejborg I, Olsen AH, Jensen MB, Rank F, Tange UB, Lynge E. Early outcome of mammography screening in Copenhagen 1991-99. Journal of Medical Screening 2002; 9:115-9.

16. Lynge E. Mammography screening for breast cancer in Copenhagen April 1991-March 1997. Mammography Screening Evaluation Group. APMIS-Suppl 1998; 83:1-44.

17. Armstrong K, Moye E, Williams S, Berlin JA, Reynolds EE. Screening mammography in women 40 to 49 years of age: a systematic review for the American College of Physicians. Annals of Internal Medicine 2007; 146:516-26.

Other relevant literature

Welch H. Should I be tested for cancer? Maybe not and here's why. Berkeley: University of California Press; 2004.

Vainio H, Bianchini F. IARC Handbooks of Cancer Prevention. Vol 7: Breast Cancer Screening. Lyon: IARC Press, 2002 (written by a working group under WHO).

Further information can be obtained by contacting the doctor

11

Appendix 3

The press release *Radiology* withdrew at the last minute

Contact: RSNA Media Relations: 1-630-590-7762

Linda Brooks	Maureen Morley
1-630-590-7738	1-630-590-7754
lbrooks@rsna.org	*mmorley@rsna.org*

Embargoed for release on August 18, 2011 at 12:01 a.m. ET

Mammography Controversy Resurfaces with Claim of Overdiagnosis
OAK BROOK, Ill. – Two articles published in the September issue of *Radiology* examine the benefits and harms of mammography screening and draw opposing conclusions.

In the articles, lead authors Karsten J. Jørgensen, M.D., a researcher at the Cochrane Collaboration in Copenhagen, Denmark, and Daniel B. Kopans, M.D., director of breast imaging at Massachusetts General Hospital in Boston, present contrasting views on the effects of screening for breast cancer with mammography.

Dr. Jørgensen writes that screening mammography has had only a negligible effect on breast cancer deaths and that universal mammography screening should be reassessed. He asserts that the benefit of screening mammography is doubtful, that overdiagnosis is substantial, and that screening increases the number of mastectomies performed. He bases his conclusions on a review of randomized controlled trials and epidemiological surveys of screening mammography around the world.

'In the United States, there has been a large increase in ductal carcinoma in situ (DCIS) and localized breast cancers but a very small decrease in cancers with metastases,' he said.

DCIS is a noninvasive breast cancer in which abnormal cells are found only inside milk ducts and not in the surrounding breast tissue. Prior to the introduction of mammography screening in the United States, DCIS accounted for two percent of all breast cancer cases. Today, DCIS accounts for approximately one in four detected breast cancers, many of which are found by screening mammography.

'Detecting DCIS is not resulting in a decrease in invasive breast cancer,' Dr. Jørgensen said. 'In fact, the incidence of early-stage breast cancer is increasing, and the incidence of late-stage breast cancer is largely unchanged. One can conclude that the increase in localized cancers that coincides with the introduction of screening is due to overdiagnosis, not early diagnosis.'

Overdiagnosis is defined as the detection of cancer that would not have been clinically identified in a woman's lifetime.

Dr. Kopans strongly disagrees. In his article, he states that early detection, although not perfect, has been repeatedly demonstrated to reduce deaths from breast cancer and that the risk of overdiagnosis is small compared to this benefit.

Dr. Kopans reports that between 1990 and 2007, the mortality rate from breast cancer in the U.S. decreased by 31 percent, principally due to the contribution of mammographic screening and improved therapies.

'Randomized controlled trials are the gold standard for evaluating the efficacy of screening in preventing deaths from breast cancer,' Dr. Kopans said. 'Meta-analyses of these trials have demonstrated a significant decrease – on the order of 20 to 25 percent – in breast cancer deaths among women invited to screening from age 40 up.'

He also writes that the incidence of invasive cancers has been decreasing in the U.S. since 1999 and that the rate of overdiagnosis attributable to screening mammography is much lower than what critics of screening mammography are reporting.

'Randomized controlled trial estimates and service screening estimates, which properly take into account the complexities of cancer incidence in the presence of screening, tend to find levels of overdiagnosis of 10 percent or less,' he said.

Because medical science currently offers no way to differentiate non-lethal cancers from progressive and potentially lethal cancers, Dr. Kopans said many women are treated with systemic therapy without knowing specifically who will benefit.

'This overtreatment is not confined to those cancers detected with mammography,' he said. 'There are also large, clinically evident cancers that are not lethal.'

There is also no way to determine which cases of DCIS detected by screening mammography will progress and become invasive. Experts estimate that approximately half of DCIS lesions progress to invasive cancer.

'Data from randomized controlled trials and the treatment of DCIS give us clear evidence that DCIS generally does have progressive potential, and that its detection and treatment are valuable,' Dr. Kopans said.

While both physicians agree that women are entitled to full disclosure on the benefits and harms of screening mammography, the debate over the value of screening mammography is likely to continue. The Cochrane Collaboration will publish an update to its 2000 review of the subject at the end of this year.

'Is Mammographic Screening Justifiable Considering Its Substantial Overdiagnosis Rate and Minor Effect on Mortality?' Collaborating with Dr. Jørgensen were John D. Keen, M.D., M.B.A., and Peter C. Gøtzsche, M.D., for The Cochrane Collaboration, an independent not-for-profit international network of scientists who prepare and update systematic reviews of research in health care and health policy.

'Mammographic Screening and 'Overdiagnosis." Collaborating with Dr. Kopans were Robert A. Smith, Ph.D., and Stephen W. Duffy, M.Sc.

Radiology is edited by Herbert Y. Kressel, M.D., Harvard Medical School, Boston, Mass., and owned and published by the Radiological Society of North America, Inc. (http://radiology.rsna.org/)

RSNA is an association of more than 46,000 radiologists, radiation oncologists, medical physicists and related scientists committed to excellence in patient care through education and research. The Society is based in Oak Brook, Ill. (RSNA.org)

For patient-friendly information on mammography, visit RadiologyInfo.org.

Index